Genetic and Phenotypic
Markers of Tumors

Genetic and Phenotypic Markers of Tumors

Edited by
Stuart A. Aaronson

National Cancer Institute
National Institutes of Health
Bethesda, Maryland

Luigi Frati
and
Roberto Verna

Institute of General Pathology
Rome, Italy

PLENUM PRESS • NEW YORK AND LONDON

Library of Congress Cataloging in Publication Data

Main entry under title:

Genetic and phenotypic markers of tumors.

"Proceedings of an international meeting on genetic and phenotypic markers of tumors, held October 13–14, 1983, in Rome, Italy "—CIP
Includes bibliographical references and index.
1. Cancer—Genetic aspects—Congresses. 2. Tumor markers—Congresses. I. Aaronson, Stuart A. II. Frati, Luigi. III. Verna, Roberto. [DNLM: 1. Genetic Marker—congresses. 2. Phenotype—congresses. 3. Neoplasms—diagnosis—congresses. QZ 241 I596g 1983]
RC268.4.G444 1984   616.99′4   84-18125
ISBN 0-306-41817-7

Proceedings of an international meeting on Genetic and Phenotypic Markers of Tumors,
held October 13–14, 1983, in Rome, Italy

© 1984 Plenum Press, New York
A Division of Plenum Publishing Corporation
233 Spring Street, New York, N.Y. 10013

PREFACE

The study of tumor markers is not only one of the most important but also one that offers one of the richest perspectives in biology and clinical oncology. The aim of scientists in this field is to adduce evidence of a property that is typical of and exclusive to tumor cells, and which is easy to determine, in order to immediately recognize, or even better, to foresee, neoplastic transformations.

Unfortunately, despite the large number of scientists and laboratories engaged in this work, the ideal tumor marker has not yet been identified. However, it is worth noting that new trends in molecular biology and immunovirology have recently opened up new avenues that may lead to the eventual resolution of this problem.

In this book, different approaches to the identification of tumor markers, from the points of view of biochemistry, immunology, and molecular biology, are compared in order to explore possible interrelationships and to stimulate scientific collaboration among scientists active in these fields, both in basic research and in clinical applications.

We wish to thank all the contributors and also the publisher, especially Dr. Robert Andrews, for making the publication of this book possible.

S.A. Aaronson
L. Frati
R. Verna

v

CONTENTS

INTRODUCTION

PHENOTYPIC MARKERS

Biochemical Markers

                    Modulation of Antigenic Expression

GENOMIC MARKERS

PHENOTYPIC AND GENETIC MARKERS OF CANCER: TURNING POINT IN RESEARCH

Luigi Frati, Enrico Cortesi, Corrado Ficorella, Vittorio
Manzari and Roberto Verna

Istituto di Patologia Generale, Università di Roma
viale Regina Elena, 324 Roma 00161 - ITALY

1. INTRODUCTION

Cancer, after cardiovascular diseases, is the second cause of
death both in Europe and U.S.A. Despite efforts and improvements
in many fields of tumor research, the surviving time of cancer
patients is strongly related to the stage of disease more than to
therapeutic strategies.

For instance, if the five-years survival for colorectal
cancer is 42% (average of all stages), the survival is about 90%
for stage I patients (Miller,1976). Therefore, screening
procedures for early diagnosis of asymptomatic patients have been
proposed, ranging from biochemistry (oncodevelopmental proteins)
to molecular biology (onc-genes), from imaging (thermography) to
the detection of so called "groups at high risk for the disease"
(identification of associated diseases, family history, HLA). From
these studies the term " marker" has been introduced for
indicating a sensitive, specific, easy to perform, recognizable
substance, related to the presence of the tumor.

The Bence Jones protein has been known for long time as the
typical marker of myeloma; from this basis other proteins
(enzymes, hormones, etc.) have been described and quantitative
analysis has shown variations of their level in body fluids

1

(blood, urine, milk, cerebrospinal fluid etc.).

The carcinoembryonic antigen (CEA), alfa fetoprotein, polyamines, enzymes, protein or isomeric proteins, cell surface markers, have been extensively studied and charged of significance. They are expression of neoplastic progression rather than of cell transformation. In fact, changes occur in phenotypic products of transformed cells and the relationship between these markers and cancer is generally restricted to a statistical and/or clinical significance without a close analysis of the molecular biology of production or disappearance. Again they are often common to many tumor types or to inflammatory diseases, and the variation of their level occurs only in clinically diagnosticable patients.

In this paper we briefly summarize data and problems about the most popular biological markers of tumors and we point attention to those markers which seem to be good candidates for an involvement in the cell transforming events.

2. SENSITIVITY AND SPECIFICITY

A marker should have the following characteristics:

a - sensitivity, to give positive results in patients bearing a
    tumor;
b - specificity for the tumor in question (hystological type,
    grade of malignancy);
c - availability in body fluid or tissue specimens (i.e. fine
    needle biopsies);
d - early appearance or loss, so that the early detection is
    significant for a very small tumor burden;
e - measurable levels which vary with the increase of tumor mass
    or recurrence of effective curve;
f - good feasibility (easy to perform, low cost, etc.).

Unfortunately the above mentioned requirements are difficult to assess for a single biological marker. The validity of each marker is dependent from its sensitivity and specificity. Sensitivity is the ability to give a positive result in patients bearing the disease (true positives), whereas specificity is the ability to give a negative result in healthy (regarding the disease) patients (true negatives).

Regarding a test, we may have the following possibilities:

-true positive (A)
-true negative (B)
-false positive (C)
-false negative (D)

Sensitivity is expressed by A/A+D (true positive/total patients). Specificity is expressed by B/B+C (true negative/total healthy patients). Predictiveness is expressed by A/A+C (true positive/true+false positive)

A test with good sensitivity has often a low specificity and this fact is more evident for tumor markers, such as oncodevelopmental antigens, which are present in patients bearing different tumors (i.e. carcinoembryonic antigen in colorectal, gastric, breast cancer, etc.). In this case predictiveness is low because of the incidence of false positives regarding that tumor (Cole and Morrison, 1980).

Simultaneous use of several tests as well as more advanced and selective methods (monoclonal antibodies as more specific binding molecules) can improve both sensitivity and specificity. Particularly, in the simultaneous use of several combined tests, significancy can be represented (Tab. 1) and the potential use of multiple markers for the management of cancer patients can be studied. Screenings of asymptomatic patients at risk by using multiple tests have been proposed as potentially more effective means for detecting early colorectal cancer (Fath Jr. and Winawer, 1983).

However, there are still very few diagnostic tests that are useful to the oncologist. Despite millions and millions of assays, results often are not reliable or useful because of technical problems, such as low selectivity, discrepancy between cost of large scale programs and early diagnosis, uncorrect clinical use (Herberman, 1983). Thus, development of new markers, preparation of monoclonal antibodies, elucidation of proteins and onc-genes sequences lead to a new step in the study of more sensitive and specific markers, such as those which are known to be related to the transforming process (Tab. 2).

Table 1. Sensitivity, Specificity and Predictiveness
for a single test and for tests' series

A-true positive	B=true negative
C=false positive	D=false negative

SINGLE TEST

Sensitivity	A / A + D
Specificity	B / B + C
Predictiveness	A / A + C

SEVERAL TESTs

Sensitivity $\dfrac{A_1+A_2+A_n}{n} / \dfrac{A_1+A_2+A_n}{n} + D$

Specificity $B / B + \dfrac{C_1+C_2+C_n}{n}$

Predictiveness $\dfrac{A_1+A_2+A_n}{n} / \dfrac{A_1+A_2+A_n}{n} + \dfrac{C_1+C_2+C_n}{n}$

Table 2. Expectation of improvement by using genomic
markers of tumors

Marker type	A	B	C
Phenotypic markers i.e. enzymes, proteins, oncodevelopmental proteins, etc.	+	+	+++
Markers related to cell transformation i.e. detection of Ig related to EBV, Oncorna viruses, etc.	ᴸ+	++	+++
Genomic markers i.e. detection of EBV, Oncorna viruses, onc-genes, etc.	+++	+++	+̲

A = Specificity   B = Sensitivity   C = Easy to perform

3. TUMOR ASSOCIATED MARKERS

Tumor Associated Antigens (TAAs) and neoplastic cell metabolites (including proteins, enzymes, hormones, carbohydrates) which are present in tumor bearing patients are included in this category. The immunological detection of new shared antigens or the finding of increased levels of proteins (such as oncodevelopmental antigens, enzymes, etc.) should be considered together since these compounds are present also in non neoplastic patients and their absence in normal tissue at any time of development is not demonstrated yet . In fact, by using sensitive techniques (RIA, ELISA), many antigens have been found in traces in normal, not embryonic cells.

Thus, TAAs and other phenotypic markers can be used by the oncologist when one of the following conditions occur:

a - quantitative differences in expression in tumor cells versus normal cells (i.e. enzymes);

b - presence in normal tissues, but only in a particular type of tumor (i.e. ectopic hormones);

c - presence in embryonic normal cells, but only in traces in adult healthy cells (i.e. AFP);

d - qualitative differences from normal proteins (i.e. isoferritin).

Low level/high level or high level/low level or typic pattern/atypic pattern between normal and tumor patients are the required findings regarding these markers. In this section we briefly discuss patterns and clinical applications of this type of tumor markers.

3.1.Oncodevelopmental proteins

The presence of tumor antigenicity in syngeneic systems has been a means for identification of tumor "diversity" and for improving tumor diagnosis and monitoring. The presence of an alpha-fetoprotein (AFP) in the sera of patients bearing primary hepatocellular tumors was the first record of a significant variation of the presence of a fetal protein in adults (Abelev et al., 1971). Thus, antigens purified from colon cancer were characterized after rabbit immunization and absorption with normal colon or blood components. These antigens were not found in adult tissues except than in malignant tumors of gastrointestinal tract and pancreas. The same antigens were found in fetal gut, liver and pancreas between 2 and 6 months of uterine life. Thus, the term " carcinoembrionic antigen" (CEA) was introduced and the progress in the measurement of traces by using RIA and ELISA methods extended the CEA-test in monitoring cancer patients (Fath and Winawer, 1983; Holyoke et al., 1982). These antigens are present in malignancies different from the original. CEAs have been found either in serum or cytosol of mammary and lung cancer, of gynecologic and urological malignancies and soft-tissue tumors (Duffy et al. 1983; Lee, 1983; Holyoke et al., 1982). The research on this field focused attention on a variety of markers and proteins such as fetal sulfoglycoprotein (FSA), colonic mucoprotein antigen (CMA), colon specific antigens (CSAs), colon specific antigen p (CSAp), pancreatic oncofetal antigen (POA), Tennessee Antigen etc, have been described. They are only in few cases cell specific, not organ or cancer specific (Goldenberg, 1982). On this field, excellent articles have been included in specific books (see General Bibliography).

The problems raising from the above presentation, according to the aim of this paper, are the following:

a - when more than a single test is performed, a test can be true
    positive when the other one is true negative and viceversa
    (e.g. CEA and CSAp correlation is about 50-60%);
b - presently RIA and ELISA tests use policlonal antibodies and
    they can be improved by the use of monoclonal antibodies;
c - the use of radioactive antibody combinations for detecting
    tumor localizations (e.g. Ig mixtures against CEA and CSAp)
    can be of great advantage;
d - the use of more than a single test can improve predictiveness
    of such markers.

3.2. Proteins

Differences in protein levels or enzyme activities between healthy and cancer patients have been described. Immunoglobulins, Ferritin and Isoferritin, Ceruloplasmin, alpha 1-Antitrypsin, beta 2-Macroglobulin, Haptoglobulin, C-reactive protein, Circulating Immune Complexes (CIC), have been measured in serum of cancer patients and they can be of help in staging or follow up. Biochemical abnormalities are different in the various tumors and the serum level of these markers correlate with tumor size. Thus, they cannot be used for early diagnosis. Only serum ferritin is a candidate for early diagnosis purpose. The level in normal subjects ranges between 10 and 200 ng/ml and higher values have been observed in about 2/3 of patients with lung cancer, but also in 15% of healthy smokers.

However, when data of lung cancer patients have been disaggregated for stage of disease, values observed in stage I (645 ng/ml; 81% elevated with cut-off level to 200 ng/ml) have been higher than in stage II (472 ng/ml; 53%) and in stage III (487 ng/ml; 57%). The fact that higher levels occur in stage I and that values in normal subjects never exceed the limit of 200 ng/ml, suggests that this test is a good candidate for early detection of lung cancer (Urushizaki and Niitsu, 1982). Except than the cases of ferritin and of Ig in myeloma, protein measurement cannot be used for early diagnosis, but only for monitoring tumor progression. The fact that about 15% of healthy smokers had high level of ferritin is suggestive for high risk patients and/or early detection of occult cancer.

3.3 Enzymes

The use of enzyme assays is very popular in clinical chemistry because easy to perform. In cancer monitoring, extent, stage, progression or regression of the disease have been related to the level of enzymes.

Tab. 3 summarizes the most important enzymes described in literature. Although research on enzymes as tumor markers is older than for other ones, they are of little help in early diagnosis

Table 3. Variation of the level of enzymes in Tumors bearing
         patients

Enzyme	Tumor	Variation
Amylase	Lung	+
Aryl Sulfatase B	Colon	+ urinary
Glycosyltransferases		
Fucosyltransferase	Breast, Colon	+
Galactosyltransferase	Colon, Ovary	+
Sialyltransferase	Massive metastatic tumors (in Lung or Liver)	+
α-Glutamyl Transpeptidase	Hepatoma, Liver Metastases	+
Hexosaminidase B	Colon	+
Histaminase	Medullary Thyroid C. Lung (Small Cell C.)	+
Lactic Dehydrogenase	Liver Metastases	+
LDH_5	Breast, Brain, Lung, Uterus Prostate, Kidney, Stomach	+
Lysozyme	Acute Myelomonocytic Leuk	+
	Acute Myeloblastic Leuk	+
Placental Alk.Phosphatase	Germ cell	+
Prostatic Acid Phosphatase	Prostate	+
Ribonuclease	Pancreas, Ovary, Epidermoid cancer	+

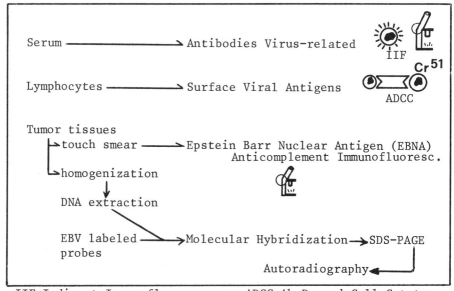

IIF=Indirect Immunofluorescence; ADCC=Ab Depend.Cell.Cytotox.

Fig. 1 - Detection of Epstein Barr Virus (EBV) infections by
         specific Immunoglobulins and DNA internal repeats

and their relevance can be restricted to a few cases (i.e. phosphatases).

3.4. Steroid receptors

   Biological basis of endrocrine therapy is the presence in the cells of specific receptors, which represent the way by which tumors are responsive or not to the administration of hormones or inhibitors. Binding capacity (for estrogen $>$ 10 fentomoles of steroid bound/mg cytosol protein) and dissociation constant (usually for estrogen-receptors complexes ranging between 10^{-10} and 10^{-11}M) should be analyzed together.

   About 60% of primary breast cancer and 50% of metastatic one are positive for estrogen receptors and about 50% of primary breast cancer is positive for progestin receptors. These positivities are related to the clinical response to endocrine therapy and positivity is also a prognostic factor. Many molecular species of receptors have been isolated and the 6S and 8S components are related to the responsiveness. Unresponsive cells show the 4S component, even under conditions of low ionic strength. Steroid receptors are present in various tumors other than those which exhibit sexual dimorphism (i.e. breast, uterus). Colorectal cancer for example is positive for estradiol. However, steroid receptors are useful for therapeutic strategies only.

3.5 Ectopic Hormones

   The production of ectopic hormones by tumors occurs frequently and RIA for hormones or precursors of hormones or hormone-like substances have been introduced. A typical example is small cell carcinoma, which often produces ACTH/LPH related molecules. Usually tumors derived from an endocrine tissue produce normal hormones, whereas ectopic hormones are heterogeneous, with a presence of high molecular weight molecules, fragments, subunits, abnormal breakdown products. Lung tumors producing ACTH-like molecules have been described. They can produce "big ACTH" (20,000 M.W.), ACTH 1-39 or ACTH 2-38 or ACTH 18-39 small M.W. components, beta (1-91) LPH and Y(1-58) LPH,

alpha   61-76 and   beta 61-91 endorphins or calcitonin, as
expression of both genomic derepression and "maturation" defects.
As tumors markers, abnormal or ectopic hormones seem to be more
interesting than hormones produced by endocrine tissues (Odell and
Wolfsen, 1978).

However, criteria to establish ectopic hormone production
have been outlined to prevent untrue evaluations:

1- arteriovenous hormone gradient across tumor mass;
2- in vitro production by the tumor;
3- demonstration of the hormone in the tumor at levels higher
   than in adjacent normal tissues;
4- quantitative and/or qualitative differences between the
   product of the tumor and the same hormone from normal endocrine
   tissue;
5- fall/rise of the level related to the regression/progression of
   the tumor.

By   these criteria, tumors derived from lung (FSH, LH,
Calcitonin,   Growth   Hormone,   Vasopressin,   HCG,   ACTH,
beta-Lipotropin),   uterus   (vasopressin),   kidney (Parathyroid
Hormone), liver (PTH, Somatomedin), thymus (ACTH, beta-MSH, PTH,
Calcitonin) have been described as ectopic hormone production.

It was suggested that   findings of ectopic hormones may
facilitate the detection of both primary and metastatic neoplasia.
As discussed by Neville (1982), various limitations, like those
found for oncofetal antigens, have restricted the role of these
markers. In fact only the assay of qualitative abnormal products
can be used for early diagnosis, but unfortunately RIA tests
generally   do   not   discriminate between normal and abnormal
polypeptide hormones. However, the monitoring of ectopic hormones
levels after primary diagnosis of tumor can be used in the
follow-up of the patient. If RIA test specific for abnormal
products shall be introduced, the significance of ectopic hormones
should be reconsidered.

3.6 Miscellaneous

Other markers have been proposed. Urinary and plasma levels of polyamines (putrescine, spermidine and spermine) have been related to tumor reduction. Increase of urinary level of putrescine 24hrs after chemotherapy, correlates with a clinical response. These markers can be used for monitoring but not for diagnosis (Russell and Durie, 1978).

Serum protein-bound carbohydrates (fucose, mannose, and galactose) or lipid-bound sialic acid have been described to be correlated respectively with the presence of lung small cell carcinoma or with various tumors as cancer of the prostate, bladder, breast, lung, colon, ovary, and in leukemia, lymphoma, Hodgkin disease and melanoma. These markers lack the required sensitivity and specificity for routine cancer detection and they can be used only for help in clinical evaluation of tumor progression. Other markers (i.e. breakdown products of tRNA: Cimino F. et al., this book) have been proposed. They are generally useful for monitoring cancer patients rather than for early diagnosis, because unrelated to the transforming events.

4. PHENOTYPIC MARKERS AS EXPRESSION OF CARCINOGENESIS

As discussed in the first part of this review article, biomarkers which are expression of neoplastic transformation seem to be inadequate for precocious biochemical diagnosis of tumors. For this purpose a marker should be more sensitive and more specific: such a marker should be expression of oncogenesis rather than a product of an established neoplasia.

New approaches in this direction seem to be:

4.1- Immunological detection of new-shared antigens

Transforming events by viruses have been joined to the advent of new specific antigens. A diagnostic procedure for detecting new shared antigens induced by Epstein-Barr virus infection is shown in Fig. 1. Membrane antigens (MA) and nuclear antigens (EBNA) of the Epstein-Barr virus can be detected in patients with Burkitt lymphoma and nasopharyngeal carcinoma. The most prevalent EBV-associated antibodies are IgA against virus capsid antigens,

VCA and IgG against early antigen (EA). Particularly the IgA-VCA antibody has been found very useful in diagnosis and identification of high-risk individuals whereas the IgG early antigen antibody was found to be of considerable prognostic value. ADCC (Antibody Dependent Cellular Cytotoxicity) is also of probable prognostic value, since high titers in the majority of patients correlate well with good survival and response to therapy and low titers with poor survival, recurrence of tumor and poor response to therapy. These antibodies would appear to be useful, very sensitive and specific precocious markers because related to the integration of the virus into the cellular DNA. This fact has been ascertained by molecular hybridization and very close relationships have been found between serological data and molecular biology (Faggioni et al., this book).

4.2 Onc-genes

   Recently, studies on the proteins encoded by onc-genes have shown that these proteins are produced in high amount in transformed cells. Transforming genes of oncogenic retroviruses (v-onc genes) have been recently described and their derivation from normal DNA sequences (c-onc genes) of normal human cells has been established. These sequences are present in the genome of various vertebrate species, so that they represent an essential requirement for cell survival and/or metabolism, differentiation and/or replication. High level expression by promoters, chromosomal rearrangement or gene amplification seem to be responsible for neoplastic transformation. Viral probes are now available and nick translated to be used as radioactive probes in detection of onc-gene amplification, or rearrangements which may lead to neoplastic transformation.

   Fig.2 shows three models of cell transformation. The final common event is a high production of the encoded proteins. In Tab. 4 protein products of onc-genes are displayed. Few of these proteins are known and they can be evaluated by RIA or by enzymatic assays (i.e. c-ras p-21, which exhibits a phosphokinase activity on threonine residues). It is worth noting that proteins encoded by onc-genes are of great significance, because they are related to the modulation of phosphokinase activity or to growth factors production or action (i.e. c-sis coding for Platelet

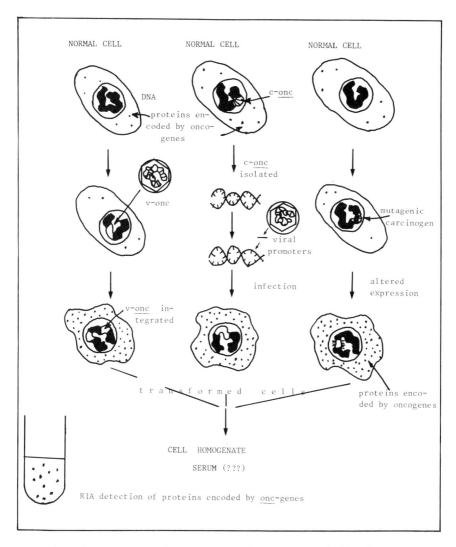

Fig. 2 — Hypotetic transforming events following
          viral or cellular oncogenes integration
          and/or mutagenic carcinogen exposure

          a. v-onc infection of normal cell
          b. virus promoter infection of normal cell
              and c-onc amplification
          c. c-onc increased expression by chemical
              carcinogens

          Proteins encoded by c-onc can be detected
          by using RIA. A significant rise of the le-
          vel is suggestive for cell transformation.

Table 4. Oncogenes trasduced by Retroviruses and probable protein products of v-onc

To detect the protein products of c-onc immunoprecipitation assay (i.e. RIA) against antigenic determinants common to v-onc
and c-onc products can be performed.
Probable protein products of v-onc   (number represents estimated m.w., esponential symbols represent v-onc) are listed:
$p21^{ras}$, $p35^{myb}$, $p29^{gag-ras}$, $p40^{erb-B}$, $p68^{gag-ros}$, $p75^{gag-erb-A}$,
$p90^{gag-yas}$, $p90^{gag-myc}$, $p85^{gag-fes}$ (Snyder-Theilen), $p95^{gag-fes}$
(Gardner-Arnstein), $p100^{gag-myc}$, $p105^{gag-fps}$, $p110^{gag-myc}$,
$p120^{gag-abl}$, $p140^{gag-fps}$, $p150^{gag-myb}$, $p180^{gag-fms}$, $p200^{gag-pol-myc}$, $pp60^{src}$

ONCOGENES TRANSDUCED BY RETROVIRUS

Viral Oncog.	Species of orig.	Tumorigenicity	Protein Products	
			Bioch. function	Subcellular loc.
v-src	Chicken	Sarcoma	PK (tyr)	Plasma membr.
v-fps/v-fcs	Chicken/Cat	"	" "	"
v-yes	"	"	" "	?
v-ros	"	"	" "	?
v-ski	"	_____	?	?
v-myc	"	Carcinoma Sarcoma Myelocytoma	DNA binding	nucleus
v-erb-A	"	?	?	cytoplasm
v-erb-B	"	Erythroleukemia Sarcoma	EGF receptor	membranes
v-myb	"	Myeloblastic leuk.	?	nucleus
v-rel	Turkey	Lymphatic leuk.	?	?
v-mos	Mouse	Sarcoma	?	cytoplasm
v-abl	Mouse/Cat	B-Cell Lymph.	PK (tyr)	Plasma membr.
v-fos	"	Sarcoma	?	?
v-Ha-ras	Rat/Mouse	"	Binds GTP	Plasma membr.
v-bas	"	Erythroleuk.	PK (thr)	"
v-Ki-ras	"	Sarcoma/Erythrol.	"	"
v-fms	Cat	"	?	membranes
v-sis	Woolly Monkey Cat	"	PDGF	Extracellular

Derived   Growth   Factor-PDGF   or   c-erb B coding for an Epidermal
Growth Factor/EGF receptor-like protein : Waterfield, 1983).

The   modification of the amount of these products is strongly
related to the transforming process as well as to the modification
of the   polypeptide   product   (Reddy,   1982 and Taparowsky, 1982).
When biochemical tests for the assay of these proteins could be of
practical use, a great advancement in very precocious diagnosis of
cancer will be obtained.

4.3 DNA derivatives of chemical carcinogens

On this field,   recently the group of C. Harris has found a
significant presence of Benzo(a)pyrene-diol-epoxide-DNA adducts
(BPDE-DNA) in peripheral white blood cells of people of certain
occupations (roofers and foundry workers), as well as in lung
tissues and alveolar macrophages of smokers. The DNA derivative
was tested by ELISA (Enzyme-Lynked-Immunoabsorbent Assay) and the
minimum level of BPDE-DNA detected was 2 fmoles/50 ng DNA, which
is equivalent to approximately one BPDE-DNA adduct per 10 bases.
It was suggested that this biochemical finding in smokers could be
related to the transforming events (Shamsuddin et al. manuscript
in preparation).

5. GENOMIC MARKERS OF TUMORS

A new approach to prevention, diagnosis and prognosis of
neoplasia are genomic markers: retrovirus infections and c-onc
genes alterations are up to date the most studied events. Actually
human T cell leukemia/lymphoma virus (HTLV) infection can be
considered as a marker of risk of neoplasia in healthy individuals
and as a negative prognostic marker in patients. There are not
practical applications for onc-genes alterations yet, both
qualitative and quantitative, but in future they will help in
patient evaluation.

Besides serology, by molecular biology we are able to find
direct evidence of virus presence in the cell and alterations in

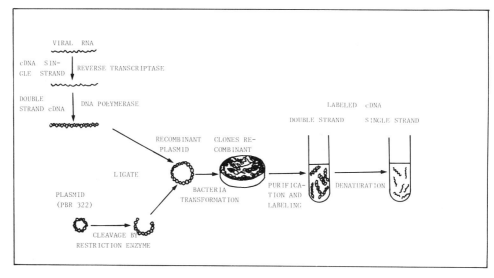

Fig. 3 - Cloning of cDNA derived from retroviruses-RNA

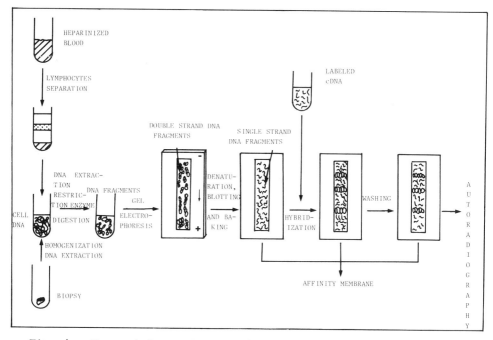

Fig. 4 - Recognition of retrovirus-DNA sequences in cellular
DNA from tumoral tissues by labeled cDNA probes

the expression of onc-genes: in fact, by DNA recombinant techniques, cDNA clones as well as genomic clones from RNA viruses and oncogenes are now available (Fig. 3). By using these probes, DNA extracted from tumor cells can be investigated for the presence of proviral DNA integrated in the genome thus demonstrating viral infection even if there is no expression, and for oncogenes amplification or recombination etc. (Fig. 4).

For their sensitivity and specificity, genomic markers represent a new approach to tumor markers which can integrate the battery of pleiotypic markers and possibly become essential to early diagnosis and tumor prevention.

GENERAL BIBLIOGRAPHY

Chu T.M. Ed., 1982
Biochemical Markers for Cancer.
Marcel Dekker Inc., New York and Basel

Colnaghi M.I., Buraggi G.L. and Ghione M.M. Eds.1982
Markers for Diagnosis and Monitoring of human cancer.
Serono Symp. Vol. 46, Acad. Press, London and New York.

Fishman W. Ed., 1983
Oncodevelopmental markers: Biologic, Diagnostic and Monitoring
Aspects.
Acad. Press, London and New York.

Chandra P. Ed., 1983
Biochemical and Biological Markers of neoplastic transformation.
NATO ASI series vol. 57, Plenum Press, New York and London.

Russel D.H. and Durie B.G.M. 1978
Polyamines as biochemical markers of normal and malignant growth.
Raven Press, New York.

REFERENCES

Abelev G.I., 1971
Alpha-Fetoprotein in ontogenesis and its association with
malignant tumors.
Adv. Cancer Res. 14, 551-558

Cimino F., Russo T., Colonna A. and Salvatore F. 1984
Pseudouridine: a biochemical marker for cancer. This book.

Cole P. and Morrison A.S., 1980
Basic issues in population screening for cancer.
J. Natn. Cancer Inst. 64, 1263-1272

Duffy M.Y. O'Connell M., O'Sullivan F., McKenna B., Allen M.A.,
McDonnell L. 1983
CEA-like material in cytosol from human breast carcinomas.
Cancer 51, 121-123

Faggioni A., Barile G., Piccoli M. and Frati L. 1984
Epstein-Barr virus markers in nasopharyngeal carcinoma This book.

Fath R.B.jr. and Winawer S.J., 1983
Early diagnosis of colorectal cancer.
Ann. Rev. Biochem. 34, 501-517.

Goffeu J., Heistarkamp N., Reynolds F.H. Jr. and Stephenson J.R.
1983:
Homology between phosphotyrosine acceptor site of human c-able
and viral oncogene products.
Nature Vol.304: 167-169

Goldenberg D.M. 1982
CEA and CSAp Markers in the detection and monitoring of colorectal
cancer.
In: Colnaghi et al. Eds. Markers for diagnosis and monitoring of
human cancer.
Serono Symp. Vol. 46, Acad. Press, London and New York pp. 141-153

Herberman R.B., 1983
Uses and limitations of Tumor Markers.

In: Fishman W.H. Ed. Oncodevelopmental markers.
Acad. Press. N.Y. pp. 409-418

Holyoke E.D., Evans J.T., Mittleman A. and Chu T.M., 1982
Carcinoembryonic antigen as a tumor marker.
In: Chu T.M. Biochemical Markers for cancer. Marcel Dekker Inc.,
New York and Basel pp. 61-80

Lee Y.T. 1983
Serial tests of carcinoembryonic antigens in patients with breast
cancer.
Am. J. Clin. Oncol. 6, 287-293

Miller D.G., 1976
The early diagnosis of cancer.
In: F. Homberger Ed. The pathophysiology of Cancer, Karger, Basel
pp.21-38

Neville A. M. 1982
Ectopic hormone production by tumors
in: Chu T.M. Ed. Biochemical Markers for cancer. Marcel Dekker
Inc., New York and Basel pp. 267-300

Odell W.D. and Wolfsen A.R. 1978
Humoral syndromes associated with cancer
Ann. Rev. Med. 29, 165-175

Reddy E.P., Reynolds R.K., Santos E. and Barbacid M. 1982
A point mutation is responsible for the acquisition of
transforming properties by the T24 human bladder carcinoma
oncogene.
Nature vol.300: 149-152

Schwartz M.K., 1982,
Enzymes as tumor markers in: Chu T.M.,Ed. Biochemical Markers for
cancer. Marcel Dekker Inc. New York and Basel pp.81-92

Taparowsky B., Suard D., Fasano O., Shinizy K., Goldforb M. and
Wigler M. 1982.
Activation of the T24 bladder carcinoma transforming gene linked
to a single amino acid change.
Nature Vol.300: 762-764

Urushizaki I. and Niitsu Y., 1982
Ferritin in diagnosis of lung cancer.
In: Colnaghi I. et al. Eds. Markers for diagnosis and monitoring
of human cancer.
Serono Symp. Vol. 46 Acad. Press, London and New York pp.111-121

Waterfield M.D., Scrace G.T., Whittle N., Strool P., Jhonsson A.,
Wastesan A., Westermark B., Mels C.H. and Dewel T.F. 1983:
Platelet Derived Growth Factor is structurally related to the
putative transforming protein p 28 sis of Simian Sarcoma virus.
Nature Vol. 304: 35-39

MULTIPLE BIOCHEMICAL MARKERS FOR CANCER: A STATISTICAL APPROACH

Paolo Marchetti, Enrico Cortesi, Corrado Ficorella, and
Luigi Frati

Istituto di Patologia Generale, Facoltà di Medicina e
Chirurgia, Università "La Sapienza", Viale Regina Elena
324, 00161, Roma, Italia

In the past few years there has been growing interest in the
identification and characterization of tumor-associated
substances, such as antigens, antibodies, enzymes, hormones, and
other proteins, that can be utilized in the diagnosis and
treatment of cancer patients. Ideally, a tumor associated marker
to aid in identifying tumor appearance and monitoring its growth,
should be available in body fluids and/or in tissue specimens
(i.e., fine needle biopsy specimens) and, obviously, undetectable
in non cancer patients, as well as specific for the type and
location of the neoplasia, and quantitatively measurable. Despite
remarkable advances recently achieved in this field, none of the
substances described up until now completely meets all these
requirements.

In regard to clinical applications, sensitivity and
specificity generally represent the most important attributes of
a tumor marker screening test. These characteristics are usually
evaluated by comparing the results given by the test in patients
with ascertained cancer and in control subjects (Thorner and
Remain, 1961). The results obtained can thus be classified into
the following four categories:
  A - cancer patients with positive test (true positive).
  B - cancer patients with negative test (false negative).
  C - non cancer patients with positive test (false positive).
  D - non cancer patients with negative test (true negative).
The sensitivity is defined as the ability of the test to reveal

the presence of a neoplasia and is expressed as the proportion of "true positive" cases as compared to all cancer patients studied. The specificity is the capacity of the test to classify as negative those subjects without tumors and is expressed as the proportion of the "true negative" cases with respect to all cancer-free subjects studied. The predictiveness furnishes the degree of reliability of the positive (or negative) responses and can be expressed as the proportion of the "true positive" (or "true negative") cases as compared to all the positive (or negative) cases. The predictive value of a positive result cannot be evaluated independently from that of a negative result. In fact, a test might have a high degree of predictiveness as far as positive results are concerned (given from $A/(A+C)$) and an elevated level of specificity ($D/(C+D)$) while having a low sensitivity ($A/(A+B)$). It is obvious that an inverse relationship between sensitivity and specificity exists. In fact, if the limit that separates the positive responses from the negatives is set high, there will be a lot of "false negative" (low sensitivity) while obtaining very few "false positives" (high specificity); on the other hand, if the chosen value is set lower, then there will be fewer "false negatives" (greater sensitivity) but more "false positives" (lower specificity). If several tests are employed in the management of the neoplastic patient, it is possible to measure the relative sensitivity of each test by expressing the proportion of positive cases identified by each test as compared to the overall cases of cancer detected by the combined tests.

In an attempt to improve the results obtainable with a single tumor marker, several investigators have explored the potential usefulness of multiple marker determination in the management of cancer patients (Maugh, 1977; Seppälä et al., 1982; Heberman, 1982). Although the current available results are encouraging and some authors (Heberman, 1982; Seppälä et al., 1982) agree that multiple biochemical and immunological tests can assist in monitoring the neoplasia, in all of these studies cut-off levels were established upon which a single case was classified as either positive or negative. The information obtainable from the quantitative assay of a tumor marker can thereby be reduced to a merely qualitative evaluation (i.e., marker "A", "B", ..., "Z" present or absent). In this way the determination of multiple markers can be utilized exclusively to recover a portion of those neoplastic patients classified as negative on the basis of a different test ("false negative"), without, however, utilizing completely the information obtainable with the different tests.

The statistical method applies well to the quantitative study of variables influenced by disturbing factors, which cannot be controlled experimentally. Among the various statistical procedures used in the analysis of several variables, we have chosen the factorial analysis (Guttman, 1956; Thurstone, 1947; Vianelli, 1960). Given "N" variables and "n" values for each one it is possible to express the observed variables in terms of a number of common factors, of single specific factors, and of residual elements. In other words, the factorial analysis deals with the elaboration of a series of data in order to identify a relatively reduced number of latent variables that can explain the covariations of a higher number of variables. The statistical theory and methodology required for the analysis of joint association of several variables in a single tumor, the type of conclusion that can be drawn from clinical and laboratory data, and the steps which must be taken to ensure that the conclusion are valid were beyond the scope of this short presentation. Based on this method, we will try to identify the degree

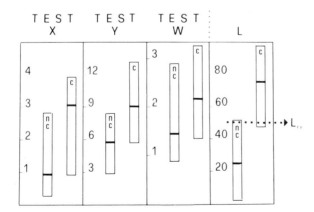

FIG. 1. Discriminant analysis of the responses to 3 different tests in cancer (C) and non cancer (n C) patients. Horizontal bars indicate the median value. L_0 indicates the optimal discriminating value.

of association between various tumor markers and different neoplasias, the extent to which the observed associations may result from bias and/or chance, and the extent to which they may be described as casual.

Once the relative importance of the various markers in the different tumors has been established, we will analyze the clinical and laboratory features for each patient, in order to identify a discriminating function for each pathological classification so that:

$L = aX + bY + \ldots + zW$

where $a,b,\ldots,z$ are the coefficients to be calculated and $X,Y,\ldots,W$ are the values of the examined characters. The identification of the "optimal discriminating level" (L) will be helpful in minimizing the number of misclassified patients (Fig. 1).

We feel that this statistical approach responds to the need of combining the various different clinical characteristics of the cancer patient in an integrated picture, which may provide highly discriminatory informations and improve the sensitivity and specificity of the detection of cancer.

REFERENCES

Guttman, L., 1956, Best possible systematic estimates for communality, Psychometrika, 122, 223-237.

Herberman, R.B., 1982, Immunological approach to the biochemical markers for cancer. In:Biochemical markers for cancer, edited by T.M. Chu, Marcel Dekker, New York, pp. 1-24.

Maugh, T.H., 1977, Biochemical markers: early warning signs of cancer, Science, 197, 543-549.

Seppälä, M., Rutanen, E.M., Lindgren, J., and Wahlström, T., 1982, Multiple markers in the management of cancer patients. In: Biochemical markers for cancer, edited by T.M. Chu, Marcel Dekker, New York, pp. 321-350.

Thurstone, L.L., 1947, Multiple factor analysis, Chicago,

University Chicago Press.

Torner, W. and Remain, Q., 1961, Principles and procedures in the evaluation of screening for disease, Public Health Monographs, 67-84.

Vianelli, S., 1960, La metodologia statistica nella analisi fattoriale. In: Lezioni di metodologia statistica per ricercatori, Istituto di Calcolo delle Probabilità, Roma, pp. 343-407.

PSEUDOURIDINE: A BIOCHEMICAL MARKER FOR CANCER

Filiberto Cimino, Tommaso Russo, Alfredo Colonna, and
Francesco Salvatore

Istituto di Scienze Biochimiche, II Facoltà di
Medicina e Chirurgia, Università degli Studi di Napoli
Via Sergio Pansini 5, 80131-Napoli, Italy

INTRODUCTION

Although some progress has been made in clarifying the
molecular basis underlying neoplastic transformation, anti-
neoplastic treatment is still based on the effort toward the
removal of all neoplastic cells. In this respect, the most
important requirement for the effectiveness of treatment is the
precocious diagnosis, possibly in the preclinical period.
Clinical, radiological and endoscopic examinations are often
poorly sensitive and in some cases invasive and dangerous, thus
efforts are focused to obtain a precocious tumor detection by
biochemical or biological assays.

Although no specific test for tumor diagnosis has been
found, many metabolites normally present in biological fluids
have been proposed as markers of tumor development (Ming Chu,
1982). Some metabolites are being used to monitor neoplastic
disease (prognosis, staging and follow-up); however, many false
negative or late positive cases are observed, together with some
false positive cases (Ming Chu, 1982).

The increased levels of modified nucleosides deriving from
the enzymatic degradation of nucleic acids observed in the urine
of neoplastic patients have been indicated as a tool to diagnose
neoplastic disease (for a review see: Salvatore, 1983a). In this
optics we have particularly studied one of these, the
pseudouridine (ψ), to evaluate its effectiveness as a biochemical
signal of neoplasia and to investigate some of its metabolic

features in tumor: the results obtained are reviewed in this paper.

PSEUDOURIDINE BIOSYNTHESIS IN NORMAL AND NEOPLASTIC CELLS

Among the modified nucleosides present in RNA, Ψ is the most abundant. In fact, almost all eukaryotic tRNA species sequenced contain 3-4 residues of Ψ per molecule, whereas Ψ content of prokaryotic species is of about 2-3 residues per tRNA molecule. From sequence studies (Gauss and Sprinzl, 1983) it can be deduced that Ψ is found in more than 15 different positions, including that of the IV loop which is quite constantly present.

Other RNA species, such as rRNA and snRNA, also contain numerous Ψ residues (see Table 1), mostly ranging between 2 to 60 Ψ per molecule, with an average of about 2 Ψ per 100 nucleotides.

Concerning its structure, Ψ differs from uridine for the glycosidic bond is between C_1' of the ribose and C_5, instead of N_1, of the uracil moiety: this C-glycosidic bond renders Ψ more stable than other nucleosides (Chambers, 1966). In mammals no enzyme is known to convert Ψ into uracil and ribose, and like all other modified nucleosides, Ψ is not reincorporated into RNA. In fact, while the "major" nucleosides can be either reutilized by various salvage mechanisms or enzymatically degraded into uric acid (purines) or into β-alanine (pyrimidines), the modified nucleosides are not converted to the correspondent triphosphates, nor further degraded. Thus these compounds have to be considered as functionless end-products of RNA catabolism, which are excreted by the cell.

Ψ biosynthesis is performed, in both mammalian and non-mammalian cells, by enzymes that catalyze the pseudouridylation of uridine residues present in RNA molecules, during the RNA maturation process. The pseudouridylation reaction, whose mechanism has not been completely clarified, occurs in eukaryotic cells at nuclear level, as it has been shown also for some tRNA methylations (Colonna and Kerr, 1980), but unlike these latter it seems to be an early event of tRNA processing (Melton et al., 1980).

An enzymatic activity (Matsushita and Davis, 1971), which catalyzes the synthesis of ΨMP from uracil and ribose-5P, has been identified in non-mammalian cells, and found in very little amount also in calf thymus: however its physiological role is quite obscure.

Table 1. Pseudouridine content of various RNAs

RNA	SIZE[a]	SOURCE	PSEUDOURIDINE RESIDUES (b)	(c)	REFERENCES
rRNA	37S	Yeast	36-37	0.8	Brand et al., 1979
"	28S	HeLa	53-59	1.12	Hughes and Madden, 1978
"	"	L-cells	50-58	1.08	" "
"	"	X.Laevis	58-66	1.24	" "
"	18S	HeLa	38-42	2.06	" "
"	"	L-cells	33-39	1.85	" "
"	"	X.Laevis	46-52	2.52	" "
"	5.8S	HeLa	2	1.29	" "
tRNA	4S	various	3-5	5.0	Gauss and Sprinzl, 1983
snRNA U1	165N	Novikoff Hepatoma	2	1.29	Busch et al., 1982
" U2	189N	"	12	6.3	" "
" U3	214N	"	2	0.9	" "
" U4	145N	"	1	0.6	" "
" U5	118N	"	3	2.5	" "
" U6	108N	"	2	2.0	" "

a molecule size is given as Svedberg units (S) or as number of nucleotides (N).
b per molecule.
c per 100 nucleotides.

Despite attempts to characterize the tRNA-Ψ-synthesizing enzymes, many of their molecular and kinetic features are still unclear. The main obstacle to perform these studies lies in the difficulty of having suitable RNA substrates, i.e. tRNAs that lack one or more Ψ residues. The availability of bacterial mutants with tRNAs lacking one Ψ in the anticodon loop permitted the purification of several tRNA-Ψ-synthases from bacterial cells (Cortese et al.,1974a; Cortese et al., 1974b; Arena et al.,1978) and from calf thymus (Green et al.,1982). It was found (Green et al.,1982) that the tRNA-Ψ-synthase belongs to a family of enzymes with sequence specificity for uridine residues in various RNAs.

Very little is known on the behaviour of these enzymes in neoplastic cells. We found, in agreement with other findings obtained in Yoshida ascites sarcoma (Fujimura and Shimizu, 1977), a two-fold increase of tRNA-Ψ- synthase activity in murine lymphomatous thymus and in chick embryo fibroblasts transformed by Rous sarcoma virus (Colonna et al., 1983a), whereas ΨMP-synthetase activity was very low both in normal and lymphomatous murine tissues (unpublished results). However, the increase of tRNA-Ψ-synthase was not correlated with the Ψ content of unfractionated tRNA isolated from tumor cells (Russo et al., 1983a, Russo and Cimino, 1983).

PSEUDOURIDINE DETERMINATION IN BIOLOGICAL FLUIDS

The presence of Ψ and other modified nucleosides in human urine was first reported more than three decades ago (Adler and Gutman, 1959). However, this research area was hampered by the lack of sufficiently sensitive techniques to analyze such compounds. Modified nucleosides were first determined in biological fluids by conventional column chromatography (Weissman et al., 1957) or by thin-layer chromatography (Randerath et al., 1972), but these procedures were unable to give precise quantitations. The sensitivity and resolution of the analysis of nucleosides in the urine improved with the introduction of gas chromatography (GLC) (Chang et al., 1974), but this method requires extensive clean-up of the samples and cannot be used without a derivatization step. A radioimmunological assay (RIA) has been developed (Levine et al., 1975), but it requires chemical modification of the nucleosides before the analysis, and the availability of specific antibodies.

More recently, the advent of high performance liquid chromatography (HPLC) has given a great impulse to the study of the excretion of modified nucleosides in physiological fluids (Gehrke et al., 1978; Colonna et al., 1983b). This method allows a rapid separation of the nucleosides as well as their quantitation with high sensitivity, precision and accuracy. Table 2 summarizes the normal values for Ψ concentration in biological fluids, determined by some of the above mentioned methods.

We have developed a method for the determination of Ψ in blood serum (Colonna et al., 1983b) based on the purification of nucleosides by affinity chromatography on phenylboronate gel column, followed by the separation and quantitation of the nucleosides by HPLC. The first step, performed after serum deproteinization, utilizes the specific affinity, at basic pH, between the ribose moiety of nucleosides and the boronate groups of the gel, so that it is possible to elute from the column, at pH 4, only the compounds with a cis-diolic structure. After concentration by liophylization the nucleosides are separated by an isocratic reverse phase HPLC on an octadecilsylane column, and the eluted compounds are identified and quantitated by absorbance measurement at 254 and 280 nm.

A reference value of 2.54 ± 0.5 nmoles of Ψ/ml of serum was obtained in a group of 30 normal human subjects. This value shows very little day by day variation and does not seem to be related to body weight when determined on samples collected in basal conditions (Salvatore et al, 1983b).

Table 2.   Pseudouridine concentration in body fluids of normal subjects.

URINE (nmol/µmol of creatinine)[a]	BLOOD (nmol/ml)[a]	METHOD	REFERENCES
8.57-27.64[b]		GLC	Tormey et al., 1980
	1.72±0.77	RIA	Levine et al., 1975
22.6±4.32		HPLC	Gehrke et al., 1979
17.7±6.36		HPLC	Salvatore et al., 1983a
26.7±9.0[c]		HPLC	Kuo et al., 1978
	2.54±0.50	HPLC	Colonna et al., 1983b
24.8±9.6		HPLC	Trewyn et al., 1982

[a] mean values ± 2 S.D., or range.
[b] calculated on the basis of creatinine mean urinary excretion of 12.3 mmoles/24 h.
[c] determined in female subjects.

We have also determined the Ψ concentration in human urine by using the method of Gehrke et al. (1978). The clearance of this compound (about 80 ml/min) suggests that it is excreted as a compound which is not reabsorbed nor secreted at tubular level.

PSEUDOURIDINE LEVELS IN BODY FLUIDS OF TUMOR PATIENTS

It has long been known that urinary modified nucleosides are increased in cancer patients (Adams et al., 1960; Park et al., 1962; Weissman et al., 1963; Hogan et al., 1970; Pinkard et al., 1972). After the early findings, several groups have studied this phenomenon using more accurate methodologies, and the results appear to be promising for a possible use of these compounds as biological tumor markers. The most interesting data are those of Walkees et al. (1975), who carried out a systematic study on more than 250 patients with various types of solid tumors, including lung, breast, gastrointestinal carcinomas, melanomas etc. They used GLC to show that the increase of urinary excretion of modified nucleosides occurs in a high percentage of cases and that it seems to be cancer-related since in 61 out of 62 non-neoplastic patients Ψ excretion was within the normal range. The same research group studied, still by means of GLC, the correlation of urinary Ψ and two other modified nucleosides, (N^2,N^2-dimethylguanosine and 1-methylinosine) with the clinical progression of breast cancer. They found that only Ψ levels are correlated with the progression of the disease or with its relapse occuring during a chemotherapeutic treatment (Tormey et al., 1980). A significant relationship between increased levels of modified nucleosides in urine of 96 patients suffering from Hodgkin's disease and the number of atypical histiocytes has been also demonstrated (Cooper et al., 1977). HPLC technology has provided a more accurate pattern of urinary modified nucleosides (Gehrke et al., 1979) and the study was extended to other malignancies with correlations between the nucleoside levels and the stage of the neoplastic disease (Speer et al., 1979). A recent contribution (Waalkes et al., 1982) has confirmed the correspondence between tumor burden and the elevation of nucleosides. Increased levels of modified nucleosides have been found in nasopharyngeal carcinoma (Trewyn et al., 1982), and in different types of acute leukemias (Heldman et al., 1983). In this last series it was observed that a significant increase of modified nucleosides in the urine occurred only during the blastic phase of chronic myelogenous leukemia.

We have investigated the levels of some modified nucleosides in the urine of patients suffering from various types of lymphoma, at various stages and before any therapeutic treatment (Cimino et al., 1982; Salvatore et al.,1983a). Of the 7 modified nucleosides studied, Ψ was the most highly and

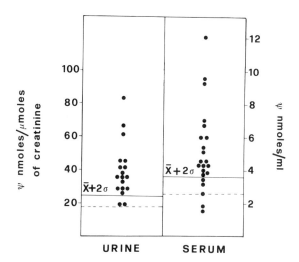

Fig. 1. Pseudouridine concentration in urine and serum of neo-
        plastic patients; from the data reported by Salvatore et
        al. (1983a) and Salvatore et al.(1983b).
        Dotted lines indicate mean normal values (X̄).

frequently increased, as well as the one that correlates best
with the progression of the disease and the response to therapy.
In another investigation (Salvatore et al., 1983b), Ψ levels were
determined in blood serum of patients bearing different types of
tumor. It was found that serum Ψ levels were significantly
increased in metastatic tumors, whereas a slight, if any,
increase was observed in localized tumors. Figure 1 summarizes
the results of Ψ determination in these two series of patients.
We also investigated the use of serum Ψ determination as a tool
for monitoring the response to treatment. Serum Ψ was evaluated
in 6 cancer patients before treatment and at the time of the
clinical evaluation of the response to therapy, or, as in one
case of non-Hodgkin lymphoma, during the chemotherapeutic
courses. In all the examined cases a satisfactory correlation was

found between the clinical response to therapy and the decrease (or increase) of Ψ serum levels.

PSEUDOURIDINE IN BIOLOGICAL FLUIDS OF ANIMALS WITH EXPERIMENTAL NEOPLASIAS

Very little is known about the mechanism(s) underlying the elevation of modified nucleosides in body fluids of cancer patients.One of the handicaps that limit investigations in this field is the difficulty of studying the phenomenon in humans. The only experimental study on this topic was performed by Borek et al. (1977). The rationale behind the experiment was based on the following considerations: i) β-AIB is the urinary end-product of thymine from both DNA and tRNA; ii) the methyl donors used for the biosynthesis of dTTP and ribothymidine in tRNA are N^5,N^{10} - methylene-tetrahydrofolate and adenosylmethionine, respectively. Thus, ^{14}C-formate and C^3H_3-methionine were administered to normal rats and to rats with tumor of the bladder. The ratio of the specific activity of the first label toward the second one in the urinary β-AIB was measured at different times, and found to be markedly decreased in tumor-bearing rats. This result was attributed to a greater turnover rate of tRNA in tumor tissue than in normal tissue.

Other studies have exploited experimental animal systems to investigate the concentration of modified nucleosides in biological fluids of cancer organisms. It was found that the urinary concentration was increased in animals bearing tumors such as Yoshida sarcoma (Shimizu and Fushimura, 1978) or 3-methyl-cholantrene-induced subcutaneous tumor (Thomale and Nass, 1982). In the latter case the increase seemed to preceed clinical evidence of the disease.

We have evaluated serum Ψ concentration in inbred mice, with spontaneous or transplanted lymphoproliferative diseases (Russo et al., 1983c). These studies (performed in collaboration with Drs. C. Gurgo and S. Bridges of the "Centro di Endocrinologia ed Oncologia Sperimentale del CNR - Napoli") focused on the AKR mouse strain, which shows a very high incidence of spontaneous thymic lymphoma (100% in female mice), with a high predictability of the onset of the disease ranging between the 7th and the 9th month of age. The disease becomes clinically and histopatho- logically evident after a "preneoplastic" period (6th month of age), during which several biochemical phenomena occur, including the generation of recombinant retroviruses, which are believed to be the etiological agents of the disease (Gross, 1970).

Table 3. Pseudouridine serum concentration in mice with spontaneous or transplanted lymphoproliferative disease (data
from Russo et al., 1983c).

	PSEUDOURIDINE nmol/ml±SD
BALB/c male mice from 1 to 11 months[a]:	6.69±1.80
BALB/c female mice from 1 to 11 months[a]:	8.10±2.49
AKR male mice from 1 to 9 months:	6.30±1.51
AKR female mice from 0.5 to 5 months:	8.55±2.15
AKR female mice of 6 months:	12.31±3.34
AKR lymphomatous mice with localized disease:	12.12±1.80
AKR lymphomatous mice with disseminated disease:	21.30±5.69

a: BALB/c mice, which have a low incidence of spontaneous
lymphomas, were examined as a control group.

As shown in Table 3, Ψ levels were found significantly and
constantly higher in lymphomatous mice than in normal ones, with
the highest values in the cases of disseminated disease. More
interestingly, a significant difference was observed between
Ψ serum levels of young normal mice (up to 5-6 months of age) and
the "preneoplastic" mice (6 month old). The latter, in fact,
showed increased Ψ levels in absence of any clinical, histopathological and biological sign of the disease, thus indicating
that serum Ψ determination can be a preclinical marker of the
lymphoma development in AKR mice.

The relationship between the increase of Ψ serum levels and
the tumor burden was studied in syngenic mice, which received a
transplantation of AKR lymphomatous thymocytes (T2 cells). During
an observation period of 25 days after transplantation a close
relationship between the increase of serum Ψ levels and the
increase of thymus and spleen weight was observed. This phenomenon does not appear to be simply linked to cell proliferation; in
fact, by using another neoplastic cell line of lymphocytic origin
(MOPC-460), whose i.v. transplantation in syngenic mice (BALB/c)
causes a disseminated myeloma, no increase of Ψ serum
concentration was observed even in presence of a very large tumor
burden. A similar behaviour was observed in hibrid mice
(AKR-BALB/c), whose Ψ serum levels increased only in the mice
transplanted with T2 tumor cells, whereas MOPC-460 cell
transplantation did not affect Ψ levels (unpublished results).
This observation suggests that the elevation of serum Ψ could be
tumor specific. The possibility that serum Ψ is a specific marker

for some neoplastic diseases is at present only a stimulating hypothesis, which deserves further studies.

The elevation of Ψ in the AKR lymphoma and not in the BALB/c myeloma could be due to differences between the two experimental systems. One such difference is the presence of retroviruses in the AKR mice, another is the different cell target for the two neoplasias (T and B lymphocytes in the AKR and BALB/c, respectively). As far as the presence of retroviruses in the AKR system is concerned, it is interesting to note that RNA oncogenic virus transcription requires a specific cellular tRNA, which functions as a primer for reverse transcriptase. For the AKR viruses, this tRNA has been identified as a tRNA^{Pro} (Harada et al., 1979), whereas for the Rous sarcoma virus is a tRNA^{Trp} (Harada et al., 1975). Both these tRNAs have an extra Ψ in the IV loop instead of ribothimidine.

It is tempting to speculate that after the tRNA molecule has functioned as a primer for reverse transcriptase it becomes a functionless molecule and as such undergoes to a faster degradation, with the result that a higher production of free Ψ takes place. Preliminary results obtained in the Authors laboratory (Esposito et al., 1983) show that when chick embryo fibroblasts are infected by RSV, a high quantity of Ψ is excreted in the cell medium, before any morphological sign of transformation is visible. If the infected CEF are comparable to thymocytes from six-month old AKR mice remains to be demonstrated.

Whatever the mechanism of serum Ψ elevation is, the results obtained with the AKR system indicate that the increase of Ψ levels is a precocious biochemical sign of the onset of the disease and that it appears to be connected with some early event of cell transformation.

AKNOWLEDGEMENTS

The experiments from Authors laboratory have been supported by grants from Progetto Finalizzato Controllo Crescita Neoplastica, CNR, Rome, Italy.

REFERENCES

Adams W. S., Davis F. and Nakatani M., 1960, Purine and
     pyrimidine excretion in normal and leukemic subjects, Am. J.
     Med. 28:726.
Adler M. and Gutman A. B., 1959, Uridine isomer (5-ribosyluracil)
     in human urine, Science 130:862.
Arena F., Ciliberto G., Ciampi S., and Cortese R., 1978,

Purification of pseudouridylate synthetase I from <u>Salmonella</u> <u>typhimurium</u>, Nucleic Acid Res. 5:4523.

Borek E., Baliga B. S., Gehrke C.W., Kuo K. C., Belman S., Troll W., Waalkes T. P., 1977, High turnover rate of transfer RNA in tumor tissue, Cancer Res. 37:3362.

Brand R. C., Klootwijk J., Siburn C. P. and Planta R. J., 1979, Pseudouridylation of yeast ribosomal precursor RNA, Nucleic Acids Res. 7:121.

Busch H., Reddy R., Rothblum L. and Choi Y. C., 1982, SnRNAs, snRNPs, and RNA processing, Ann. Rev. Biochem. 51:617.

Chambers R. W., The chemistry of pseudouridine, 1966, Prog. Nucleic Acid Res. Mol. Biol. 5:349.

Chang S.Y., Lakings D. B., Zumwalt R. W., Gehrke C. W. and Waalkes T. P., 1974, Quantitative determination of methylated nucleosides and pseudouridine in urine by gas-liquid chromatography, J. Lab. Clin. Clin. Med. 83:816.

Cimino F., Costanzo F., Russo T., Colonna A., Esposito F., Salvatore F., 1982, Modified nucleosides from transfer ribonucleic acid as tumor markers, in:"The Biochemistry of S-Adenosylmethionine and related compounds", E. Usdin, R. T. Borchardt, C.R. Creveling, eds., MacMillan, London.

Colonna A. and Kerr S. J., 1980, The nucleus as the site of tRNA methylation, J. Cell. Physiol. 103:29.

Colonna A., Duilio A., Russo T., Salvatore F., and Cimino F., 1983a, tRNA pseudouridine synthase activity in malignant cells. Abstracts of 15th F.E.B.S. Meeting, Bruxelles, p. 243.

Colonna A., Russo T., Esposito F., Salvatore F., Cimino F.,1983b Determination of pseudouridine and other nucleosides in human blood serum by high performance liquid chromatography, Anal. Biochem. 130:19.

Cooper I. A., Wray G. R. and Murphy T. L., 1977, Urinary excretion patterns of tRNA degradation products: a marker of Hodgkin's cell metabolism? Europ. J. Cancer 13:1309.

Cortese R., Kammen H. O., Spengler S. J., and Ames B. N., 1974a, Biosynthesis of pseudouridine transfer ribonucleic acid, J. Biol. Chem. 249:1103.

Cortese R., Landsberg R., Von der Haar R. A., Umbarger H. E. and Ames B. N., 1974b, Pleiotropy of His T mutants blocked in pseudouridine synthesis in tRNA: leucine and isoleucine-valine operon, Proc. Natl. Acad. Sci. U.S.A., 71:1857.

Esposito F., Ammendola R., Russo T., and Cimino F., 1983, Abstract of 29th Meeting of S.I.B., Saint Vincent, Italy, p. 509.

Fujimura S. and Shimizu M., 1977, Enhanced activity of tRNA pseudouridine synthetase in Yoshida ascites sarcoma. Biochim. Biophys. Res. Commun. 79:763.

Gauss D.H. and Sprinzl, 1983, Compilation of tRNA sequences, Nucleic Acid Res., 11:rl.

Gehrke C. W., Kuo K. C., Davis G. E., Suits R. D., Waalkes T. P.,

E. Borek, 1978, Quantitative high-performance liquid
    chromatography of nucleoside in biological materials.
    J. Chromatogr. 150:455.
Gehrke C. W., Kuo K. C., Waalkes T. P., Borek E., 1979, Pattern
    of urinary excretion of modified nucleosides, Cancer Res.
    39:1150.
Green C. J., Kammen H. O., and Penhoet E. E., 1982, Purification
    and properties of a mammalian tRNA pseudouridine synthase,
    J. Biol. Chem. 257:3045.
Gross L., 1970, "Oncogenic viruses", Pergamon Press, London.
Harada F., Sawyer R. C., and Dahlberg J. E., 1975, A primer
    ribonucleic acid for initiation of in vitro Rous sarcoma
    virus deoxyribonucleic acid synthesis, J. Biol. Chem.
    2500:3483.
Harada F., Peters G. G., and Dahlberg J. E., 1979, The primer
    tRNA for Moloney murine leukemia virus DNA synthesis, J.
    Biol. Chem. 254:10979.
Heldman D. A., Grever M. R., Trewyn R. W., 1983, Differential
    excretion of modified nucleosides in adult acute leukemia,
    Blood 61:291.
Hogan A., Creuss-Callaghan A. and Fennelly J. J., 1970, Studies
    of pseudouridine change in chronic lymphatic leukemia during
    therapy, Ir. J. Med. Sci. 3:505.
Hughes D. G. and Maden B. E. H., 1978, The pseudouridine contents
    of the ribosomal ribonucleic acids of three vertebrate
    species, Biochem. J. 171:781.
Kuo K. C., Gehrke C. W., Mc Cune R. A., Waalkes T. P. and Borek
    E.,1978, Rapid, quantitative high-performance liquid column
    chromatography of pseudouridine, 145:383.
Levine$_2$L., Waalkes T. P., and Stolbach L., 1975, Serum levels of
    N^2,N^2-dimethylguanosine and pseudouridine as
    determined by radioimmunoassay for patients with
    malignancy, J. Natl. Cancer Inst. 54:341.
Matsushita T., and Davis F. F., 1971, Studies on pseudouridylic
    acid synthetase from various sources. Biochim. Biophys.
    Acta 238:165.
Melton D. A., De Robertis E. M., and Cortese R., 1980, Order and
    intracellular location of the events involved in the
    maturation of the spliced RNA, Nature 284:143.
Ming Chu T., 1982,"Biochemical markers for cancer", Marcel Dekker
    Inc., New York and Berlin.
Park R. W., Holland J. F. and Jenkins R., 1962, Urinary purines
    in leukemia, Cancer Res. 22:469.
Pinkard K. J., Cooper I. A., Motterman R. and Turner C. N., 1972,
    Purine and pyrimidine excretion in Hodgkin's disease, J.
    Natl. Cancer Inst. 49:27.
Randerath K., Yu C. T. and Randerath E., 1972, Base analysis of
    ribopolynucleotides by chemical tritium labeling: a
    methodological study with model nucleosides and purified
    tRNA species, Anal. Biochem. 48:172.

Russo T., Bridges S., Gurgo C., Salvatore F., and Cimino F., 1983a, Determination of pseudouridine present in tRNA and in acid soluble extract of thymic murine lymphoma. Abstracts of 15th F.E.B.S. Meeting, Bruxelles, p. 313.

Russo T. and Cimino F., 1983b, High performance liquid chromatography analysis of nucleoside composition of tRNA. Abstracts of 3rd International Symposium on HPLC of Proteins, Peptides and polynucleotides, p. 24.

Russo T., Colonna A., Salvatore F., Cimino F., Bridges S., and Gurgo C., 1983c, Serum pseudouridine as a biochemical marker in the development of AKR mouse lymphoma. Cancer Res.,in press.

Salvatore F., Colonna A., Costanzo F., Russo T., Esposito F., and F. Cimino, 1983a, Modified nucleosides in body fluids of tumor-bearing patients, Recent Results Cancer Res. 84:360.

Salvatore F., Russo T., Colonna A., Cimino L., Mazzacca G., and Cimino F., 1983b, Pseudouridine determination in blood serum as tumor marker, Cancer Detec. Prev. 6: in press.

Shimizu M., and Fushimura S., 1978, Studies on the abnormal excretion of pyrimidine nucleosides in the urine of Yoshida ascites sarcoma-bearing rats, Biochim. Biophys, Acta 517: 277.

Speer J., Gehrke C. W., Kuo K. C., Waalkes T. P., Borek E., 1979, tRNA breakdown products as markers for cancer, Cancer 44:2120.

Thomale J., and Nass G., 1982, Elevated urinary excretion of RNA catabolites as an early signal of tumor development in mice. Cancer Letters 15:149.

Tormey D. C., Waalkes T. P., Gehrke C. W., 1980, Biological markers in breast carcinoma. Clinical correlation with pseudouridine, N^2,N^2-dimethylguanosine and 1-methylinosine, J. Surg. Oncol. 14:267.

Trewyn R. W., Glaser R., Kelly D. R., Jakson D. G., Graham W. P., and Speicher C. E., 1982, Elevated nucleoside excretion by patients with nasopharyngeal carcinoma, Cancer 49:2513.

Waalkes T. P., Gehrke C. W., Zumwalt R. W., Chang S. Y., Lakings D.B., Tormey D. C., Ahmann D. L., Moertel C. G., 1975, The urinary excretion of nucleosides of ribonucleic acid by patients with advanced cancer, Cancer 36:390.

Waalkes T. P., Abeloff M. D., Ettinger D. S., Woo K. B., Gehrke C. W., Kuo K. C., Borek E., 1982, Biological markers and small cell carcinoma of the lung. A clinical evaluation of urinary ribonucleosides, Cancer 50:2457.

Weissman B., Bromberg P. A. and Guttman A. B., 1957, The purine bases of human urine. Separation and identification. J. Biol. Chem. 224:407.

Weissman S. M., Lewis M. and Karon M., 1963, Pseudouridine metabolism. Excretion of pseudouridine and other nitrogenous metabolites in chronic leukemia, Blood 22:657.

SERUM LIPID ASSOCIATED SIALIC ACID IN DIFFERENT HUMAN MALIGNANCES:

PRELIMINARY RESULTS

L. Santamaria[1], N. Katopodis[2], G. Santagati[1], A. Bianchi[1],
R. Pizzala[1], and C.C. Stock[2]

[1]C. Golgi Institute of General Pathology, Centro Tumori
Medical Clinic; Institute of Pharmacology II, University
of Pavia, USSL 77, 27100 Pavia, Italy
[2]Sloan Kettering Institute for Cancer Research, New York,
NY 10021; N-K Laboratories, Stamford, CT 06901, USA

INTRODUCTION

The documentation of alteration in the metabolism of tumor
cell surface glycoproteins and sialoglycolipids[1,2] has encouraged
the study of these components as possible tumor marker in blood.
Recent studies show that mean values for total bound sialic
acid[3,4,5,6] or protein bound sialic acid[7,8] were higher in cancer
patients than in normal subjects. Sialic acid levels correlated
with stage of disease[9,7], tumor burden[5,10], degree of metastasis
and recurrence of disease[11]. In some cases protein-bound sialic
acid showed only limited correlation with the clinical disease
status of the patient[8]. A serious limitation of this procedure was
the finding that sialic acid levels were also elevated in other
inflammatory or chronic diseases[9,5,12] resulting in false positive
findings.

Interest in sialoglycolipids (gangliosides) as markers in cancer
was generated by the discovery that circulating levels of these
components were elevated in tumor bearing animals in a pattern
consistent with the concept that lipid bound sialic acid (LSA) was
of tumor origin[13,14]. In other animal experiments, elevated LSA

41

levels were reported in mice bearing transplanted mammary tumors[15], in dogs with various spontaneous tumors[16], and in leukemic AKR/J mice[17].

Increases in serum/plasma lipid bound sialic acid or lipid associated sialic acid have been reported in cancer patients in general[18] and in patients with breast cancer[15], prostate cancer[19], bladder cancer[19], or melanoma[22].

LSA has not been studied extensively in human tumors but alterations in sialoglycolipids have been reported in brain tumors[20], gastric and colonic carcinomas[21], malignant melanomas[22] and leukemic leukocytes[23].

Recently, Katopodis and Stock[24] developed a simple reliable procedure for determining LSA in serum or plasma; this method assays lipid associated sialic acid (LSA), rather than individual serum gangliosides concentration in plasma or serum, and its speed allows rapid screening of patients with suspected malignancy and their follow-up regarding variation of blood level of LSA in conjunction with therapeutic effect of therapy. Their results indicate that measurement of LSA may be more useful and discriminating than measurement of total sialic acid, so we have employed this procedure to investigate the role of LSA as a tumor marker.

The present study regards serum LSA levels in patients bearing breast, gastric, lung cancers, leucoses and limphomas. Such patients were from general hospitals in the Pavia area.

MATERIALS AND METHODS

The method used is the one developed by Katopodis et al.[18] and improved by Katopodis and Stock[24]. Blood samples were clotted, separated, and assayed within few hours from drawing or stored at -80 C in freezer, until assayed, to avoid loose of detectable LSA[8]. Such blood samples were from 42 patients as follows: 13 with primary breast cancer, 7 with primary gastric cancer and 6 with primary lung cancer, 4 with non-Hodgkin's lymphoma, 2 with Hodgkin's lymphoma, 3 with lymphocytic leucosis and 2 with myelocytic leucosis, and from 20 normal subjects with no evidence of disease, as control. Statistical analysis was carried out using range, mean, and standard deviation.

RESULTS

Results, as reported in Figure 1, show a relevant increase in LSA blood level in a spectrum of malignances broader than in other tumor marker tests. The average value of LSA blood level in the total tumors is above 50% higher than normals. The most elevated values respect to normal (20.76 $\pm$ 3.45 mg/100 ml serum) were found in lymphomas (+87.9%), next in lung cancer (+72.4%), leucosis (+57%), gastric cancer (+36.7%) and breast cancer (+31.5%). The average LSA level increase in cancer patients was found to be +61%.

DISCUSSION

The above data are in general agreement with those published as carried out in USA[24,25,26]. Our values of normals, however, are about 25% higher than those reported in other laboratories; nevertheless, pathological values are higher but with the same order of magnitude. This may be explained with minor differences in running the test, as far as basic chemicals origin.

The overall picture of the data confirms that serum LSA may be a non - specific marker in cancer. In this connection, should be recalled that LSA values in blood serum from patients with benign breast disease are not significantly different from the normals[26].

Such a marker appears to be quite definite in patients bearing lymphomas, leukemias and lung cancer. In the case of breast cancer and gastric cancer a few false negatives may be detected.

Ongoing studies indicate that monitoring cancer patients with LSA determination is helpful in that LSA levels rise immediately after surgery, fall again within 2-4 weeks postoperatively in case of success, whereas persistent elevations or their developments are associated with failing of therapy[19]. Decrease in LSA values is registered also after radiation and/or chemotherapy in patients with Hodgkin's disease[25].

Limitations of the LSA test may be due to the above false negatives data in a few types of cancer. On the whole, however, such a test appears to deserve further studies to contribute to the detection, monitoring and possibly the assessment of the clinical status of cancer patients.

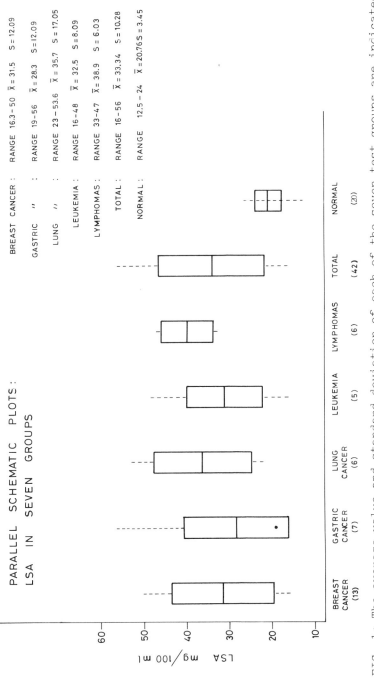

FIG. 1: The average value and standard deviation of each of the seven test groups are indicated on a rectangle. The cancer groups appear to have both greater spread of LSA values and larger LSA values than do the normals.

SUMMARY

Lipid-bound sialic acid (LSA), as a non-specific tumor marker, was evaluated in serum from 42 patients bearing breast, gastric, lung cancers, leukemias and lymphomas. The data showed increase of LSA levels.

AKNOWLEDGEMENTS

This research project is under the auspices of the Ministero della Sanità, Dir. Gen. Serv. Med. Soc. Div. IV; Roma.

REFERENCES

1. S. I. Hakomori, Glycolipids of tumor cell membrane. Adv. Cancer Res. 18: 265-315 (1974).
2. V. N. Nigam, A. Cantero, Polysaccharides in cancer:glycoproteins and glycolipids. Adv. Cancer Res. 17:1-80 (1973).
3. A. Hogan-Ryan, J. J. Fennelly, J. Jones, B. Cantevell, M. J. Duffy, Serum sialic acid and CEA concentration in human breast cancer. Br. J. Cancer 41:587-592 (1980).
4. H. K. B. Silver, K. A. Karim, F. A. Salinas, Development of an improved assay for N-acetil neuraminic acid (NANA) using high performance liquid chromatography (Abstr) Proc. Am. Ass. Cancer Res. 22:185 (1981).
5. H. K. B. Silver, D. M. Rangel, D. L. Morton, Serum sialic acid elevations in malignant melanoma patients. Cancer 41:1497-1499 (1978).
6. R. J. Shamberger, Sialic acid in cancer patients (Abstr). Proc. Am. Ass. Cancer Res. 22:21 (1981).
7. A. J. Moss, N. K. Bissada, C. M. Boyd, W. C. Hunter, Significance of protein-bound neuraminic acid level in patients with prostatic and bladder carcinoma. Urology 13:182-184 (1979).
8. J. E. Mrochek, S. R. Dinsmore, D. C. Tormey, T. P. Waalkes, Protein-bound carbohydrates in breast cancer: liquid chromatographic analysis for mannose, galactose,fucose and sialic acid in serum. Clin. Chem. 2:1516-1521.
9. R. A. L. MacBeth, J. G. Bekasi, Plasma glycoprotein in various diseases states including carcinoma. Cancer Res. 22:1170-1176 (1962).
10. H. K. B. Silver, K. A. Karim, E. L. Archibald, F. A. Salinas, Serum sialic acid and sialyltransferase as monitor of tumor burden in malignant melanoma patients. Cancer Res. 39:5036-5042 (1979).

11. O. Kirikuta, R. Bojan Comes, R. Cristian, Significance of serum fucose, sialic acid, haptoglobine and phospholipide levels in the evolution and treatment of breast cancer. Arch. Geschivultforsch 49:16-112 (1979).

12. A. Lipton, H. A. Harvey, S. Delong et Al., Glycoproteins and human cancer 1. Circulating levels in cancer serum. Cancer 43:1766-1771 (1979).

13. A. M. Dnistrian, V. P. Skipski, M. Barclay, E. S. Essner and C. C. Stock: Gangliosides of plasma membranes from normal rat liver and Morris Hepatoma. Biochem. Biophis. Res. Comm. 64:367-375 (1975).

14. V. P. Skipski, N. Katopodis, J. S. Prendergast and C. C. Stock, Gangliosides in blood serum of normal rats and Morris hepatoma 5123 tc-bearing rats. Biochem. Biophis. Res. Comm. 67:1122-1127 (1975).

15. F. M. Kloppel, T. W. Keenan, M. J. Freeman, D. J. Moore, Glycolipids-bound sialic acid in serum: increased levels in mice and human bearing mammary carcinomas. Proc. Natl. Acad. Sci. 74:3011-3013.

16. F. M. Kloppel, C. P. Franz, D. J. Moore, R. C. Richardson, Serum sialic acid levels increase in tumor bearing dogs. Am. J. Vet. Res. 39:1377-1380 (1978).

17. E. E. Lengle, Increased level of lipid bound sialic acid in thymic lymphocytes and plasma from leukemic AKR/J mice. J. Natl. Cancer. Inst. 62:1565-1567 (1979).

18. N. Katopodis, Y. Hirshaut and C. C. Stock, Spectrophotometric assay of total lipid-bound sialic acid in blood plasma of cancer patients and asymptomatic healty individuals. Proc. Am. Assoc. Cancer. Res. 21:182 (1980).

19. U. Dunzendorfer, N. Katopodis, A. N. Dnistrian, C. C. Stock, M. K. Schwartz, W. E. Jr. Withmore, Plasma lipid bound sialic acid in patients with prostate and bladder cancer. Investigative Urology 19, 3 194-196 (1981).

20. D. Kostic and F. Bucheit, Gangliosides in human brain tumor. Life Sci. 9:589-596 (1970).

21. A. Keranen, M. Lempinen and K. Puro, Gangliosides pattern and neuraminic acid content of human gastric and colonic carcinoma. Clin. Chem. Acta 70:103-112 (1976).

22. J. Portoukalian, G. Zwingelstein, J. F. Dore, 4th International symposium on malignant melanoma- Lyon- France- (1976).

23. J. Hildebrand, P. A. Stryckmans and J. Vanouche, Gangliosides in leukemic and non-leukemic human leukocites. Biochem.

Biophis. Acta 260:272-278 (1972).

24. N. Katopodis and C. C. Stock, Improved method to determine
     lipid bound sialic acid in plasma or serum. Res. Comm.
     Chem. Pathol. Pharm. 30:171-180 (1980).

25. N. Katopodis, Y. Hirshaut, N. L. Geller and C. C. Stock,
     Lipid associated sialic acid test for the detection of
     human cancer. Cancer Res. 42:5270-5275 (1982).

26. A. M. Dnistrian, K. Morton, N. Katopodis, A. Fracchia and
     C. C. Stock, Serum lipid-bound sialic acid as a marker in
     breast cancer. Cancer 50:1815-1819 (1982).

HETEROGENEITY OF BINDING SITES FOR TRIPHENYLETHYLENE ANTIESTROGENS IN ESTROGEN TARGET TISSUES

Alberto Gulino and Jorge Raul Pasqualini

C.N.R.S. Steroid Hormone Research Unit
Foundation for Hormone Research
26 boulevard Brune, 75014 Paris, France

INTRODUCTION

Most of the interest in understanding the mechanism of action of triphenylethylene antiestrogens (Fig. 1) arises from their ability to induce weak estrogenic effects, to antagonize many of the actions of estrogens and to induce the remission of human breast cancer particularly during the post-menopausal period (Legha et al., 1978). In particular, these compounds are able to suppress estrogen-induced uterine growth (Jordan et al., 1977) and to antagonize estrogen-induced growth of human breast cancer cells which contain estrogen receptor (Lippman et al., 1976). In this regard, triphenylethylene antiestrogens are used for understanding the mechanism by which estrogens regulate cell growth. However, triphenylethylene antiestrogens are also able to inhibit the growth of estrogen sensitive and estrogen receptor containing human breast cancer cells, even in the absence of estrogens (Lippman et al., 1976). The attempt to understand the mechanism of action of both estrogen and antiestrogens awaits the elucidation of the molecular events and interactions which occur at the subcellular and cellular level. In recent years, multiple interactions of triphenylethylene antiestrogens have been reported at the subcellular level : a) the interaction with the estrogen receptor system (Terenius, 1971 ; Lippman et al., 1976 ; Horwitz and McGuire, 1978), and b) the binding of these compounds to specific binding sites distinct from the estrogen receptor in several experimental models such as the chick oviduct (Sutherland and Foo, 1979), rat uterus (Faye et al., 1980), fetal guinea pig uterus (Gulino and Pasqualini, 1980), human mammary cancer (Sutherland and Murphy, 1980) and human myometrium (Kon, 1983). The aim of this paper is to summarize the data so far known about the interactions of triphenylethylene antiestrogens with target cells at the subcellular level.

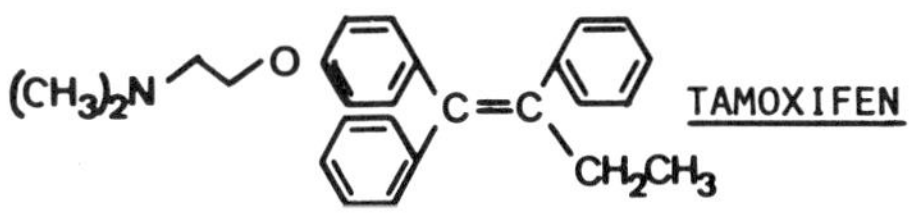

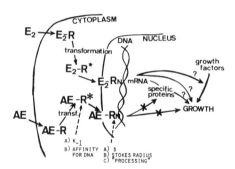

Figure 1. Structure of the antiestrogen Tamoxifen.

For this purpose, the interactions of triphenylethylene antiestrogens with the estrogen receptor system and their eventual implications in mediating antiestrogen actions on cancer cells are briefly reported. Furthermore, the partial characterization of triphenylethylene antiestrogen-specific binding sites and their possible role in modulating the distribution and the action of antiestrogens will be described. We will particularly describe the characteristics of the triphenylethylene antiestrogen-specific binding sites we have observed in the fetal uterus of guinea pig, which we have previously reported to be a useful model for the study of estrogen and anti-estrogen action (Gulino and Pasqualini, 1980 ; Pasqualini and Nguyen, 1980 ; Pasqualini et al., 1980 ; Sumida and Pasqualini, 1980), and we will compare their characteristics with those of fetal uterine estrogen receptor and of triphenylethylene antiestrogen-specific binding sites described in other models.

Figure 2. Model of the mechanism of action of estrogens and anti-estrogens. E_2 : estradiol ; R : estrogen receptor ; Rn : nuclear estrogen receptor ; AE : antiestrogen. The broken arrows indicate the characteristics which differentiate the estrogen receptor-antiestrogen complex from the estrogen receptor-estradiol complex (from Horwitz and McGuire, 1978 ; Rochefort and Borgna, 1981 ; Eckert and Katzenellenbogen, 1982 ; Evans et al., 1982).

TRIPHENYLETHYLENE ANTIESTROGENS AND THE ESTROGEN RECEPTOR SYSTEM

Figure 2 summarizes some of the molecular events which mediate estrogen action in target cells. The principal event is the binding of estradiol to cytoplasmic receptor proteins, which is followed by the transfer of the activated complex to the nucleus, its binding to the chromatin, the synthesis of specific mRNA by activation of RNA polymerase activity and the subsequent synthesis of specific proteins. Antiestrogens have been shown to interact directly with the estrogen receptor in uterus and breast cancer cells and to translocate estrogen receptor to the nucleus (Jordan et al., 1977 ; Horwitz and McGuire, 1978). The nuclear antiestrogen-receptor complex appears to be only partially active in promoting specific biological responses and is effective in blocking the action of estrogens (Lippman et al., 1976 ; Horwitz et al., 1978 ; Westley and Rochefort, 1980). This suggests that antiestrogen-receptor complex and its interaction with chromatin might be different from those of estra-diol-receptor complex. Such differences have indeed been found for nuclear receptor of human breast cancer cells (sedimentation co-efficient, Stokes radius, nuclear "processing") (Horwitz and McGuire, 1978 ; Eckert and Katzenellenbogen, 1982) and of rat uterus (salt extractibility) (Baudendistel and Ruh, 1976). A difference in the "activation" process of cytoplasmic estrogen receptor by antiestrogens and estradiol has also been reported (Rochefort and Borgna, 1981 ; Evans et al., 1982). Whether the differences in the actions of est-radiol and antiestrogens on target cells are due to differences in interactions with the estrogen receptor system is not however fully elucidated. As reported in Table 1, several findings suggest a role of estrogen receptors in mediating antiestrogen action on the growth of cancer cells. However, the exclusive role of estrogens and estrogen receptors in the control of cancer cell proliferation has not yet been fully elucidated, and findings from several laboratories suggest that additional events could mediate the inhibitory effect of anti-estrogens on cancer growth (Table 1).

THE FETAL UTERUS OF GUINEA PIG AS A MODEL FOR THE STUDY OF ANTI-ESTROGEN ACTION

Biological Responses to Triphenylethylene Antiestrogens in the Fetal Uterus of Guinea pig

We have previously reported that the fetal uterus of guinea pig contains high amounts of estrogen receptors (Pasqualini and Nguyen, 1976). Estrogens are also able to induce several biological responses in this fetal organ (Pasqualini and Nguyen, 1980 ; Sumida and Pasqualini, 1980). The responsiveness of the fetal uterus to

Table 1. A) Antiestrogen-induced Inhibition of Cancer Cell growth
            is Mediated by Estrogen Receptor

---

1. Correlation between affinity for estrogen receptor and biolo-
    gical potency in vitro of different antiestrogens (Coezy et
    al., 1982).

2. Lack of antiestrogen activity in estrogen receptor-negative
    breast cancer cells (Lippman et al., 1976).

3. Estradiol can reverse the effect of tamoxifen (<10 μM)
    (Lippman et al., 1976 ; Sutherland et al., 1983).

B) Antiestrogen-induced Inhibition of Cancer Cell growth
            not Mediated by Estrogen Receptor

---

1. Estradiol does not reverse the effect of tamoxifen (≥ 10 μM)
    (Sutherland et al., 1983).

2. Antiestrogen can inhibit the growth of some estrogen receptor-
    negative breast cancer cells in culture (Green et al., 1981).

3. Some estrogen receptor-negative tumors respond to tamoxifen
    therapy (Patterson et al., 1982).

---

triphenylethylene antiestrogens is shown by the induction and the
modulation of several estrogenic responses by tamoxifen. The activity of tamoxifen in this fetal organ is particularly complex since
it is able to provoke a uterotrophic effect similar to that induced
by estradiol, while its effect on the increase of the levels of
progesterone receptor is weaker with respect to estradiol (Gulino
and Pasqualini, 1980). Finally tamoxifen also possesses antagonistic
effects, since it antagonizes the estradiol-induced increase of the
acetylation of nuclear histones of the fetal uterus (Pasqualini et
al., 1983). The administration of tamoxifen to fetal guinea pigs
results in a depletion of uterine cytoplasmic estrogen receptors
and in an increase of estrogen receptors in the nuclear fraction,
suggesting that the antiestrogen is able to transfer the estrogen
receptor into the nucleus of this fetal organ (Gulino and Pasqualini,
1980).

    In order to investigate further the subcellular interactions
of triphenylethylene antiestrogens with the fetal uterus of guinea
pig, the binding of tamoxifen in this fetal organ has been studied,
as described in the following sections.

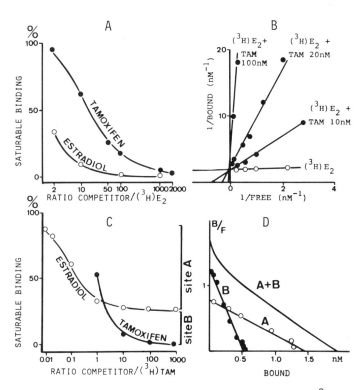

Figure 3. A) Effect of tamoxifen on the binding of [^{3}H]estradiol (E$_2$) (4 nM) to fetal uterine estrogen receptor in the guinea pig. B) Lineweaver-Burk plot of the specific binding of [^{3}H]E$_2$ to cytoplasmic receptor in the presence of tamoxifen. C) Effect of estradiol and tamoxifen on the binding of [^{3}H]tamoxifen (15 nM) in the cytosol of fetal guinea pig uterus. D) Scatchard analysis (Scatchard, 1949) of the binding of [^{3}H]tamoxifen to site A (O), and to site B (●) evaluated as previously described (Gulino and Pasqualini, 1980).

Heterogeneity of Binding Sites for Triphenylethylene Antiestrogens Evidence for Triphenylethylene-specific Binding Sites distinct from Estrogen Receptor

Affinity of tamoxifen for cytoplasmic binding sites in the fetal uterus of guinea pig. The availability of tritiated anti-estrogens has recently allowed a better understanding of the inter-action of triphenylethylene antiestrogens with target cells. We have used [3H]tamoxifen to study the binding of this antiestrogen in the cytosol of the fetal uterus of guinea pig. As indicated in Figures 3 A and B tamoxifen is able to compete with [3H]estradiol for cyto-plasmic estrogen receptor in the fetal uterus of guinea pig. The relative binding affinity of tamoxifen for estrogen receptor is about 10 % that of estradiol (apparent Kd : 1.3 nM). In contrast estradiol only partially displaces [3H]tamoxifen binding in fetal uterine cytosol (about 70 % of the total saturable binding) as shown in Figure 3C and indicated as site A. This figure also indi-cates that the affinity of estradiol for [3H]tamoxifen binding sites (site A) is about 10 times higher that that of tamoxifen itself, in agreement with the differences observed in estimated relative binding affinities for the estrogen receptor of estradiol and tamoxifen in studies using [3H]estradiol (Fig. 3A-B), which suggests a mutually competitive binding of tamoxifen and estradiol to estrogen receptor (site A). But this study also suggests the existence of a saturable specific tamoxifen binding site (site B) distinct from the estrogen receptor.

The presence of distinct binding sites for tamoxifen is also suggested by Scatchard analyses of [3H]tamoxifen binding in fetal uterine cytosol (Fig. 3D) which shows the presence of two classes of binding sites with different affinities. The first one, site A, displaced by estradiol, has a concentration of 1.800 ± 100 fmol/mg protein and a Kd of 1.8 ± 0.4 nM, and the second one, site B, per-sists after saturation of estrogen receptors by estradiol (655 ± 55 fmol/mg protein and Kd 0.4 ± 0.01 nM). Parallel Scatchard analyses of [3H]estradiol binding show the presence of a single class of binding sites (1.600 fmol/mg protein) with an affinity for estradiol (Kd : 0.13 ± 0.05 nM) about 10 times higher than the affinity of [3H]tamoxifen for site A. These data suggest that site A corresponds to the estrogen receptor.

Determination of the sedimentation coefficient of tamoxifen-site A and tamoxifen-site B complexes. The identity between site A and estrogen receptor has been further supported by sedimentation analyses of [3H]tamoxifen cytoplasmic complexes of the fetal uterus of guinea pig, which have been carried out using glycerol gradients containing 0.4 M KCl. Figure 4A shows that [3H]tamoxifen-site B complex sediments more rapidly (sedimentation coefficient about 25 S) than the [3H]tamoxifen-site A complex (4 S). Sedimentation analyses of both [3H]estradiol-estrogen receptor complex and [3H]tamoxifen-

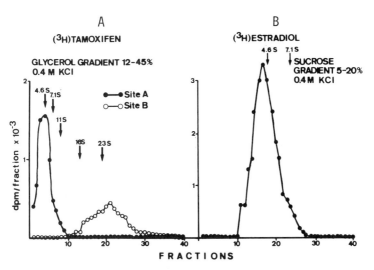

Figure 4. Density gradient analysis of [³H]tamoxifen and [³H]estradiol cytoplasmic complexes in the fetal guinea pig uterus. A) Cytosol (180.000 x g for 30 min supernatant) labelled with [³H]tamoxifen was layered on 12-45 % glycerol gradients containing Tris-HCl 0.01 M, 0.4 M KCl, 10 mM molybdate, 0.5 mM dithiothreitol, pH 7.4 and centrifuged 13 h at 30.000 rpm in a Beckman SW 40 rotor at 4°C. B) [³H]estradiol labelled cytosol was centrifuged at 4°C for 90 min at 60.000 rpm in a Beckman Vti 60 rotor, on a 5-20 % sucrose gradient containing Tris-HCl 0.01 M, 0.4 M KCl, 10 mM molybdate, 0.5 mM dithiothreitol, pH 7.4. Saturable binding is represented. Arrows show the sedimentation coefficients of bovine serum albumine (4.6 S), human γ globuline (7.1 S), Catalase (11 S) and 16 and 23 S RNAs.

site A complex in 0.4 M KCl-containing sucrose gradients produced 4 S sedimenting macromolecules (Fig. 4B and unpublished results, respectively).

Ion-exchange chromatography of [³H]tamoxifen-site A and [³H]-tamoxifen-site B complexes. Ion-exchange chromatography on DEAE-Trisacryl of [³H]tamoxifen and [³H]estradiol cytoplasmic complexes of the fetal uterus of guinea pig resulted in the elution of both [³H]tamoxifen-site A complex and [³H]estradiol-estrogen receptor complex by 0.18 M KCl, while [³H]tamoxifen-site B was eluted by 0.08 M KCl (Fig. 5).

Association and dissociation kinetics of tamoxifen binding in fetal uterine cytosol. As previously reported (Gulino and Pasqualini,

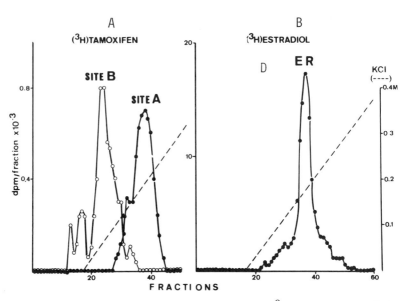

Figure 5. DEAE-Trisacryl chromatography of [^{3}H] tamofixen (A) and
[^{3}H] estradiol (B) cytoplasmic complexes in the fetal uterus of
guinea pig. DEAE-Trisacryl chromatography was carried out as described previously (Screpanti et al., 1982). [^{3}H]tamoxifen and [^{3}H]-
estradiol cytoplasmic complexes obtained as described in Figure 4,
have been eluted by a 0-0.4 M KCl gradient. Saturable binding is
represented. ER : estrogen receptor.

1982), the association kinetics of [^{3}H]tamoxifen to site A and site
B are similar, the association rate constant (k_{+1}) of the antiestrogen to site A being $1.03 \pm 0.5 \times 10^5$ M^{-1}sec^{-1} and that to site
B $0.95 \pm 0.16 \times 10^5$ M^{-1}sec^{-1}.   In contrast, the dissociation kinetics of [^{3}H]tamoxifen from site A and site B underline a further
difference between the two binding sites. In fact, tamoxifen disso-
ciates more slowly from site B at both 4°C (k_{-1} : $0.81 \pm 0.14 \times$
10^{-4}sec^{-1}) and 26°C (k_{-1} : $3.0 \pm 0.4 \times 10^{-4}$sec^{-1}) than from site A
(k_{-1} at 4°C : $8.3 \pm 2 \times 10^{-4}$sec^{-1} and k_{-1} at 26°C : 126×10^{-4}sec^{-1})
(Gulino and Pasqualini, 1982).

Binding specificity of estrogen receptor and antiestrogen
binding sites. Estrogen receptor and site B can also be distinguished
by their different binding specificity. Site B is specific for triphenylethylene antiestrogens because several tamoxifen derivatives
and other triphenylethylene antiestrogens can inhibit the binding
of [^{3}H]tamoxifen to site B (Gulino and Pasqualini, 1982). In contrast
site B does not bind natural and synthetic estrogens nor other
steroids such as cortisol, testosterone and progesterone (Gulino

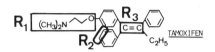

		R	BINDING AFFINITY %	
			AEBS (SITE B)	ER (SITE A)
TAMOXIFEN			100	100
R_1	N-DES-METHYL-TAM	$CH_3HN(CH_2)_2O$	32	100
	METABOLITE E	OH	0	60
	ICI 145680	$OCH_2CHOHCHCH_3$	0	100
	COMPOUND 7	$O(CH_2)_2NHC(NH)NH_2 \cdot HNO_3$	55	200
	COMPOUND 13	$O(CH_2)_2N(CH_2CH_2)_2O$	1174	10
R_2	MONO-OH-TAM	C_4 : OH	10	900
	DI-OH-TAM	C_3 AND C_4 : OH	0.5	500
R_3	METABOLITE A	$\underset{\text{OH H}}{>C-C<}$	35	3
TRIPHENYLETHYLENE NUCLEUS	LY 117018		19	5000

Figure 6. Binding affinities of triphenylethylene antiestrogens for antiestrogen binding site (AEBS) and estrogen receptor (ER) in the fetal guinea pig uterus, rat uterus and MCF-7 breast cancer cells (from Gulino and Pasqualini, 1982 ; Miller and Katzenellenbogen, 1983 ; Sudo et al., 1983).

and Pasqualini, 1982) in agreement with results found by other authors (Sutherland and Foo, 1979 ; Faye et al., 1980 ; Sutherland et al., 1980 ; Kon, 1983 ; Miller and Katzenellenbogen, 1983 ; Sudo et al., 1983).

In order to investigate which regions of the triphenylethylene molecule are important for binding to the different intracellular binding sites, the study of the affinity of different triphenyl-ethylene derivatives for antiestrogen specific binding sites and for the estrogen receptor has been undertaken by our and other laboratories. The results are summarized in Figure 6 which shows

that modifications of the aminoether side chain greatly modify the
affinity of triphenylethylene antiestrogens to both the antiestrogen
binding site and the estrogen receptor. However, the same modifications of the aminoether side chain differentially modify the affinity of triphenylethylene for the antiestrogen binding site and the
estrogen receptor, so that the affinity for the estrogen receptor
is increased and that for the antiestrogen binding site decreased.
Similar results have been observed after hydroxylation of tamoxifen
on the phenyl ring, which increases the affinity for estrogen receptor and decreases that for the antiestrogen binding site. LY
117018 also has a higher affinity for estrogen receptor but a lower
affinity for the antiestrogen binding site with respect to tamoxifen.
In contrast, the hydroxylation and saturation of the ethylene chain
interconnecting the phenyl rings decrease the affinity for both the
estrogen receptor and the antiestrogen binding site. These results
suggest that the stereospecificity of estrogen receptor and of the
antiestrogen binding site are very different.

"In vitro" binding of [^{3}H]tamoxifen cytoplasmic complexes to
isolated nuclei of the fetal uterus of guinea pig. The ability of
[^{3}H]tamoxifen cytoplasmic complexes to bind to uterine nuclei was
tested using a "cell free" system (Gulino and Pasqualini, 1982).
The tamoxifen-estrogen receptor complex does not bind to uterine
nuclei at 3°C, but this binding occurs at 30°C. On the other hand,
the tamoxifen-site B complex does not bind at any temperature to
uterine nuclei. It is concluded that tamoxifen can translocate the

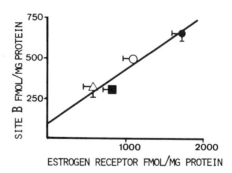

Figure 7. Correlation between site B and estrogen receptor
levels in the uterine cytosol of fetal (●), neonatal (○), immature (■) and adult (△) guinea pigs (from Gulino and Pasqualini,
1982).

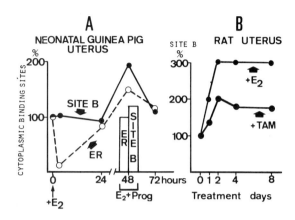

Figure 8. Hormonal regulation of antiestrogen binding site levels.
A) Six-day-old guinea pigs were given s.c. 30 ng/g b.w. of estradiol
(E_2) and estrogen receptor (ER) and site B levels were measured as
previously described (Gulino and Pasqualini, 1983). Columns indicate
ER and site B levels 48 h after the administration of E_2 plus progesterone (15 µg/g b.w.) (data from Gulino and Pasqualini, 1983).
B) Antiestrogen specific binding site levels in the rat uterus after
E_2 and tamoxifen (TAM) pellet implants (data from Winneker and Clark,
1983). The results are expressed as percentage of values observed
in control animals assigned the value of 100 %.

estrogen receptor to the nucleus by a temperature-dependent process,
while it cannot translocate its specific binding site (site B).

    Localization of triphenylethylene antiestrogen-specific binding
sites in different tissues. Correlation with estrogen receptor levels.
The finding of triphenylethylene antiestrogen-specific binding sites
in organs containing estrogen receptor raises the question of the
relationship between these sites and estrogen receptors. In the
preceding sections, we have shown that several characteristics differentiate cytoplasmic site B in the fetal uterus of guinea pig as
well as the triphenylethylene antiestrogen-specific binding sites
observed in other models from estrogen receptor, suggesting that
the antiestrogen binding site and the estrogen receptor do represent distinct molecular entities.

In order to investigate a possible relationship between site B and estrogen receptor, we have examined its presence in fetal organs of guinea pig containing no estrogen receptor (heart) or very low levels (lung, 20 fmol/mg protein). Although site B can be found in these tissues, significantly lower levels of site B have been observed in these two fetal organs compared to the fetal uterus (Gulino and Pasqualini, 1982). Sutherland et al. (1980) have also observed higher levels of triphenylethylene antiestrogen-specific binding sites in the cytosol of organs containing higher levels of estrogen receptors in the rat. Other authors fail to find any significant difference in triphenylethylene antiestrogen-specific binding sites between estrogen target and non target organs in humans (Kon, 1983) and rats (Sudo et al., 1983). Taken together these data suggest that the presence of triphenylethylene antiestrogen-specific binding sites is not generally limited to estrogen target organs. However, a relationship between site B and estrogen receptor could indeed exist because we have found a positive correlation between the levels of site B and estrogen receptor in the uterus of guinea pig during development from the fetal until the adult age (Fig. 7).

   Regulation of triphenylethylene antiestrogen-specific binding site levels. The correlation we have found between uterine site B and estrogen receptor levels led us to investigate whether factors which are known to modulate the levels of estrogen receptors, such as estradiol and progesterone (Clark and Peck, 1979), are also able to modify site B levels. Since the effects of estradiol and progesterone on estrogen receptor replenishment is a response acquired during the neonatal period in the guinea pig, we have chosen newborn guinea pigs to study the control by estradiol and progesterone of both uterine estrogen receptor and site B levels (Gulino and Pasqualini, 1983). A single injection of estradiol to the animal induces a significant increase in both cytoplasmic estrogen receptor and cytoplasmic and nuclear site B of the neonatal uterus 48 h after hormone administration (Fig. 8A). Progesterone has an antagonistic effect on the estradiol-induced increase in cytoplasmic estrogen receptors and also antagonizes the estradiol-induced increase in site B in the neonatal uterus (Fig. 8A). The stimulation of site B levels by estradiol has recently been confirmed by Winneker and Clark (1983) in the uterus and liver of immature rats (Fig. 8B). It is noteworthy that the effect of tamoxifen on triphenylethylene antiestrogen-specific binding site levels in the uterus of immature rats is lower than that of estradiol (Figure 8B).

   Binding of tamoxifen in serum. Besides having an intracellular binding site, we have reported that tamoxifen shows an additional saturable binding in the fetal serum of guinea pig (Gulino and Pasqualini, 1980). This binding site does not bind estradiol. Furthermore, the affinity of tamoxifen for this binding site is significantly lower (Kd : 8.8 $\pm$ 2 nM) than that of tamoxifen for intracellular site B. More recently the presence of a binding site

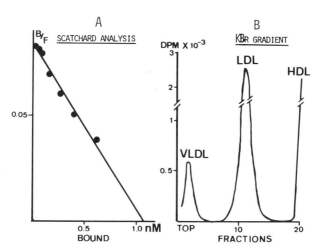

Figure 9. Characteristics of tamoxifen binding in fetal guinea pig serum. A) Scatchard analysis of [3H]tamoxifen binding in 1:20 diluted serum. Saturable binding is represented. B) Potassium bromide density gradient centrifugation profile showing the fractionation of serum lipoproteins (very low density lipoproteins, VLDL ; low density lipoproteins, LDL ; high density lipoproteins, HDL) and [3H]tamoxifen binding sites. Potassium bromide gradients, prepared in agreement with the method previously described (Terpstra et al., 1981 ; Winneker et al., 1983), containing [3H]tamoxifen labelled serum, were centrifuged at 230.000 x g for 7 h in a Beckman SW60 rotor at 4°C. Saturable binding is reported.

for tamoxifen in serum has also been reported by Winneker et al. (1983) in rats and characterized as being a low density lipoprotein. We have confirmed these data in the fetal serum of guinea pig, as indicated in figure 9 which shows that most of [3H]tamoxifen specific binding co-migrates with low density lipoproteins.

CONCLUSIONS

We have shown that the triphenylethylene antiestrogen [3H]-tamoxifen binds to two distinct binding sites in the fetal uterus of guinea pig : the first one corresponds to the estrogen receptor and the second one, site B, is specific for the triphenylethylene class of antiestrogens and does not bind estrogens. Even though several characteristics differentiate these two binding sites, both site B and estrogen receptor levels are under the control of estradiol and progesterone. Most of the characteristics we have described for site B are shared by the antiestrogen specific binding site reported by other authors in other experimental models (Sutherland and Foo, 1979 ; Faye et al., 1980 ; Sutherland et al., 1980 ; Kon, 1983 ; Miller and Katzenellenbogen, 1983 ; Sudo et al., 1983). The only difference is the slightly higher affinity of tamoxifen for fetal uterine site B (Kd 0.4 nM) with respect to the affinity of tamoxifen for the antiestrogen binding site observed in other models (range Kd 1-4 nM). This suggests that similar antiestrogen specific binding sites exist in several animal species.

The role played by the antiestrogen binding site in human breast cancer is totally unknown at present. However, the control of both the antiestrogen binding site and the estrogen receptor by estradiol and progesterone (Gulino and Pasqualini, 1983 ; Winneker and Clark, 1983) could suggest that estrogen receptor-mediated bioactivities and the function of antiestrogen binding sites could be mutually related. If this is the case it could support a new approach to the investigation of additional markers of hormone dependency in human breast cancer.

Sutherland has recently suggested that antiestrogen specific binding sites could be involved in the growth inhibiting and cytotoxic action of antiestrogens in human breast cancer cells because clomiphene derivatives, which have a high affinity for estrogen receptor but which show only a limited binding to antiestrogen specific binding sites, fail to induce the estradiol-irreversible cytotoxic effect on MCF-7 cells (Murphy and Sutherland, 1983).

Finally, antiestrogen-specific binding sites could control the intracellular distribution of antiestrogens and in this way they could regulate the availability of antiestrogens for estrogen receptor. Further studies are required before the role of antiestrogen specific binding sites can be delineated.

ACKNOWLEDGEMENTS

        Part of the expenses of this work was supported by the "Centre National de la Recherche Scientifique", France (Equipe de Recherche du C.N.R.S. N°187) and by the "Ligue Française contre le Cancer".

REFERENCES

Baudendistel, L. J., and Ruh, T. S., 1976, Antiestrogen action : differential nuclear retention and extractibility of the estrogen receptor, Steroids, 28:223.

Clark, J. H., and Peck, Jr., E. J., 1979, "Female Sex Steroids, Receptors and Function," Springer-Verlag, Berlin – Heidelberg.

Coezy, E., Borgna, J. L., and Rochefort, H., 1982, Tamoxifen and metabolites in MCF-7 cells : correlation between binding to estrogen receptors and inhibition of cell growth, Cancer Res., 42:317.

Eckert, R. L., and Katzenellenbogen, B. S., 1982, Physical properties of estrogen receptor complexes in MCF-7 human breast cancer cells – Differences with antiestrogen and estrogen, J. Biol. Chem., 257:8840.

Evans, E., Baskevitch, P. P., and Rochefort, H., 1982, Estrogen receptor. DNA interaction : differences between activation by estrogen and antiestrogen, Europ. J. Biochem., 128:185.

Faye, J. C., Lasserre, B., and Bayard, F., 1980, Antiestrogen specific, high affinity, saturable binding sites in rat uterine cytosol, Biochem. Biophys. Res. Commun., 93:1225.

Green, M. D., Whybourne, A. M., Taylor, I. W., and Sutherland, R. L., 1981, Effects of antioestrogens on the growth and cell kinetics of cultured human mammary carcinoma cells, in: "Non-Steroidal Antioestrogens," R. L. Sutherland, and V. C. Jordan, eds, Academic Press, Sidney.

Gulino, A., and Pasqualini, J. R., 1980, Specific binding and biological response of antiestrogens in the fetal uterus of the guinea pig, Cancer Res., 40:3821.

Gulino, A., and Pasqualini, J. R., 1982, Heterogeneity of binding sites for tamoxifen and tamoxifen derivatives in estrogen target and non target fetal organs of guinea pig, Cancer Res., 42:1913.

Gulino, A., and Pasqualini, J. R., 1983, Modulation of tamoxifen-specific binding sites and estrogen receptors by estradiol and progesterone in the neonatal uterus of guinea pig, Endocrinology, 112:1871.

Horwitz, K. B., and McGuire, W. L., 1978, Nuclear mechanism of estrogen action. J. Biol. Chem., 253:8185.

Horwitz, K. B., Yoshiro, K., and McGuire, W. L., 1978, Estrogen control of progesterone receptor in human breast cancer : role of estradiol and antiestrogen, Endocrinology, 103:1742.

Jordan, V. C., Dix, C. J., Rowsby, L., and Prestwich, G., 1977, Studies on the mechanism of action of the non steroidal antioestrogen tamoxifen (ICI 46.474) in the rat, Mol. Cell. Endocrinol., 7:177.

Kon, O. L., 1983, An antiestrogen-binding protein in human tissues, J. Biol. Chem., 258:3173.

Legha, S. S., Davis, A. L., and Muggia, F. M., 1978, Hormonal therapy of breast cancer : new approaches and concepts, Ann. Intern. Med., 88:69.

Lippman, M. E., Bolan, G., and Huff, K., 1976, The effects of est-
    rogens and antiestrogens on hormone-responsive human breast
    cancer in long-term tissue culture, Cancer Res., 36:4595.
Miller, M. A., and Katzenellenbogen, B. S., 1983, Characterization
    and quantitation of antiestrogen binding sites in estrogen
    receptor-positive and negative human breast cancer cell lines,
    Cancer Res., 43:3094.
Murphy, L. C., and Sutherland, R. L., 1983, Antitumor activity of
    Clomiphene analogs in vitro : relationship to affinity for the
    estrogen receptor and another high affinity antiestrogen
    binding site, J. Clin. Endocr. Metab., 57:373.
Pasqualini, J. R., and Nguyen, B. L., 1976, Mise en évidence des
    récepteurs cytosoliques et nucléaires de l'oestradiol dans
    l'utérus de foetus de cobaye, C.R. Acad. Sci., (Série D)
    (Paris) 283:413.
Pasqualini, J. R., and Nguyen, B. L., 1980, Progesterone receptors
    in the fetal uterus and ovary of the guinea pig : evolution
    during fetal development and induction and stimulation in
    estradiol-primed animals, Endocrinology, 106:1160.
Pasqualini, J. R., Cosquer-Clavreul, C., and Gelly, C., 1983, Rapid
    modulation by progesterone and tamoxifen of estradiol effects
    on nuclear histone acetylation in the uterus of the fetal
    guinea pig, Biochim. Biophys. Acta, 739:137.
Pasqualini, J. R., Sumida, C., Gulino, A., Nguyen, B. L., Tardy, J.,
    and Gelly, C., 1980, Recent data on receptors and biological
    action of estrogens and antiestrogens in the fetal uterus of
    guinea pig, in: "Hormones and Cancer," S. Iacobelli, R. J. B.
    King, H. R. Lindner, and M. E. Lippman, eds, Raven Press, New
    York.
Patterson, J., Furr, B., Wakeling, A., and Battersby, L., 1982, The
    biological physiology of Nolvadex (Tamoxifen) in the treatment
    of breast cancer, Breast Cancer Res. and Treat., 2:363.
Rochefort, H., and Borgna, J. L., 1981, Differences between the
    activation of the estrogen receptor by estrogen and anti-
    estrogen, Nature, 292:257.
Scatchard, G., 1949, The attractions of proteins for small molecules
    and ions, Ann. N. Y. Acad. Sci., 51:660.
Screpanti, I., Gulino, A., and Pasqualini, J. R., 1982, The fetal
    thymus of guinea pig as an estrogen target organ, Endocrino-
    logy, 111:1552.
Sudo, K., Monsma, Jr., F. J., and Katzenellenbogen, B. S., 1983,
    Antiestrogen binding sites distinct from the estrogen receptor :
    subcellular localization, ligand specificity and distribution
    in tissues of the rat, Endocrinology, 112:425.
Sumida, C., and Pasqualini, J. R., 1980, Dynamic studies on estrogen
    responses in fetal guinea pig uterus : effect of estradiol
    administration on estradiol receptor, progesterone receptor
    and uterine growth, J. Receptor Res., 1:439.
Sutherland, R. L., and Foo, M. S., 1979, Differential binding of
    antiestrogens by rat uterine and chick oviduct cytosol. Biochem.

Biophys. Res. Commun., 91:183.

Sutherland, R. L., and Murphy, L. C., 1980, The binding of tamoxifen to human mammary carcinoma cytosol, Europ. J. Cancer, 16:1141.

Sutherland, R. L., Green, M. D., Hall, R. E., Reddel, R. R., and Taylor, I. W., 1983, Tamoxifen induces accumulation of MCF-7 human mammary carcinoma cells in the G_0/G_1 phase of the cycle, Europ. J. Cancer Clin. Oncol., 19:615.

Sutherland, R. L., Murphy, L. C., Foo, M. S., Green, M. D., Whybourne, A. M., and Krozowski, Z. S., 1980, High affinity antioestrogen binding site distinct from the oestrogen receptor, Nature, 288: 273.

Terenius, L., 1971, Structure-activity relationships of antiestrogens with regard to interaction with 17β-estradiol in the mouse uterus and vagina, Acta Endocrinol. (Copenh.), 66:431.

Terpstra, A. H. M., Woodward, C. J. H., and Sanchez-Muniz F. J., 1981, Improved techniques for the separation of serum lipoproteins by density gradient ultracentrifugation : visualization by prestaining and rapid separation of serum lipoproteins from small volumes of serum, Anal. Biochem., 111:149.

Westley, B., and Rochefort, H., 1980, A secreted glycoprotein induced by estrogen in human breast cancer cell lines, Cell, 20:353.

Winneker, R. C., and Clark, J. H., 1983, Estrogenic stimulation of the antiestrogen specific binding site in rat uterus and liver, Endocrinology, 112:1910.

Winneker, R. C., Sylvia, C. G., and Clark, J. H., 1983, Characterization of a triphenylethylene antiestrogen binding site on rat serum low density lipoproteins, Endocrinology, 112:1823.

FAILURE TO DEMONSTRATE PLASMA HORMONE ABNORMALITIES IN WOMEN WITH

OPERABLE BREAST CANCER

I. Ricciardi[°], S. De Placido[*], C. Pagliarulo[*], G. Delrio[°],
F. Citarella[°], L. De Sio[*], M. D' Istria[°], S. Fasano[°],
G. Petrella[*], A. Contegiacomo[*], R. V. Iaffaioli[*], and
A. R. Bianco[*]

[*]Istituto di Oncologia, II Facoltà di Medicina
Università di Napoli; [°]Istituto di Biologia Generale
Facoltà di Medicina, Università di Napoli, Italy

INTRODUCTION

The endocrine profile of patients with breast cancer has been the object of extensive studies during the past several years. Abnormal secretion of a variety of hormones has been described on different occasions in patients with breast cancer (Gambrell, 1982; Henderson et al., 1982; Kirschner et al., 1982; Kwa and Wang, 1977; Ohgo et al., 1976), and has been considered a possible risk factor. However, conclusive evidence has not yet been presented to show that the cancer patients are significantly different in endogenous hormone profiles from their healthy counterparts. The main purpose of the present study was to critically reevaluate this controversial issue and possibly identify hormonal changes in a large population of patients with operable breast cancer not present in a comparable population of normal healthy women.

MATERIAL AND METHODS

A total of 120 patients with clinical stage I-II breast cancer, aged 20-70, were included in the study. Sixty patients were premenopausal, sixty postmenopausal. An equivalent number of normal pre- and postmenopausal healthy women, matched by age, parity, weight, socioeconomic status and with no family history of breast cancer, was used as a control. None of individuals under study was on any form of endocrine medication and administration of other drugs was avoided during the study period. Endocrine evaluation was performed before mastectomy in breast cancer patients, and included determination by radioimmunoassay of plasma follicle stimulating hormone (FSH), luteinizing hormone (LH), prolactin (Prl), thyroid stimulating hormone (TSH), estrone (E_1), estradiol-17-beta (E_2), progesterone (P), and testosterone (T). Blood of hormone determinations was drawn between 9.00 a.m. and 11.00 a.m.; in premenopausal women blood sample were obtained in the mid-follicular phase (day 7-10) of each menstrual cycle for all of the hormones except progesterone, which was assayed in the mid-luteal phase (day 20-21).

In 20 pre- and 20 postmenopausal women, randomly selected amoung our breast cancer patients, the pattern of noctural Prl secretion was studied by continuous blood withdrawal from 12.00 p.m. to 10.00 a.m. Blood samples were obtained through an indwellig propylene catheter placed in a forearm vein and connected to a portable peristaltic pump set to deliver a blood flow of 5 ml per hour. Prl determinations were done on blood samples collected during the period of each hour. The patients were allowed to sleep throughout the night and a sleep record was maintained on each patient during the whole study period.

In 20 additional randomly selected patients, 10 pre- and 10 postmenopausal, plasma FSH and LH, and Prl and TSH concentrations were measured under either basal conditions or following stimulation with gonadotropin releasing hormone (GnRH) and thyrotropin releasing hormone (TRH), respectively. The stimulatory tests were performed by injecting 100 mcg of GnRH and 200 mcg of TRH, respectively, i.v., and by collecting blood samples at 0, +15, +30, +60, +90, and +240 minutes. As controls an equivalent number of pre- and postmenopausal healthy women were used.

All serum samples were stored at $-20°$ C until used for hormone determination. Peptide hormone assay were performed by the use of commercial kits (Sorin, Saluggia, Italy); steroid hormones were assayed by the use of antisera generously provided by the Antiserum National Service of the National Research Council (CNR) of Italy. Labelled steroids of high specific activity were obtained from Amersham International (Buckingamshire, England). The inter- and intra assay coefficients of variation were < 9% and <7%; respectively.

The data are expressed as the mean of the individual values $\pm$ one standard deviation (SD). Statistical analysis was done by the use of the Student's $\underline{t}$ test.

RESULTS

The results of hormone determinations under basal conditions are summarized in tables 1 and 2. Serum concentrations of $E_1 + E_2$, P, T, FSH, LH, Prl, TSH were not significantly different in breast cancer patients and controls. Progesterone determinations in the

Table 1.   Plasma estrogen, progesterone, and testosterone concentrations in breast cancer and normal women

Individuals	$E_1 + E_2$ (pg/ml)	P (ng/dl)	T (ng/dl)
Normal			
Premenopause	218 + 97	540 + 355	32 + 9.4
Postmenopause	41 + 18	37 + 21	34 + 10
Breast cancer			
Premenopause	201 + 125	525 + 383	26 + 10
Postmenopause	49 + 17	45 + 26	22 + 8.3

Table 2.   Plasma gonadotropin, prolactin and thyroid stimulating hormone concentrations in normal and breast cancer women

Individuals	FSH (mUI/ml)	LH (mUI/ml)	Prl (ng/ml)	TSH (uUI/ml)
Normal				
Premenopause	9.3+3.4	12.5+5.7	13.1+6.2	1.3+0.2
Postmenopause	79.0+31.2	45.2+15.7	7.3+3.5	2.1+0.4
Breast cancer				
Premenopause	7.5+5.5	11.1+8.2	14.0+5.9	1.9+0.4
Postmenopause	71.6+29.9	39.1+13.5	6.2+2.7	1.1+0.3

presumed secretory phase of the menstrual cycle showed a 30%
incidence of anovulation in breast cancer patients which was not
different from the 27% observed in normal premenopausal women.

Single determinations of plasma Prl in cancer patients showed
levels not significantly different from controls. When the pattern
of noctural secretion of Prl was studied by the technique of
continuous blood sampling, noctural secretory peaks tended to
occur in either late night or early morning and were clearly
related to the onset of sleep. In general, a secretory peak was
observed 2-4 hours after sleep began. Late occurring peaks could
clearly be explained by the difficulty of some patients to attain
sleep probably because of the procedure of blood withdrawal. In
fact, in two premenopausal patients who failed to reach sleep a
Prl peak was not observed at all during the whole study period.
However, a comparison of the two areas under the normalized Prl
secretory curves showed that they were not significantly different
in pre- and postmenopausal breast cancer patients.

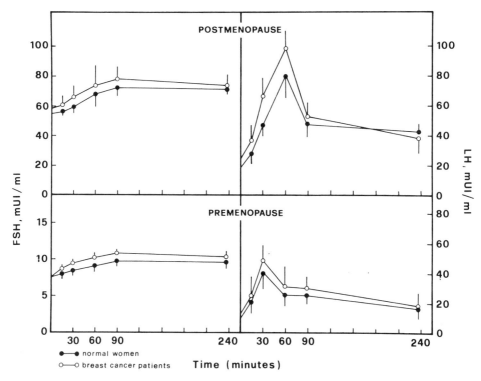

Fig. 1.   Release into plasma of FSH and LH in pre- and postmeno-
          pausal normal and breast cancer women following GnRH
          injection.

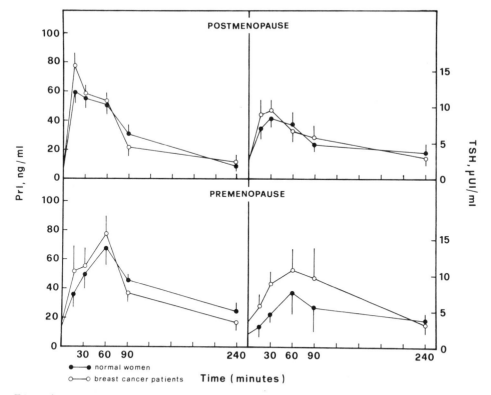

Fig. 2. Release of Prl and TSH into plasma in pre- and postmenopausal normal   and breast cancer women after TRH
injection.

    The results of the stimulatory tests with releasing factors
are shown in Figs. 1 and 2. They clearly indicate that the release
of FSH, LH, Prl and TSH is identical in breast cancer patients and
in normal women.

DISCUSSION

    We have demonstrated that serum concentration and secretion
of a variety of peptide and steroid hormones in women with stage
I-II   breast   cancer,   evaluated   preoperatively,   are   not
significantly different from those found in matched normal
individuals. Levels of estradiol, a potent stimulator of normal
(McGuire, 1975) and malignant (Porte, 1974) mammary tissue, have
been reported to be elevated in women with breast cancer (Cole et
al., 1978; England et al., 1974; Kirschner,1977) and in daughters

of women with breast cancer (Henderson et al., 1982). We found normal E_1+E_2 serum concentrations in pre- and postmenopausal women with breast cancer, and these findings are supported by the data of McFayden et al. (1976). Progesterone also influences normal as well as malignant (Porter, 1974; Horwitz et al., 1975) breast tissue growth and metabolism, and it has been suggested (Sherman et al., 1974) that estrogen-progesterone imbalance may play a role in the development of breast cancer. Abnormally elevated serum progesterone levels in postmenopausal women with breast cancer have been reported by Smethutst et al. (1975), although this observation was not supported by others (Malarkey et al., 1977). Our data showed no significant differences between breast cancer and healthy women.

The role of male steroid hormones on normal and malignant breast tissue is not clear. Grattarola et al. (1975) reported elevated urinary testosterone levels in women with breast cancer studied preoperatively. Testosterone levels remained elevated in patients who eventually developed metastatic disease. McFayden et al. (1976) described increased 8-hour plasma testosterone levels in six postmenopausal breast cancer patients, and Malarkey et al. (1977) demonstred a significant elevation of the 24-hour mean serum concentration testosterone in premenopausal breast cancer patients in the luteal phase of their menstrual cycle but not in postmenopausal patients. Our data showed similar concentrations of testosterone in pre- and postmenopausal women with breast cancer and in normal controls.

Secretion of FSH, LH and TSH under basal conditions and followig stimulation by releasing factors did not differ significantly in breast cancer patients and in controls.

Abnormalities of Prl secretion have been reported on several occasions in patients with breast cancer (Malarkey et al., 1977; Mc Guire et al., 1975; Ohgo et al., 1976; Sheth et al., 1975). In a study in Guernsey islands, Kwa et al. (1977) observed a transient but significant elevation of plasma Prl early at night in unaffected daughters of women with breast cancer during the luteal phase of their menstrual cycle. Malarkey et al. (1977) reported marked elevations of preoperative mean 24-hour Prl levels in some of their premenopausal patients which contrasted with the significantly depressed nocturnal Prl secretion of postmenopausal breast cancer patients, although a convincing explanation for these discrepancy was not given. Our data demonstrate that the pattern of nocturnal Prl secretion did not vary significantly between postmenopausal and premenopausal breast cancer patients evaluated in mid-follicular phase of the menstrual cycle. In addition, Prl response to TRH stimulation was identical in pre- and postmenopausal breast cancer patients and in normal women, indicating that breast cancer patients do not differ significantly from normal women. Similar conclusions have been recently suggested by Bruning et al. (1983), who questioned Kwa's statement that the early evening Prl peak can be used to identify individual risk in first degree relatives of breast cancer patients. They also emphasized the existence of considerable fluctuations of Prl and steroid hormone concentrations even within a few hours and suggested that "spot" sample values are of little significance unless they are compensated by large numbers of patients. In our study the size of the population under investigation was chosen bearing these short-comings in mind.

We believe that the results of our study, by combining the data from hormone determinations both under basal and stimulated conditions, have failed to demostrate, in breast cancer patients, significant alterations in the secretion of polypeptide and steroid hormones known to somehow influence growth and development of the mammary gland. We therefore conclude that, although a proportion of breast cancers are hormone dependent, endogenous hormone profiles cannot be used to identify persons at risk for the development of the disease.

Supported by CNR Special Project "Control of Neoplastic Growth", grant no. 80.1535.96.

REFERENCES

Bruning, P .F., Bonfrer, H., Dejong-Bakker, M., Hart, A. A. M., and Kwa, H. G., 1983, Prolactin and steroid hormones in premenopausal women at risk for breast cancer, Proc. 3rd EORTC Breast Cancer Working Conf., Amsterdam, April 27-29.
Cole, P., Cramer, D., Yen, S., Pattenbarger, R., McMahon, B., and Brown, J., 1978, Estrogen profiles of premenopausal women with breast cancer, Cancer Res., 38:745.
England, P.C., Skinner, L. G., Cottrel, K. M., and Seilwood,R.A., 1974, Serum oestradiol-17 in women with benign and malignant breast disease, Brit. J. Cancer, 30:571.
Gambrell, R. D., 1982, Role of hormones in the etiology and prevention of endometrial and breast cancer, Acta Obstet. Gynaecol.Scand. (suppl.), 106:37.
Grattarola, R., Secreto, G., and Recchione, C., 1975, Androgens in breast cancer. III. Breast cancer recurrences years after mastectomy and increased androgen activity, Am. J. Obst. Gynecol., 118:173.
Henderson, B. E., Gerkins, V., Rosario, I., Casagrande, J., and Pike, M. C., 1975, Elevated serum levels of estrogen and prolactin in daughters of patients with breast cancer, N. Engl. J. Med., 293:790.
Henderson, B. E., Ross, R. K., and Pike, M. C., 1982, Endogenous hormones as a major factor in human breast cancer, Cancer

Res. (suppl.8), 42:3232.

Horwitz, K. B., McGuire, W. L., Pearson, O. H., and Segaloff, A., 1975, Predicting response to endocrine therapy in human breast cancer. A hypothesis. Science, 189:726.

Kirschner, M. A., 1977, The role of hormones in the etiology of human breast cancer, Cancer, 39:2716.

Kirschner, M. A., Schneider, G., and Ertel, N. H., 1982, Obesity, androgens, estrogens and cancer risk, Cancer Res., (suppl.8), 42:3281.

Kwa, H. G., and Wang, D. Y., 1977, An abnormal luteal-phase evening peak of plasma prolactin in women with a family history of breast cancer, Int. J. Cancer, 20:12.

Malarkey, W. B., Schroeder, L. L., Stevens, V. C., James, A. G., and Lanese, R. R., 1977, Twenty-four hour preoperative endocrine profiles in women with benign and malignant breast disease, Cancer Res., 37:4655.

Malarkey, W. B., Schroeder, L. L., Stevens, V. C., James, A. G., and Lanese, R. R., 1977, Disordered noctural prolactin regulation in women with breast cancer, Cancer Res.,37:4650.

McFayden, W. H., Prescott, I. J., Goom, G. V., Forrest, A. P. M., Golden, M. P., Fahmy, D. R., and Griffiths, K., 1976, Circulating hormone concentrations in women with breast cancer, Lancet, 7:1100.

McGuire, W. R., Carbone, P. P., Seans, M. E., and Escher, G. C., 1975, Estrogen receptor in human breast cancer. An overview, in:"Estrogen receptors in human breast cancer", W.L. Mc Guire, P. P. Carbone, E. P. Wollmer, eds., Raven Press, New York, N. Y. Ohgo, S., Kato, Y., Chihara, K., and Imura, H., 1976, Plasma prolactin responses to thyrotropin releasing hormone in patients with breast cancer, Cancer, 37:1412.

Porter, J. C., 1974, Hormonal regulation of breast development and activity, J. Invest. Dermatol., 63:85.

Sheth, N. A., Ranadive, K. J., Suraiva, J. N., and Sheth, A. R., 1975, Circulating levels of prolactin in human breast cancer, Brit. J. Cancer, 32:160.

Sherman, B. M., and Korenman, S. G.,1974, Inadeguate corpus luteum function. A pathophysiological interpretation of human breast cancer epidemiology, Cancer, 33:1306.

Smethutst, M., Alexander, K., and Williams, D. C., 1975, Plasma progestrerone levels in postmenopausal women with breast cancer. IRCS Medical Science. Cancer, endocrine system, metabolism and nutrition, Obstet. Gynecol., 3:89.

CELL-TYPE-INDEPENDENT ACCUMULATION OF PHOSPHATIDIC ACID

INDUCED BY TRIFLUOPERAZINE IN STIMULATED HUMAN PLATELETS,

LEUKOCYTES, AND FIBROBLASTS

Marco Ruggiero, Gabriella Fibbi, Mario Del Rosso,
Simonetta Vannucchi, Franca Pasquali, and
Vincenzo Chiarugi

Laboratory of Molecular Biology
Institute of General Pathology
University of Florence
Viale Morgagni 50
50134 Florence, Italy

It is generally believed that receptor-stimulated breakdown of
phosphatidylinositol (PI) is implicated in transmembrane cell signaling whereby activation of a variety of cell surface receptors brings
about a rise in intracellular calcium (Michell, 1975; Nishizuka, 1983;
Irvine et al., 1983). The breakdown of polyphosphated phosphoinositides is characterized by the rapid interconversion of short-lived
intermediates (suggesting the so-called "phosphatidylinositol cycle"),
where diacylglycerol (DG) is phosphorylated to phosphatidic acid (PA)
by a DG-kinase, which is in turn reconverted to PI via CDP-diglycer-
ide-inositolphosphatidyl transferase.

Phosphoinositide hydrolysis has been proposed by Michell to be
coupled with the opening of calcium gates, but the authentic role of
each intermediate of the cycle in cell signaling is still a matter
for discussion. The evidence so far obtained clearly points to DG
and PA as major effectors: the former was identified by Castagna et
al. (1982) as a specific stimulator of proteinkinase C (a calcium-
phospholipid-dependent kinase of paramount importance in cell signaling), while the latter was suspected to be a calcium ionophore and
an important marker of receptor-mediated signaling whose general
involvement in cell biology is worth being clarified. Lapetina et
al. (1982) furnished the first evidence that the antipsychotic drug

---
Supported by Progetto Finalizzato della Crescita Neoplastica Consiglio
Nazionale delle Ricerche.

75

trifluoperazine (TFP) is able to induce a PA accumulation in stimulated platelets. In this short report we provide evidence that this effect is not a prerogative of cells that react rapidly to stimuli, such as platelets, but that it occurs at the same level and in the same time span, as a response to stimulation, also in leukocytes and fibroblasts.

Human foreskin fibroblasts, as well as human leukocytes and platelets, were labeled with ^{32}P-inorganic phosphate and ^{3}H-arachidonate. Then they were treated with various drugs, subjected to stimulation with phorbol ester or thrombin, and then analyzed for their PA content. As shown in Table I, all three types of cells have very low levels of endogeneous PA. This level is poorly affected by stimulation after a 1-minute time course (that is, a time span generally sufficient to reveal other effects of stimulation such as a rise of free arachidonate (FA) and the phosphorylation of a 44-kilodalton protein).

A possible explanation for this lack of effect on PA could be the bypassing of the PA cycle by phorbol ester (Nishizuka, 1983), or, more likely, the rapid interconversion of this intermediate, as it seems to be in the case of thrombin-treated platelets. As a matter of fact, stimulation of leukocytes and fibroblasts with the chemoattractant peptides or bradykinin, respectively, was slightly effective in inducing a measurable accumulation of PA in the absence of TFP (data not shown). TFP, and chlorpromazine as well, produces a dramatic increase in the accumulation of PA (Figure 1). This accumulation effect is abolished by serine esterase inhibitors, but not by glucocorticoids or nonsteroid antiinflammatory drugs (NSAID), and this could indicate that a serine esterase (presumably a PI-specific phospholipase C) is necessary to free the DG and make it available for the DG-kinase. Steroid and nonsteroid antiinflammatory drugs do not prevent such an early signal, being conceivably more active in later metabolic steps of the arachidonate cascade.

The accumulation effect induced by TFP was completely independent of the type of cell or stimulator used, and all these facts lead us to the following conclusions:

1. The interconversion of phosphoinositides to PA seems to be a general route in the very early steps of cell signaling, at least in connective tissue cells.
2. The time course of accumulation induced by TFP seems to be independent of fast or slow cellular reaction to stimulation.
3. This important event in receptor-mediated stimulation is not measurable without the use of a phenotyazin drug, which presumably blocks a calmodulin-dependent enzyme mediating the further metabolic fate of the phosphatidate.

Table 1. Effects of various drugs on the level of PA, free arachidonate (FA), and phosphorylation of a 44-kilodalton protein in the early response to stimuli (1 minute)

| | Type of cells | | | | | | | | |
| | Fibroblasts | | | Leukocytes | | | Platelets | | |
Drugs	PA	FA	44K	PA	FA	44K	PA	FA	44K
None	49	43	37	65	71	45	90	38	27
TPA	57	358	187	61	345	389	68	198	237
TPA+PMSF	69	40	85	41	87	43	78	98	37
TPA+TFP	1478	59	67	699	78	86	1007	87	101
TPA+TFP+PMSF	168	67	96	39	89	65	123	98	78
TPA+Dexa	143	203	176	76	105	198	79	107	116
TPA+Dexa+TFP	1298	110	58	654	70	47	987	53	21
TFP	237	51	38	301	77	54	201	50	34
TPA+Indomethacin	107	403	201	89	332	245	89	327	183

Values correspond to radioactivity of the material scraped from the
TLC plates or slices of acrylamide slabs. For the present experiment all the cells were labeled simultaneously for two hours with
5 µCi/ml of ^{32}P-inorganic phosphate and 1 µCi/ml ^{3}H-arachidonate
(New England Nuclear). Approximately the same biomass of cells
(measured as wet packed cells) was used for the three different types
of cells, corresponding to 2×10^{6} leukocytes and fibroblasts and 10^{9}
platelets incubated in 10 ml of F-10 medium. The cells were treated
with drugs, stimulated, and then extracted with chloroform/methanol,
as reported in the legend of Fig. 1. PA and FA spots were scraped
and counted after chromatography with different appropriate solvents
as reported by Lapetina et al. (1979) and identified by comigration
with authentic standards (Sigma Chem., U.S.). The interfacial proteins, obtained after extraction of lipids, were dialyzed, liophylized,
and dissolved in the appropriate buffer for slab gel acrylamide electrophoresis following Laemli (1970).

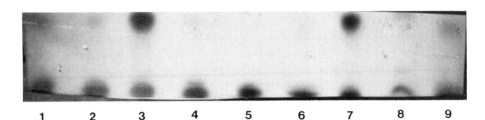

Fig. 1.   Autoradiography of a thin-layer chromatography plate where phospholipids from stimulated fibroblasts labeled with ^{32}P-inorganic phosphate were run.

Semiconfluent human foreskin fibroblasts grown in F-10 medium plus 10% calf serum were labeled with ^{32}P-inorganic phosphate (50 μCi per plate) for three hours. The culture plates were then treated with the various drugs at the concentrations indicated below and incubated for an additional ten minutes. The stimulator – tetradecanoyl phorbol myristate acetate (TPA) at a final concentration of 10^{-6} – was allowed to work for one minute. Then 10 ml of 2/1 v/v chloroform/methanol was added, the mixture rapidly shaken, and the organic phase separated by centrifugation and cold-dried under nitrogen flow. PA was separated from the bulk/phospholipids essentially following Lapetina et al. (1979), but improving on their method by using Linear K Preadsorbent silica gel plates (Wathman, U.K.), which allow a better resolution of PA from other phospholipids at the start owing to the stacking effect of the preadsorbent. The PA spot was directly visualized with a very sensitive detection method (Chiarugi et al., 1983), processed for autoradiograph and quantitized by scraping and counting the radioactivity by liquid scintillation.

(1) TPA 10^{-6}; (2) TPA + phenyl methyl sulfonyl fluoride (PMSF) 10^{-4}; (3) TPA + TFP 10^{-5}; (4) TPA + TFP + PMSF; (5) No compound added; (6) TPA + Dexamethasone 10^{-4}; (7) TPA + Dexa + TFP; (8) TFP; (9) TPA + Indomethacin 10^{-4}.

REFERENCES

Castagna, M., Takai, Y., Kaibuchi, K., Sano, K., Kikkawa, U., and
    Nishizuka, Y. (1982): Direct activation of calcium-activated,
    phospholipid-dependent protein kinase by tumor-promoting phorbol
    esters, J. Biol. Chem. 257:7847-7851.
Chiarugi, V., Ruggiero, M., and Ricoveri, W. (1983): A rapid and
    simple method to detect nanogram amounts of arachidonic acid
    metabolites by thin layer chromatography, J. Chromotography,
    in press.
Hirasawa, K., Irvine, R.F., and Dawson, M.C. (1982): Proteolytic
    activation can produce a phosphatidylinositol phosphodiesterase
    highly sensitive to Ca^{2+}, Biochem. J. 206:675-678.
Laemli, U.K. (1970): Cleavage of structural proteins during the
    assembly of the head of bacteriophage T4, Nature, 227:680-685.
Lapetina, E.G. (1979): Platelet-activating factor stimulates the
    phosphatidylinositol cycle, Biochim. Biophys. Acta, 573:394-402.
Michell, R.H. (1982): Is phosphatidylinositol really out of the
    calcium gate? Nature, 296:492-493.
Nishizuka, Y. (1983): Phospholipid degradation and signal transla-
    tion for protein phosphorylation, Trends Bioch. Sci. 1:13-16.
Vannucchi, S., Fibbi, G., Del Rosso, M., Cappelletti, R., Pasquali,
    F., and Chiarugi, V. (1982): Adhesion-dependent heparin produc-
    tion by platelets, Nature, 296:492-493.

PROTEASE INHIBITORS IN 3T3 CELLS

Gabriella Fibbi, Vincenzo Chiarugi, and
Mario Del Rosso

Institute of General Pathology
University of Florence
Viale Morgagni 50
50134 Florence, Italy

A 44K anti-thrombin-like protease inhibitor, termed protease-nexin, has recently been discovered in the culture medium of human fibroblasts (Baker et al., 1980). It forms heparin-dependent covalent complexes with the catalytic site of serine proteases. The action of heparin consists in accellerating the formation of the complex by inducing a shape change in the inhibitory site of protease-nexin, which confers to this molecule the affinity for the protease. In the present study we show that 3T3 cells shed into the culture medium at least two inhibitors of exogenous urokinase, which form covalent complexes with the serine-protease. The same study, carried out with 3T3-SV transformed cells, shows a ten fold decrease in the production of both inhibitors.

BALB/c-3T3 and 3T3-SV transformed mouse fibroblasts were grown in DMEM supplemented with 10% fetal calf serum (FCS) and cultured in an atmosphere of 5% CO_2. Standard urokinase (Serono) was purified by affinity chromatography on Sepharose CH-4B substituted with p-aminobenzamidine. Purified urokinase was then labelled with tritium using the

Supported by Ministero Pubblica Istruzione (60% and 40%).

potassium borohydride method. Conditioned medium was
obtained from cell cultures that had been in serum-free
conditions after confluence for 48 h. Since previous obse
vations by this group (Chiarugi et al., 1982) had shown
the contemporary presence of both protease-inhibitor and
protease in the same medium, the conditioned media were
first eluted from a column of Sepharose CH-4B-p-aminobenza
midine, to retain endogenous proteases. Non retained material was then concentrated ten-fold by ultrafiltration.
The inhibitory activity present in this material was evaluated by inhibition of fibrinolysis on fibrin plates,
according to Nilsson et al. (1978). In brief, 5 ul of
conditioned medium was added to increasing amounts of urokinase and then incubated on fibrin films in a humidified
chamber at 37°C. The amount of urokinase whose fibrinolytic activity was completely inhibited by the same amount
of medium, was a measure of the inhibitor present in the
conditioned medium. The concentrated conditioned medium
was then incubated 2 h at 37°C with the amount of ^{3}H-labe-
led urokinase suggested by the fibrinolytic tests in the
presence of heparin (1 ug/ml) to speed up the formation of
the complex. The modification of the gel-chromatogram of
^{3}H-urokinase after incubation with the conditioned medium
was evaluated by gel-chromatography on Sephacryl S-200.
The activity present in the eluted fractions was measured
by fibrinolytic tests.

    The gel-chromatogram of ^{3}H-labeled urokinase is show
in fig. 1a. The molecular weight of our urokinase resulte
54K, and the fibrinolytic activity coeluted with the radi
activity. Fig. 1b shows the modification of the chromato-
gram after incubation of ^{3}H-urokinase with the medium of
3T3 cells in the conditions described above. The fibrinolytic activity was absent in the peak fractions. Running
the chromatography under disaggregating conditions in 4.0
M guanidinium chloride (Fig. 1c) did not cause any change
of the chromatographic pattern, but the excluded material
eluted in the 130K complex. It is therefore possible to
conceive of a covalent binding of urokinase with two inhibitors, whose apparent molecular weight result 45 and 75K
respectively. A ten fold decrease of both inhibitors is
observed in the medium of 3T3-SV transformed cells (fig.1

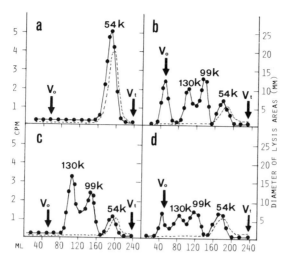

Fig. 1. Gel-chromatography analysis of Sephacryl S-200 of
^{3}H-labeled urokinase before (a) and after incubation (b) with medium of normal cells. (c) Modification of the pattern in 4.0 M guanidinium chloride.
(d) The same experiment as in section b, using
medium of 3T3-SV transformed cells: in this case
the sample applied was concentrated five-fold to
obtain a comparable pattern. The dotted lines
indicate the fibrinolytic activity of fractions.

Data obtained by Teng and Chen (1976) indicate that the
mitogenic action of serine-proteases require the binding of
the mitogen to a cell receptor and the subsequent cleavage
of one or more key proteins of the cell surface. The proteo-
lysis of the pericellular matrix can be buffered by protease-
nexin-like molecules and modulated by cell-surface heparan-
sulphate, as suggested by previous studies by this group
(Chiarugi et al., 1982). The decrease of nexin molecules
in the transformed cells, shown in the present study, as
well as the general increase of plasminogen activator is
a common phenomenon of neoplasia (Wilson et al., 1980) and
can account for the increased auto-stimulation of growth
of transformed cells. We have shown the existence of two
protease inhibitors (75K and 45K, respectively) in the 3T3
cell system. Other authors (Kawano et al., 1980) have been

able to show two inhibitors of the same molecular weight, produced by the human placenta. The possibility of having a contamination of the covalent protease inhibitor alfa$_2$-antiplasmin (as suggested by Holmberg et al., 1978) can be excluded in our experimental conditions, since experiments were performed after a 48 h culture in serum-free medium.

REFERENCES

Baker J.B., Low D.A., Simmer R.L. and Cunningham D.D. "Protease-nexin: a cellular component that links thrombin and plasminogen activator and mediates thei binding to cells" - Cell 21, 37-45 (1980).

Chiarugi V., Del Rosso M., Vannucchi S., Fibbi G. and Pasquali F. "Studies on glycosaminoglycan-dependent protease inhibitors" in Extracellular Matrix. Academ press, Eds. Susan Hawkes and J. Wang, 353-359 (1982)

Holmberg L., Lecander I., Persson B. and Åstedt B. "An inhibitor from placenta specifically binds uro-kinase and inhibits plasminogen activator released from ovarian carcinoma in tissue culture" - Biochim. Biophys. Acta, 544, 128-137 (1978).

Kawano T., Morimoto K and Uemura Y. "Partial purification and properties of urokinase inhibitor from human placenta" - The J. of Biochem., 67, 333-342 (1970).

Nilsson I.M., Hedner U. and Pandolfi M. "The measurement c fibrinolytic activities" in: Markwardt F. ed. Handb of Experimental Pharmacology, Berlin (1978).

Teng N.N.H. and Chen L.B. "Thrombin-sensitive surface pro of cultured chick embryo cells" - Nature, 259, 578-580 (1976).

Wilson L., Becker M.L.B., Hoal E.G. and Dowdle E.B. "Molecular species of plasminogen activators secret by normal and neoplastic human cells" - Cancer Res. 40, 933-938 (1980).

HETEROGENEITY OF EXTRAMITOCHONDRIAL FORMS OF ASPARTATE AMINO-TRANSFERASE AND MALATE DEHYDROGENASE IN YOSHIDA ASCITES HEPATOMA CELLS

Pier Paolo Gazzaniga

Institute of General Pathology
University La Sapienza, Rome

Isozyme patterns of experimental both solid and ascites rat hepatomas have been extensively investigated in recent years. For many enzymes, such as hexokinase (Sato and Sugimura, 1973), pyruvate kinase (Farina et al., 1974), alcohol dehydrogenase (Cederbaum and Rubin, 1976), glycogen phosphorilase (Sato et al., 1976), acid and alkaline phosphatases (Emmelot and Bos,1969; Kaneko et al., 1972), malate dehydrogenase (Otani and Morris, 1971), aspartate and alanine aminotransferase (Otani and Morris, 1971), tyrosine aminotransferase (Aviram and Hershko, 1977), S-adenosyl-methionine synthetase (Liau et al., 1979; Tsukada and Okada, 1980) evidence has been given that the disappearance of some enzymatic components that are typical of the normal adult rat liver and appearance of new, frequently foetal-type isozymes generally correspond to the degree of dedifferentiation and to the growth rate of the tumor.

Since these phenotypic features of tumors have to be related to distortions of gene regulation and expression, which leads to misprogrammed protein synthesis, it was noteworthy to investigate the behaviour of the atypical isozymes after treatment with drugs that at different levels affect protein synthesis.

In this preliminary report we present the following data:

1. In Yoshida AH 100 strain ascites tumor, at the 8th and 10th day from the transplantation, the isozyme patterns which can be obtained by means of ion exchange DEAE chromatography of acid phosphatase, aspartate and alanine aminotransferase, malate dehydrogenase, glucose-6-phosphate dehydrogenase and β-glucuronidase are very similar to those of normal adult rat liver (Gazzaniga, 1975; Gazzaniga, 1979).

2. Two atypical isozymes, of aspartate aminotransferase and malate dehydrogenase respectively were present in about 60% of the Yoshida cells extracts obtained at the 10th day after the inoculum.

3. Both these abnormal isozymes were demonstrable in a very low amount only in two Yoshida cells extracts from rats that after the transplantation received ethionine intraperitoneally. Ethionine has been preliminarily used because it has been shown (Gazzaniga, 1975) that it seems to selectively affect the extramitochondrial isozyme of aspartate aminotransferase of normal rat liver, to which the atypical form that we have found in Yoshida cells could be referred for the elution profile.

Material and methods

About 10^6 Yoshida cells, AH 100 strain, were injected intraperitoneally in male Wistar rats of about 150-180 grams body weight; the animals were killed by decapitation after 8 or 10 days from the inoculum. In a second group of rats, after the Yoshida cells transplantation, L-ethionine was given intraperitoneally, 0.25 g/Kg, corresponding to 1,5 mmol/Kg b.w., for 8 days: these animals were killed after 10 days from the inoculum. The ascites fluid was collected, diluted with 3 volumes of a cold phosphate buffer pH 7,4, and centrifuged at 300 g for 5 minutes. After washing three times with the same buffer, the cells were disrupted by means of a Mullard MSE sonic disintegrator at 20.000 cps and 4°C for 10 minutes. Centrifugation at 10.000 g for 10 minutes followed, then the supernatant fluid was dyalized for 12 hours against 0.005 mol/l Tris-phosphate buffer pH 8.0.

Columns of 30 x 1,4 cm were packed with a 2% suspension of DEAE cellulose in the same starting buffer; chromatography was

carried out at 4°C, with a limit buffer Na Cl 0.40 mol/l as elsewhere described (Gazzaniga, 1972). The elution fractions, each
of 5 ml volume, were analyzed for protein content according to
Lowry et al., with bovine serum albumin as a standard and for
the following enzymatic activities: acid phosphatase (EC 3.1.3.2),
aspartate aminotransferase (EC2.6.1.1), alanine aminotransferase
(EC 2.6.1.2), malate dehydrogenase (EC 1.1.1.37), glucose-6-pho-
sphate dehydrogenase (EC 1.1.1.49), β-glucuronidase (EC 3.2.1.
31). Procedures of the enzyme assays have been described elsewhere (Gazzaniga, 1972). Activities of the enzyme components
have been expressed as μmol of transformed substrate/min/g of
protein, at 37°C.

Results and Discussion

The activity values of the chromatographic fractions of the
assayed enzymes, expressed in μmol/min/g of protein, are reported in Table 1.

The isozyme elution profiles strictly correspond to those of
normal liver from adult Wistar rats (Gazzaniga, 1975 and 1979);
activity values of the single isozymes were from 1/10 (for acid
phosphatase) and 1/5 (for malate dehydrogenase) to about 1/3
(for alanine aminotransferase and β-glucuronidase) and 1/2
(for aspartate aminotransferase and glucose-6-phosphate dehydrogenase) of those that can be calculated in normal rat livers.
No significant change in comparison with normal liver has been
observed in the activity ratios between the different forms of
the same enzyme. The activity values found in Yoshida cells
collected after 8 and 10 days respectively from the inoculum
were similar, except for both mitochondrial and cytoplasmic
forms of acid phosphatase which showed a significant decrease
at the 10th day.

In 8 of 13 Yoshida cells extracts we have found an atypical
form of aspartate aminotransferase, that was eluted at 45-100
mmol chloride concentration and accounted for about 30-40% of
the total activity of the enzyme; in ethionine-treated rats
this form was present in only two extracts, less than 10 % in
amount, while the normal cytoplasmic one, that is eluted at 15-
35 mmol chloride concentration, was significantly increased
(see Table 1).

Table 1. Activity values of some isozymes of Yoshida tumor cells from rats untreated and treated with ethionine.

Enzyme	Fraction		Chloride elution mmol/l	Activity (μmol/min/g of protein)	
				Untreated	Treated with ethionine
Acid phosphatase	I	(lys.)	unadsorbed	32.9 ± 9.3	41.0 ± 10.4
	II	(cyt.)	45 - 100	18.8 ± 4.7	14.8 ± 4.5
Aspartate aminotransferase	I	(mit.)	unadsorbed	52.6 ± 14.5	44.0 ± 7.8
	II	(cyt.)	15 - 35	69.9 ± 16.1	131.3 ± 26.1
	Atypical		45 - 100	48.9 ± 13.4 (+)	-
Alanine aminotransferase	I		60 - 120	60.3 ± 7.8	43.2 ± 5.4
	II		130 - 200	84.1 ± 11.9	60.9 ± 13.6
Malate dehydrogenase	I	(mit.)	unadsorbed	53.6 ± 8.4	81.5 ± 14.5
	Atypical		10 - 25	46.6 ± 7.1 (++)	-
	II	(cyt.)	40 - 110	64.4 ± 11.0	112.3 ± 27.4
Glucose 6-phosphate dehydrogenase	I		60 - 90	1.3 ± 0.3	1.7 ± 0.4
	II		120 - 210	7.5 ± 1.7	11.3 ± 3.0
	III		270 - 370	4.3 ± 0.8	2.8 ± 1.0
β-Glucuronidase	I	(micros.)	65 - 90	0.8 ± 0.3	1.1 ± 0.3
	II	(lys.)	100 - 145	3.7 ± 1.1	3.1 ± 1.2

Untreated: 13 columns; treated with ethionine: 9 columns. (+)Mean of 8 and (++) of 7 extracts.

Moreover, in 7 of these 8 extracts, we have found an abnormal cathodic form of malate dehydrogenase, which was eluted at 10-25 mmol chloride concentration and accounted for about 30 % of the total malate dehydrogenase activity; it similarly lacked in ethionine-treated rats, with a corresponding increase of the cytoplasmic typical form, eluted at 40-110 mmol chloride concentration.

Evidence of the anodic behaviour of the atypical form of aspartate aminotransferase, in contrast with the cathodic one of the atypical form of malate dehydrogenase, provides considerable support for the view that the present data should not be referred to aggregation of typical isozymes with some abnormal cellular protein, whose synthesis could be selectively affected by ethionine.

It is our purpose a biochemical characterization of these atypical molecular forms in order to determine if they are to be considered as distinct isozymes; the effects on the isozyme patterns of Yoshida ascites tumor of protein synthesis inhibitors other than ethionine will also be investigated.

REFERENCES

1. Aviram M. and Hershko A., 1977: Interconversion of multiple forms of tyrosine aminotransferase in vitro and in vivo in cultured hepatoma cells. Bioch. Bioph. Acta, 498, 83.

2. Cederbaum A.J. and Rubin E., 1976: Kinetic properties of alcohol dehydrogenase in hepatocellular carcinoma and normal tissues of rat. Cancer Res., 36, 2274.

3. Emmelot P. and Bos C.J., 1969: A survey of enzyme activities displayed by plasma membranes isolated from normal and pre-neoplastic livers and primary and transplanted hepatomas of the rat. Int. J. Cancer, 4, 705.

4. Farina F.A., Shatton J.B., Morris H.P. and Weinhouse S., 1974: Isozymes of pyruvate kinase in liver and hepatomas of the rat. Cancer Res., 34, 1439.

5. Gazzaniga P.P., 1972: Rat liver isozymes in cloudy swelling. Enzyme, 14, 25.

6. Gazzaniga P.P., 1975: Rat liver isozymes in acute carbon tetrachloride and ethionine poisoning. Enzyme, 20, 193.

7. Gazzaniga P.P., 1979: Rat liver isozymes in acute and chronic
   thioacetamide poisoning. Arch. De Vecchi, 63, 1.

8. Kakizoe T., Kawachi T. and Sugimura T., 1976: β-glucuronidase isozyme patterns of experimental hepatomas of rats. Gann, 67, 289.

9. Kaneko A., Dempo K., Onoè T. and Isaka H., 1972: Deviations in
   isozyme patterns of acid phosphatase and esterase and in ultra-
   structures of Yoshida ascites hepatomas from rat hepatocytes.
   Gann, 63, 747.

10. Liau M.C., Chang C.F. and Becker F.F., 1979: Alteration of S-
    adenosylmethionine synthetases during chemical hepatocarcino-
    genesis and in resulting carcinomas. Cancer Res., 39, 2113.

11. Otani T.T. and Morris H.P., 1971: Comparison of activity and
    isozyme patterns of four enzymes from hepatomas of different
    growth rates. J. Nat. Cancer Inst., 47, 1247.

12. Sato K., Satoh K., Sato T., Imai F. and Morris H.P., 1976: Iso-
    zyme patterns of glycogen phosphorilase in rat tissues and
    transplantable hepatomas. Cancer Res., 36, 487.

13. Sato S. and Sugimura T., 1973: Presence of fast-moving type
    IV hexokinase isozyme in Morris hepatoma. Gann, 64, 359.

14. Tsukada K. and Okada G., 1980: S-adenosylmethionine synthetase
    isozyme patterns from rat hepatoma induced by N-2-fluorenyl-
    acetamide. Bioch. Bioph. Res. Commun., 94, 1078.

BIOLOGY AND IMMUNOLOGY OF HUMAN CARCINOMA CELL POPULATIONS

J. Schlom, D. Colcher, P. Hand, D. Wunderlich, M. Nuti,
R. Mariani-Costantini, D. Stramignoni, J. Greiner,
S. Pestka, P. Fisher, and P. Noguchi

National Institutes of Health, National Cancer Institute
Bethesda, Maryland

The rationale for the studies overviewed here was to utilize membrane-enriched extracts of human metastatic mammary tumor cells as immunogens in an attempt to generate and characterize monoclonal antibodies (MAbs) reactive with determinants that would be maintained on primary as well as metastatic human mammary carcinoma cells. Multiple assays have been employed to reveal the range of reactivities and diversity of the various antibodies.

Some of the MAbs generated showed a strong selective reactivity for some non-breast carcinomas, especially colon carcinoma. In an attempt to overcome the antigenic heterogeneity observed among cells within carcinoma masses, recombinant interferon was used and was shown to enhance specific cell surface tumor antigen expression.

Generation of Monoclonal Antibodies

Mice were immunized with membrane-enriched fractions of human metastatic mammary carcinoma cells from either of two involved livers of two different patients. Spleens of immunized mice were fused with non-immunoglobulin (Ig) secreting NS-1 murine myeloma cells to generate 4,250 primary hybridoma cultures. Supernatant fluids from hybridoma cultures were first screened in solid phase radioimmunoassays (RIAs) for the presence of Ig that is reactive with extracts of metastatic mammary tumor cells from involved liver versus normal liver; eleven double cloned hybridoma cell lines were chosen for further study. The isotypes of all eleven antibodies were determined; ten were IgG of various subclasses and one was an IgM.

The eleven MAbs could be divided into three major groups based on their differential reactivity to tumor extracts in solid phase

RIA (Colcher, et al., 1981). All eleven antibodies were negative when tested against similar extracts from normal human liver, a rhabdomyosarcoma cell line, the HBL-100 cell line derived from cultures of human milk cells, mouse mammary tumor and fibroblast cell lines, disrupted mouse mammary tumor virus and mouse leukemia virus, purified carcinoembryonic antigen (CEA) and ferritin. Two MAbs were used as positive controls in all these studies: (a) W6/32, a commercially available anti-human histocompatibility antigen (Barnstable et al., 1978) and (b) B139, which was generated in our laboratory against a human breast tumor metastasis, and which demonstrates reactivity to all human cells tested.

To determine if the MAbs bind cell surface determinants, each was tested for binding to live cells in culture. The monoclonals grouped together on the basis of their binding to both metastatic cell extracts could be further separated into three different groups on the basis of their differential binding to breast cancer cell line surface determinants. Many of the monoclonals also bound to the surface of selected non-breast carcinoma cell lines. None of the eleven MAbs, however, bound to the surface of sarcoma or melanoma cell lines, nor to the surface of over 24 cell lines derived from apparently normal human tissues (Colcher, et al., 1981; Horan Hand, et al., 1983).

To further define specificity and range of reactivity of each of the MAbs, the immunoperoxidase technique was employed on formalin fixed tissue sections. All the monoclonals reacted with carcinoma cells of both infiltrating ductal and lobular primary mammary carcinomas. The percentage of primary tumors that were reactive varied for the different monoclonals and in many of the positive primary and metastatic mammary carcinomas, not all tumor cells stained. A high degree of selective reactivity with mammary tumor cells, but not with apparently normal mammary epithelium, stroma, blood vessels, or lymphocytes of the breast was also observed.

Experiments were then carried out to determine if the eleven MAbs could detect mammary carcinoma cell populations in regional nodes and at distal sites. Since the MAbs were all generated using metastatic mammary carcinoma cells as antigens, it was not unexpected that the MAbs all reacted, but with different degrees, to various metastases. None of the monoclonals reacted with normal lymphocytes or stroma from any involved or uninvolved nodes. The MAbs were then tested for reactivity to normal and neoplastic non-mammary tissues. Most of the monoclonals showed reactivity with selected non-breast carcinomas such as adenocarcinoma of the colon, but showed no staining of sarcomas and lymphomas. MAbs B72.3, B6.2, and B38.1 were chosen for further study since they recognized noncoordinately expressed antigens in different breast tumor cells and lesions; these monoclonals reacted with approximately 45, 75, and 56 percent, respectively, of 39 infiltrating duct carcinomas tested via the immunoperoxidase technique. MAb B38.1 also reacted to several normal epithelial tissues such as sweat glands. The major reactivity to normal tissues of MAb B6.2 was subsets of circulating polymorphonuclear leukocytes. Thus far, MAb B72.3 has demonstrated the most selective degree of reactivity for normal versus tumor tissues. However, fetal tissue has not yet been carefully examined nor has every tissue type in the body. It would be naive to assume that any antigenic determinant consisting of a few amino acids would be expressed only on carcinoma cells, and at no time during development in the embryo, or at various stages of cell differentiation within the spectrum of adult tissues.

Since MAb B72.3 (an IgG1) displayed such a restricted range of reactivity for human mammary tumor versus normal cells, this antibody was used for further studies in immunoperoxidase assays. Using 4 ug of MAb per slide the percent of positive primary breast tumors was 46% (19/41); 62% (13/21) of the metastatic lesions scored positive. Several histologic types of primary mammary tumors scored positive (Nuti, et al., 1982). Metastatic breast carcinoma lesions that were positive were in axillary lymph nodes, and at the distal sites of skin, liver, lung, pleura and mesentery. A variety of non-breast cells and tissues were tested and were negative; these included uterus, liver, spleen, lung, bone marrow, colon, stomach, salivary gland, lymph node and kidney (Nuti, et al. 1982).

Mammary Carcinoma Tissue as Immunogen for the Preparation of MAbs to Carcinoembryonic Antigen (CEA)

MAbs were also generated to membrane-enriched fractions of human mammary carcinoma metastases and screened for reactivity with purified CEA. The differential binding properties of two of these antibodies (B1.1 and F5.5) to CEA and to breast and non-breast tumors was investigated (Colcher, et al., 1983). Both B1.1 (IgG2a) and F5.5 (IgG1) precipitated iodinated CEA, resulting in a radiolabeled peak at approximately 180,000d. No precipitation of purified CEA was obtained using MAbs B6.2, B72.3 nor with any of the other MAbs described above.

Extracts of breast tumor metastases were assayed for reactivity with monoclonals B1.1, B6.2, and B72.3 by solid phase RIA. The appropriate immunoreactive fractions were then pooled and labeled with [125]I. MAb B72.3 immunoprecipitated a complex of four bands with molecular weights of approximately 220,000; 250,000; 285,000; and 400,000. B1.1 immunoprecipitated a heterogenous component with an average estimated molecular weight of 180,000. B6.2 immunoprecipitated a 90,000d component.

Antigenic Heterogeneity, Modulation, and Evolution Within Human
Mammary Carcinoma Cell Populations

Phenotypic variation was usually observed in the expression
of tumor associated antigens (TAAs) within a given mammary
tumor (Horan Hand et al., 1983). One pattern sometimes observed
was that one area of a mammary tumor contained cells with TAAs
reactive with a particular MAb, while another area of the same
tumor contained unreactive cells. A more common type of
antigenic heterogeneity was observed among cells in a given
area of a tumor mass. Tumor cells expressing a specific TAA
were seen directly adjacent to tumor cells negative for the
same antigen.
     In an attempt to elucidate the phenomenon of antigenic
heterogeneity in human mammary tumors, model systems were
examined. The MCF-7 human mammary tumor cell line was tested
for the presence of TAAs using the cytospin/immunoperoxidase
method. The cell line was shown to contain various subpopulations
of cells as defined by variability in expression of TAA reactive
with MAb B6.2, i.e., positive MCF-7 cells are seen adjacent to
cells which scored negative (Horan Hand et al., 1983).
     Studies were then conducted to determine if the antigenic
heterogeneity observed in MCF-7 cells was (i) the result of at
least two stable genotypes or phenotypes, or (ii) was the
reflection of a modulation of cell surface antigen expression of
a single phenotype, or (iii) the result of both phenomena. In
experiments designed to monitor cell surface antigen expression
with different phases of cell growth, it was observed that MCF-7
cells at contact inhibition expressed less antigen on their
surfaces, as detected by MAb B6.2, than cells in active proliferation. Using fluorescent activated cell sorter analyses, it
has been shown that at least two of the monoclonal antibodies
developed (B6.2 and B38.1) are most reactive with the surface of
MCF-7 cells during S-phase of the cell cycle (Kufe, et al., 1983).
     To further understand the nature of antigenic heterogeneity
of human mammary tumor cell populations, MCF-7 cells were cloned
by end-point dilution and ten different clones were obtained and
assayed for cell surface TAAs (Horan Hand et al., 1983). The
parent MCF-7 culture reacts most strongly with MAbs B1.1 and B6.2
and least with monoclonal B72.3. One clone exhibited a similar
phenotype to that of the parent, but at least three additional
major phenotypes were observed among the other clones. To
determine the stability of the cell surface phenotype of the MCF-7
clones, each line was monitored through a four month period and
assayed during log phase at approximately every other passage.
While some of the MCF-7 clones maintained a stable antigenic
phenotype throughout the observation period, a dramatic change in
antigenic phenotype, i.e., antigenic evolution, was observed in
some of the clones (Horan Hand et al., 1983).

Radiolocalization of Human Mammary Tumors in Athymic Mice by a Monoclonal Antibody

With the development of the hybridoma technology, homogenous populations of MAbs to TAAs can now be utilized in either lymphangiography, to detect mammary tumor lesions in nodes of the axilla and internal mammary chain, or to detect distal metastases. In the studies described here, MAb B6.2, which may be useful in lymphangiography procedures was utilized. B6.2 IgG was purified and F(ab')$_2$ and Fab' fragments were generated by pepsin digestion All three forms of the antibody were radiolabeled and assayed to determine their utility in the radioimmunolocalization of transplanted human mammary tumor masses (Colcher, et al., 1983).

The IgG and its fragments were labeled with ^{125}I using the iodogen method to specific activities of 15-50 uCi ug. The labeled antibody was shown to bind to the surface of live MCF-7 cells and retained the same specificity as the unlabeled antibody. Better than 70 percent of the antibody remained immunoreactive in sequential saturation solid phase RIAs after labeling.

Athymic mice bearing the Clouser transplantable human mammary tumor were injected with 0.1 ug of ^{125}I- MAb B6.2. The ratio of radioactivity/mg of tissue in the tumor compared to that of various tissues rose over a 4 day period and then fell at 7 days. The tumor to tissue ratios were 10:1 or greater in the liver, spleen and kidney at day 4. Ratios of the counts in the tumor to that found in the brain and muscle were greater than 50:1 and as high as 110:1. When the mammary tumor bearing mice were injected with ^{125}I-F(ab')$_2$ fragments of B6.2, higher tumor to tissue ratios were obtained. The tumor to tissue ratios in the liver and spleen were 15-20:1 at 96 hours. This is probably due to the faster clearance of the F(ab')$_2$ fragments, as compared to the IgG. Athymic mice bearing a human melanoma (A375), a tumor that shows no surface reactivity with B6.2 in live cell RIAs were used as controls and were negative for non-specific binding of the labeled antibody or antibody fragments to tumor tissue. Similary, no localization was observed when either normal murine IgG or MOPC-21 IgG1 (the same isotype as B6.2 from a murine myeloma), or their F(ab')$_2$ fragments, were radiolabeled and inoculated into athymic mice bearing human mammary tumor or melanoma transplants.

Studies were than undertaken to determine whether the localization of the ^{125}I-labeled antibody and fragments in the tumors was sufficient to detect using a gamma camera. Mice were injected with ^{125}I-B6.2 F(ab')$_2$ fragments. Due to the rapid clearance of the fragments, a significant amount of radioactivity was observed in the two kidneys and bladder at 24 hours (Fig. 1A); tumors were also clearly positive (Fig. 1A). The activity was cleared from the kidneys and bladder by 48 hours and the tumor to background ratio increased over the 4 day period of scanning, with little background, and good tumor localization observed at 96 hours (Fig. 1B). No localization was observed with the radiolabeled B6.2 F(ab')^2 fragments in the athymic mice bearing the control A375 melanoma (Fig. 1C).

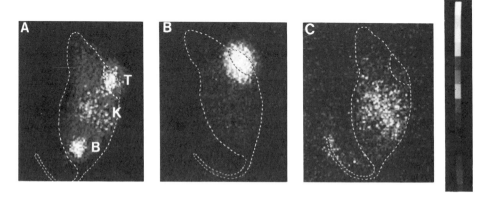

Fig. 1. Gamma camera scanning with ^{125}I–labeled MAb B6.2
F(ab')^2 of athymic mice bearing transplanted human tumors.
Mice bearing a transplantable human mammary tumor (Clouser,
Panels A and B) or a human melanoma (A375, Panel C) were
innoculated with approximately 30 uCi of ^{125}I–B6.2 F(ab')^2 The
mice were scanned after various time intervals (24 hrs., Panel
A; 96 hrs., Panels B and C) until an equal number of counts
were detected in each field.

MAbs to human colon, lung, and breast carcinomas have been generated in a number of laboratories. A surprising finding in these studies has been the large number of antigenic cross reactivities observed among these three major carcinoma groups. The studies reported here are designed to define the range of reactivities of monoclonals B72.3, B6.2, and B1.1 to colon adenocarcinomas versus benign colon lesions and normal colon epithelium.

Reactivity of MAbs with malignant and benign colon lesions

Purified IgG of monoclonal B1.1 was reacted with fixed, 5 micron tissue sections of malignant and benign colon lesions at concentrations of 10, 1, and 0.1 ug/ml of purified IgG per slide using the avidin-biotin complex (ABC) method of immunoperoxidase staining (Stramignoni, et al., 1983). The characteristic dark reddish-brown positive reaction was contrasted with that of the blue hematoxylin counterstain. Scoring of carcinomas was based on the percent of carcinoma cells in samples that were positive, as well as the intensity of the stain.

Using 10 ug/ml of MAb B1.1, 94% (15 of 16) colon carcinomas from different patients scored positive (Fig. 2A). All the positive carcinomas contained greater than 25% reactive cells with three of the tumors having 100% of their cells positive. A heterogeneity of antigenic expression in terms of luminal versus cytoplasmic reactivity in a given tumor mass was usually observed. Approximately two thirds of coexistant adenoma lesions and normal colon epithelium were also positive. The majority of adenomas from non-carcinoma patients scored positive. Using lower dilutions of B1.1 (1 ug/ml and 0.1 ug/ml), the majority of colon carcinoma specimens remained positive. Some of the adenomas in non-carcinoma patients also remained positive, scoring from 71% positive at 1 ug/ml, to 44% positive at 0.1 ug/ml.

Using 10 ug/ml of MAb B72.3, 14 of 17 (82%) of colon carcinomas demonstrated a variable number of positive staining cells (Fig. 2B). The majority of the carcinomas that were positive, had more than 50% of tumor cells present reacting. The cellular location of the reactivity also varied within a given tumor mass; luminal reactivity was often observed in glandular structures, with cytoplasmic staining in less differentiated structures. As a negative for the specificity of the staining observed, parallel slides with PBS (instead of primary antibody B72.3), isotype identical IgG (MOPC-21), as well as normal murine IgG were used; all of these gave negative results.

Adenomas in patients with colon carcinoma were also examined for expression of antigen reactive with MAb B72.3; only one of ten such lesions showed a positive reaction. This lesion was immediately adjacent to a carcinoma and had less than 5% cells positive. All other adenomas and adjacent normal epithelium in carcinoma patients were negative, with one exception in which

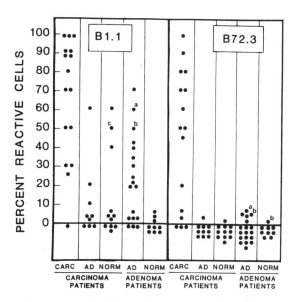

Fig. 2. Reactivities of MAbs B1.1 and B72.3 with Colon
Carcinomas. The scoring of immunoperoxidase staining with MAb
B1.1 (Panel A) and MAb B72.3 (Panel B) used at 10ug/ml is based
on a semiquantitative rating by two pathologists (Stramignoni
et al., 1983). The first three columns of each panel show the
reactivity of formalin fixed carcinomas (CARC), adenomas (AD),
and normal epithelium (NORM) in carcinoma-bearing patients; the
next two columns show the reactivity of formalin fixed adenomas
(AD) and normal epithelium (NORM) of adenoma-bearing patients.
The lesions from the 18 adenoma patients studied could be
divided into two groups: 10 were classified as tubular adenomas
and 8 as tubulovillous adenomas. (a) tubular adenoma in a
patient with "probable recurrence" of colon carcinoma; (b)
tubulovillous adenoma with atypia and diagnosis of in situ
carcinoma; (c) colon cancer patient with ulcerative colitis.

less than 1% of the cells scored positive. Adenomas from
patients without apparent carcinoma were examined using 10
ug/ml monoclonal B72.3. None of the 18 lesions showed reactivity
with greater than a few percent of adenoma cells positive.
Five of the 18 samples, however, did show staining in a few
percent of adenoma cells.

Malignant and benign colon lesions were then examined
using ten fold less (1 ug/ml) MAb B72.3. At this antibody
dilution, 50% (8/16) carcinomas showed a positive reaction; one
of 10 adjacent adenomas showed a focal reactivity of less than
one percent of adenomatous cells. None of 16 adenomas from non-
carcinoma patients, and none of normal epithelium from 19
carcinoma or adenoma patients reacted at this antibody dilution.
Thus, a positive reactivity with MAb B72.3 at this dilution
appears to be an even stronger marker for malignancy.

As mentioned above, monoclonals B1.1 and B6.2 can be
distinguished on the basis of the molecular weight of the
proteins precipitated from tumor cells. From reactivity patterns
on tumor and normal tissues, it has been difficult thus far to
distinguish the reactivities of these two monoclonals. Used at
10 ug/ml, MAb B6.2 reacted with all of 15 colon carcinomas
tested, with 3 of the tumors showing 100% reactivity. Three of
ten adenomas, as well as 2 of 11 normal epithelia, adjacent to
carcinoma lesions were positive. Using 10 ug/ml of B6.2 per
slide, 65% (11/17) adenomas from noncarcinoma patients also
scored positive.

Using 1 ug/ml of monoclonal B6.2 per slide, 14 of 15 (93%)
of carcinoma lesions scored positive. Two of ten adenomas in
carcinoma patients and 5 of 16 (30%) of adenomas from noncarcinoma
patients also were positive. However, with the exception of
one lesion, all adenomas had less than 10 percent tumor cells
positive. Using 0.1 ug/ml of B6.2, 8/15 carcinomas were positive
while three of 18 adenomas were positive with only a few percent
of cells reacting. Thus, monoclonal B6.2 could clearly be
distinguished from monoclonal B1.1 on the basis of its more
selective reactivity with colon carcinoma versus adenomas or
normal colon epithelium. The reactivity of B6.2, however, was
not as selective for carcinomas as was that observed for
monoclonal B72.3 (Stramignoni, et al., 1983).

Colon carcinomas and adenomas were also antigenically
phenotyped into several distinct groups based on their reactivity
with the three monoclonal antibodies employed in this study.
Large retrospective studies using fixed tissue sections can now
be conducted to determine if a given antigenic phenotype
correlates with a specific biologic property such as response
to a specific therapeutic modality or prognosis.

Recombinant Interferon Enhances Tumor Antigen Detection

Previous studies with MAbs have shown a great deal of
antigenic heterogeneity among cells within both primary and

metastatic human breast and coloncarcinoma lessions. If MAbs
are to be used successfully for the in situ detection or therapy
of human carcinoma lesions, this phenomenon of antigenic heterogeneity must be modified so that most or all cells of a tumor
mass express a given TAA. One approach to enhance the expression
of TAAs on the surface of cancer cells would be the use of
those substances which (a) have been shown to alter states of
cell differentiation, and (b) have potential clinical applicability.
Native interferon (Imai, et al., 1981) and recombinant human
leukocyte clone A interferon (IFN) (Pestka, 1983) meet the
above two criteria. Because of its homogeneity, stability, and
extensive degree of characterization (Pestka, 1983) IFN was
thus evaluated for its ability to enhance the detection of TAAs
on the surface of human carcinoma cells by MAbs (Greiner et
al., 1983).

IFN was first titrated on the human mammary carcinoma cell
line MCF-7 for its ability to enhance the detection of TAAs as
well as normal cell surface antigens. A solid phase RIA with
live cells (Hand, et al., 1983) and various concentrations of
purified monoclonal Ig were used to detect antigen expression.
As seen in Figure 3, 10 100, or 1000 U/ml of IFN enhanced the
detection of the 90K (Fig. 3C), the 180K CEA (Fig. 3D) and the
220-400K (Fig. 3E) TAAs by MAbs B6.2, B1.1, and B72.3,
respectively, in a dose dependent manner. MAbs W6/32 and B139,
directed against two antigens found on the surface of normal
and neoplastic human cells were used as controls. As seen in
Figure 3A, IFN enhanced the cell surface binding of MAb W6/32
but had no effect on the surface binding of MAb B139 (Fig. 3B).
Addition of 5,000 and 10,000 U/ml of IFN resulted in less
effective binding of all the MAbs than with 1000 U/ml. The
effect of time of exposure of cells to IFN was also examined.
The enhanced expression of TAA was first detected within 4 to
12 hrs after the addition of 1000 U/ml IFN; optimal enhancement
was observed 16 to 24 hours after IFN addition. IFN was then
analyzed for its ability to enhance the detection of TAAs on
the surface of the human colon carcinoma cell line WiDr. Ten
to 1000 U/ml IFN enhanced the binding of MAbs B6.2 (Fig. 3H)
and B1.1 (Fig. 3I) in a dose-dependent manner. The 220-400K
TAA is not expressed on the surface of WiDr cells, and various
levels of IFN up to 1000 U/ml failed to elicit any B72.3 binding
(Fig. 3J). While IFN enhanced the binding of MAb W6/32 to the
surface of WiDr (Fig. 3F) and MCF-7 cells (Fig. 3A), it enhanced
the binding of MAb B139 only to WiDr (Fig. 3G), and not to
MCF-7 cells (Fig. 3B).

The effect of ten, 100 and 1000 U/ml of IFN on the growth
of MCF-7 and WiDr cells was monitored. Incubation of cells in
growth medium containing 10 or 100 U/ml IFN for 6 days had no
appreciable effect on cell growth; incubation with 1000 U/ml
IFN for 6 days reduced the total cell number by 46%. However,
no effect on cell number was observed 1, 2, or 4 days following
IFN addition at any dose level. Since all determinations of

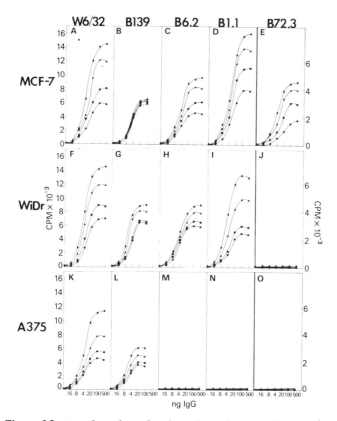

Fig. 3. The effect of molecularly cloned interferon (IFN) on the expression of human tumor associated and normal cell surface antigens. The live cell solid phase RIA used has been described previously (Horan Hand, et al., 1983). Cells (5×10^4) were added to 96 well microtiter plates. After 24 hrs at 37°C, in medium with or without IFN, medium was removed and MAb was added. After one hr at 37°C, cells were washed 2x and 75,000 cpm of ^{125}I-labeled goat anti-mouse IgG was added. After 1 hr at 37°C, cells were washed and the cpm bound were determined. Panels A-E are MCF-7 human mammary carcinoma cells; Panels F-J are WiDr colon carcinoma cells; Panels K-O are A375 melanoma cells (Flow 4000 human embryonic kidney, and WI-38 human embryonic lung cell gave similar results.) Monoclonal IgGs were affinity purified and used at the amounts indicated. MAb W6/32 (Panels A,F,K), MAbs B139 (Panels B,G, L), B6.2 (C,H,M), B1.1 (D,I,N) and B72.3 (E,J,O) have been previously described (Colcher, et al., 1981). IFN was obtained and purified as previously described (Peska, 1983). The specific activity of the preparation used was 2×10^8 U/mg protein when tested on MDBK (bovine kidney) cells. Amounts of IFN per ml used were 10 U (boxes), 100 U (triangles), 1000 U (diamonds). Control buffer RPMI 1640 containing 1% BSA is denoted by circles.

surface antigen expression were made 24 hours after addition of
IFN and in many cases similar results were observed using 100
or 1000 U/ml, the enhanced TAA expression appears to be
independent of changes in cell proliferation.

Studies were carried out to determine if various concentrations
of IFN would induce the expression of the 90K, 180K, and 220-
400K TAAs on normal as well as noncarcinoma neoplastic cells
not normally expressing these surface antigens. Three cell
lines were chosen for these studies: WI-38 (normal human
embryonic lung), Flow 4000 (normal human embryonic kidney), and
A375 (human melanoma). All three cell lines were previously
shown to be negative for the expression of the three TAAs
(Colcher, et al., 1981; Horan Hand, et al., 1983) and remained
so following exposure to various concentrations (10-1000 U/ml)
of IFN (see Fig. 3 M-O). IFN did, however, increase the
expression of the normal cell surface antigens that bind MAbs
B139 (Fig. 3L) and W6/32 (Fig. 3K).

The enhanced binding of MAbs to TAAs on the surface of
human breast and colon carcinoma cells mediated by IFN could be
due to (i) the increased expression of TAAs on a subpopulation
of cells already expressing the TAAs, or (ii) the induction of
the expression of a given TAA on a population of cells not
previously expressing the antigen, or (iii) a combination of
both phenomena. To explore these possibilities, MAb Bl.1 was
reacted with WiDr human colon carcinoma cells in the presence
or absence of 1000 U/ml IFN and the cells were analyzed via
fluorescent activated cell sorting. The background analysis of
WiDr cells in the absence of addition of MAb Bl.1, with or
without IFN is shown in Fig. 4A. Fig. 4B shows a heterogenous
population of cells, depicted as a spectrum of fluorescence
intensities (X-axis), expressing various levels of the cell
surface 180K antigen. Following a 24 hr incubation with 1000
U/ml IFN a dramatic shift is observed (Fig. 4C) in both the
percentage of cells expressing the 180K antigen (vertical
Z-axis), and the fluorescence intensity per cell (X-axis). No
difference in DNA content of cells (Fig. 4, Y-axis) was observed
after IFN treatment. Thus, following the addition of IFN,
computer analysis revealed more than 98% of tumor cells now
bound MAb Bl.1.

One of the potential clinical applications of MAbs is the
use of radiolabeled immunoglobulins to detect micrometastases
in regional nodes and at distal sites. MAbs B6.2 and B72.3
have already been used to detect human carcinoma transplants in
athymic mice (Colcher, et al., 1983). One of the major
considerations of radiolocalization studies is reducing the
amount of radiolabeled MAb required to bind and detect a given
tumor mass in situ; the use of lower levels of labeled MAb
would increase "signal to noise" ratios and thus make detection
of smaller lesions more efficient. Accordingly, we investigated
the effect of IFN on the amount of MAb B72.3 required to bind

Fig. 4. Flow cytometric analyses of MAb B1.1 binding the
surface of WiDr carcinoma colon cells following treatment with
recombinant interferon (IFN). Each figure is a three-dimensional
isometric display of DNA content (Y axis), fluorescence intensity,
i.e., cell surface 180K antigen expression (X axis), with the
Z axis representing the number of cells. WiDr cells (10^7) were
incubated for 24 hrs at 37°C with or without 1000 units/ml IFN.
The cells were then harvested, washed and incubated for 2 hours
at 4°C in medium containing 2 ug MAb B1.1 per 10^6 cells. The
cells were then washed with PBS and incubated with fluorescinated
sheep anti-mouse antibody for 60 minutes at 4°C. The cells
were washed, centrifuged at 500 x g and resuspended at a
concentration of 10^6 cells/0.3 ml. The cells were then fixed
by adding 0.7 ml of ice-cold 100% ethanol while vortexing.
After fixing in ethanol for 24 hours, the cells were pelleted,
resuspended, and stained for 4 hours at room temperature, 10^6
cells/ml in PBS with propidium iodide (PI,18 ug/ml) and
ribonuclease A (2000 units/ml). The stained cells were analyzed
on an Ortho Cytofluorograf System 50H with blue laser excitation
of 200 milliwatts at 488 nm. Under these conditions PI bound
to nuclear DNA fluoresces red while surface immunofluorescence
bound to the 180K antigen fluoresces green. Data from 25,000
cells was stored on an Ortho Model 2150 computer system and
used to generate the figures shown here. A. WiDr cells stained
for DNA content, but with no MAb B1.1. B. WiDr cells stained
for both nuclear DNA and MAb B1.1 binding.   C. WiDr cells
treated with 1000U IFN for 24 hours and stained as in B.

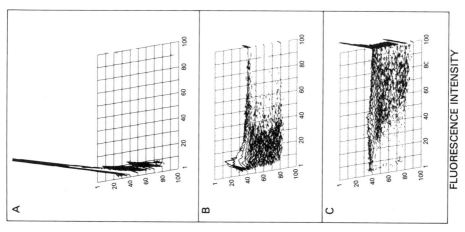

DNA CONTENT

FLUORESCENCE INTENSITY

a reference number of cpm to the surface of MCF-7 mammary tumor
cells. Ninety-four ng of MAb 72.3 were required to bind 1000
cpm to 5 x 10^4 MCF-7 cells, whereas this could be reduced to
4 ng of MAb B72.3 following exposure of the same number of
cells to 1000 U/ml of IFN. This 24-fold reduction in the amount
of MAb required to give an equally efficient signal for surface
binding of a MAb may have potential clinical application for
the in situ detection of carcinoma lesions with radiolabeled
MAbs or in the use of MAbs for immunotherapy. In addition, the
ability of recombinant interferon to selectively enhance the
expression of monoclonal-defined TAAs in carcinoma cell lines
may prove useful in defining the role of specific TAAs in the
expression of the transformed phenotype.

Acknowledgements

We wish to thank R. Riley, D. Poole, D. Simpson, J.
Howell, J. Collins, and A. Sloan for expert technical
assistance in these studies. We also thank Dr. M. Weeks
for many helpful suggestions in the preparation of this
manuscript.

REFERENCES

Barnstable, C., Bodmer, W., Brown, G., Galfre, G., Milstein, C., Williams, A. and Ziegler, A, 1978, Production of monoclonal antibodies to group A erythrocyles, HLA and other human cell surface antigens - new tools for genetic analysis, Cell, 14:9.

Colcher, D., Horan Hand, P., Nuti, M., and J. Schlom, 1981, A spectrum of monoclonal antibodies reactive with human mammary tumor cells, Proc. Natl. Acad. Sci. U.S.A., 73:3199.

Colcher, D., Horan Hand, P., Nuti, M., and Schlom, J., 1983, Differential binding to human mammry and nonmammary tumors of monoclonal antibodies reactive with carcinoembryonic antigen, J. Cancer Invest., 1:127.

Colcher, D., Zalutsky, M., Kaplan, W., Kufe, D., Austin, F., and Schlom, J., 1983, Radiolocalization of human mammary tumors in athymic mice by a monoclonal antibody, Cancer Res., 43:736.

Greiner, J., Horan Hand, P., Noguchi, P., Fisher, P., Pestka, S., and Schlom, J., 1983, Recombinant interferon enhances detection of human breast and colon carcinoma associated antigens by monoclonal antibodies, Science, (Submitted for publication).

Horan Hand, P., Nuti, M., Colcher, D., and Schlom, J., 1983, Definition of antigenic heterogeneity and modulation among human mammary carcinoma cell populations using monoclonal antibodies to tumor-associated antigens, Cancer Res., 43:728.

Imai, K., Ng, A., Glassy, M, and Ferrone, S., 1981, Differential effect of interferon on the expression of tumor-associated antigens and histocompatibility antigens on human melanoma cells: relationship to susceptibility to immune lysis mediated by monoclonal antibodies J. Immunol., 127:505.

Kufe, D., Nadler, L., Sargent, L., Shapiro, H., Horan Hand, P., Colcher, D., and Schlom, J., 1983, Biological behavior of human breast carcinomaassociated antigens expressed during cellular proliferation, Cancer Res., 43:851.

Nuti, M., Colcher, D., Horan Hand, P., Austin, F., and Schlom, J., 1981, Generation and characterization of monoclonal antibodies reactive with human primary and metastatic mammary tumor cells, in "Monoclonal Antibodies and Development in Immunoassay," A. Albertini and R. Ekins, ed., Elsevicr/North Holland Biomedical Press, North Holland.

Nuti, M., Teramoto, Y., Mariani-Costantini, R., Horan Hand, P., Colcher, D., and Schlom, J., 1982, A monoclonal antibody (B72.3) defines patterns of distribution of a novel tumor associated antigen in human mammary carcinoma cell populations, Int. J. Cancer, 29:539.

Pestka, S, 1983, The human interferons - from protein purification and sequence to cloning and expression in bacteria: before, between, and beyond, Arch. Biochem. Biophys., 221:1.

Stramignoni, D., Bowen, R., Atkinson, B. F., and Schlom, J., 1983, Differential reactivity of monoclonal antibodies with human colon adenocarcinomas and adenomas, Int. J. Cancer, 31: 543.

MONOCLONAL ANTIBODIES AGAINST BREAST CANCER

M.I. Colnaghi, S. Mènard, R. Mariani-Costantini, S. Canevari,
S. Miotti, G. Della Torre, S. Orefice, and S. Andreola

Istituto Nazionale per lo Studio e la Cura dei Tumori
Via G. Venezian 1, 20133 Milano

The application of classical hybridoma technology to the study of human mammary carcinoma resulted in the generation of a variety of monoclonal antibodies that identify several antigens associated with this type of tumor (1-3). Monoclonal reagents with selected specificities are therefore available in increasing number, and their potential for applications in the diagnosis and characterization of breast cancer is under investigation.

Even monoclonal reagents not specific for cancer cells may prove useful in complementing conventional diagnostic procedures in clinical oncology, provided they are able to discriminate between tumor cells and normal cells in specific sites. Such reagents might be accepted for detection of tumor cells in lymph nodes, bone marrow and serous effusions, assays on circulating markers and elimination of neoplastic cells from bone marrow.

We recently reported the generation of murine monoclonal antibodies against the human breast carcinoma line MCF-7. One of these monoclonals designated MBr1 (Table 1), has been shown to identify a determinant on the sugar moiety of a glycolipidic complex expressed in neoplastic and normal breast epithelial cells (4, 5).

The reactivity shown by different histotypes of breast carcinoma is shown in Table 2. Immunohistologic antigen detection was comparable in ductal and lobular histotypes and in mammary Paget's disease. The incidence of staining appeared slightly higher in tubular carcinomas whereas a high proportion of mucinous, medullary and papillary tumors was negative. Three

Table 1. Immunohistochemical reactivity of MBr1 with breast tissues
          and breast tumors

Tissue	No. examined cases	Cell type	% MBr1 positive cases
Adult female resting breast	80	Epithelium Myoepithelium	83 0
Breast with lactational changes	2	Epithelium	100
Primary breast carcinoma	50 29	Ductal Lobular	66 72
Metastatic breast carcinoma	17	Nodal metastatic cells	71

carcinomas with metaplasia (chondroid, spindle cell and squamous)
and two carcinoids of the breast resulted unreactive (data not
shown). Reactions of tumor cells were markedly heterogeneous. With
regard to the number of positive cells in tumor sections, the
cases studied could be divided in four groups: 1) unreactive (-);
2) focally reactive (+, i.e. with small clusters of cells or
isolated cells positive in few high power fields); 3) reactive
(++, i.e. with a measurable percentage, up to 50%, of positive
neoplastic cells); 4) diffusely reactive (+++, i.e. with more than
50% of positive neoplastic cells).

    A "patchwork" heterogeneity pattern (6, 7) was most frequently
observed (Fig. 1a). Potentially metastatic neoplastic emboli
within mammary veins or lymphatics revealed such pattern of
heterogeneity. In few cases, however, MBr1 reactivity appeared
concentrated in well defined areas of the tumor, whereas the
adjacent neoplastic tissue was either unreactive or focally
reactive.

    The cytological distribution of the labeling revealed a
spectrum of variations related to different tumor types or to
areas with different differentiation within the same neoplastic
lesion. In well differentiated ductal carcinomas, or wherever
tumors formed glandular structures, apical and secretion product
staining predominated (Fig. 1b). In moderately to poorly

Table 2. Heterogeneity of MBr1 immunohistochemical reactivity in
primary breast carcinomas

Histology	Percentage				Positive/ Total	%
	−	+	++	+++		
Ductal	34	16	14	36	33/50	66
Lobular	28	14	17	41	21/29	72
Tubular	20	0	0	80	4/5	80
Paget's disease	31	25	25	19	11/16	69
Mucinous	50	50	0	0	3/6	50
Medullary	80	20	0	0	1/5	20
Papillary	67	33	0	0	1/3	33

differentiated ductal carcinomas and in lobular carcinomas, circumferential membrane and cytoplasmic staining were prominent. A marginal pattern of labeling was often seen in tight clusters of ductal carcinoma cells infiltrating lymphatic spaces. In lobular carcinomas, intracytoplasmic lumina (ICL) were well defined by dark diaminobenzidine reaction product. Malignant cells of mammary Paget's disease had cytoplasmic, membrane and ICL staining. In medullary carcinomas, small clusters of tumor cells only had intense cytoplasmic staining, whereas the bulk of the tumor was unreactive. In mucinous carcinomas, few nests of tumor cells, surrounded by epithelial mucin, had marginal labeling associated to focal staining of the adjacent mucin. Focal apical reactivity was detected in one out of three papillary carcinomas tested.

The correlation between the reactivity of metastatic cells in axillary lymph nodes and that of primary tumors is shown in Table 3. The data revealed concordant reactivity in 34/40 cases (85%). In six cases, (15%), metastases were unreactive whereas primary tumors stained, but in no cases with reactive metastases the primary tumor was unreactive.

Metastatic cells in lymph nodes had a degree of heterogeneity in their reactions which was comparable to that of the primary tumor (Fig. 2). Even in diffusely reactive cases, foci of

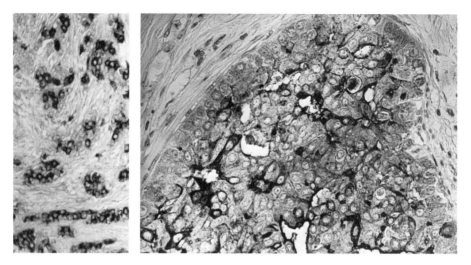

Fig. 1.   a) "Patchwork" immunostaining in an infiltrating lobular
          carcinoma: immunoreactive cells adjacent to immuno-
          negative cells (avidin–biotin complex immunoperoxidase
          stain, x 660).
          b)   Predominantly apical reactivity at luminal surfaces
          in   an   intraductal   carcinoma   (avidin–biotin   complex
          immunoperoxidase stain, x 1050).

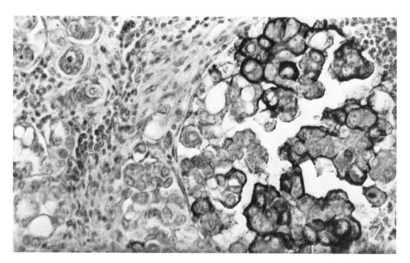

Fig. 2.   "Patchwork"   immunostaining   heterogeneity   in   ductal
          carcinoma cells metastatic in an axillary lymph node
          (avidin–biotin complex immunoperoxidase stain, x 1030).

Table 3. MBr1 immunohistochemical reactivity in nodal metastases and in primary breast carcinomas (metastasis/primary): concordant reaction in 34/40 cases (85%)

-/- (%)	-/+ (%)	+/- (%)	+/+ (%)
11 (27)	6 (15)	0 (0)	23 (58)

unreactive tumor cells were present. Patterns of labeling distribution included circumferential membrane (Fig. 2), cytoplasmic and, in metastatic lobular carcinomas, ICL staining. Marginal staining was focally observed in tight clumps of malignant cells within lymphatics adjacent to metastatic lymph nodes or in nodal sinuses.

The specificity of MBr1 as defined by the assays and targets reported in Table 4, is summarized in Table 5.

Table 4. Assays and target material used for defining the specificity of MBr1

Assays
Solid phase radioimmunoassay, immunofluorescence, ABC immunoperoxidase - Electronmicroscopy immunoperoxidase

Material
  Cell Lines

Carcinoma: Breast (MCF-7, SK-BR-3), ovary (SW626), stomach (KatoIII), colon (HT-29), bladder (VM-CUB-3), kideny (A498, A704)
Sarcoma: SaOS, SW684
Melanoma: MeWo, Me20, Me9556

  Lymphoid Cells: Daudi

  Normal Tissues and Corresponding Tumors
Kidney, bladder, prostate, liver, gall-bladder, lung, larynx, stomach, pancreas, intestine, ovary, uterus, testis, skin, sweat and sebaceous glands, mammary gland, adrenal gland, salivary gland, thyroid, muscle, connective tissue, cartilage, bone marrow, spleen, lymph nodes, thymus, blood cells, cerebral cortex, peripheral nerves, FCS proteins, total milk proteins, casein, lactoferrin, whey proteins

Table 5. Reactivity of MBr1 on the material described in Table 4

	Positive reaction on
Cell lines	MCF-7, SK-BR-3
Normal tissues	Breast epithelium, salivary glands, exocrine pancreas, distal and collecting renal tubules, some epithelia of the reproductive system, sweat glands
Tumors	75% most common histological types of breast carcinoma 20% other carcinomas

    MBr1 was shown to react with metastatic breast cancer cells in tissue sections and to discriminate between cancer cells and normal cells in bone marrow biopsies and in pleural and peritoneal effusions from breast cancer patients (8).

    MBr1 is currently studied in view of potential clinical applications in the areas reported in Table 6.

Table 6. Possible application of monoclonal antibodies in clinical oncology

In vitro	
Diagnosis:	Detection of metastatic tumor cells in lymph nodes, bone marrow, pleural and peritoneal effusions, by immunohistochemical examination
	Detection of circulating tumor markers by radioimmuno-assay
	Differential diagnosis by immunohistochemical techniques
Therapy:	Elimination of neoplastic cells from bone marrow to be reinjected after high dose chemotherapy
In vivo	
Diagnosis:	Radioimmunodetection of small nests of tumor cells
Therapy:	Killing of residual tumor cells by MAb linked toxins, drugs or radionuclides

In a preliminary study, 39 bone marrow samples were examined. The results obtained by conventional histology were compared to those obtained by immunofluorescence (IF) with MBr1. In 17 cases a bone marrow involvement was diagnosed by conventional histology and confirmed by positive IF with MBr1. Of 22 cases that scored negative by conventional histology, 7 scored positive by IF. No positive cells were found in numerous bone marrow samples from non tumor patients or patients with non epithelial tumors examined as controls. It would appear, therefore, that MBr1 may improve the conventional diagnostic procedures employed to detect bone marrow micrometastases.

On the basis of these results, MBr1 is now under investigation in a clinical trial aimed at clarifying the prognostic value of MBr1. Bone marrow samples were obtained from T_1 and T_2 patients at mastectomy and analyzed by IF. The patients were monitored to correlate disease recurrences with the presence of bone marrow micrometastases at the time of surgery. At present we have examined 31 bone marrow biopsies from T_1-T_2 N_0 or N_{1A} patients, and we have found that 32% of the cases had MBr1 positive cells.

The application of our monoclonal antibody in immunocyto-diagnosis was also considered. First of all we verified the reactivity of MBr1 on nonneoplastic cells commonly present in body fluids. We used pleural and peritoneal effusions from noncancer patients and from patients with cancers other than breast and ovary (MBr1 cross reacts with ovarian carcinoma). When tested by direct IF with MBr1, there was no labeling of cells of any type, irrespective of whether the effusions were cytologically positive or negative. We subsequently examined 46 pleural effusions from breast cancer patients and 19 effusions from patients with other pathologies (nonneoplastic diseases or tumors other than carcinoma). We used both conventional cytology and IF with MBr1 monoclonal antibody.

The results are given in Table 7. Twelve effusions from breast cancer patients were negative by both cytology and IF. Of 27 effusions cytopathologically diagnosed as positive, 17 only had cells positive with MBr1. The negativity of the other 10 cases may be explained by the fact that a subset of breast cancer failed to react with MBr1 as determined by immunohistochemistry on tissue sections (Table 1 and 2). Seven cases were found negative by cytological examination but were positive by IF with MBr1. Positivity was confirmed by further clinical, pathological and electronmicroscopic examinations.

Table 7. Immunofluorescence on cells from pleural effusions of
         cancer patients with MBr1 monoclonal antibody

Pathology	No effusions tested	Cytological diagnosis	MBr1 reactivity	Final diagnosis[1]
Breast carcinoma	46	12 negative	12 negative	
		27 positive	17 positive	
		7 negative	7 positive	7 positive
Other carcinomas	22	11 negative	11 negative	
		11 positive	2 positive	
Other pathology	19	17 negative	17 negative	
		2 positive	0 positive	

[1] Final diagnosis formulated after further clinical, pathological
and electronmicroscopic examination: 37% false negative cases
detected by MBr1.

In order to precisely identify the cells labeled, an electron
microscopic immunoperoxidase test was carried out on cells from
effusions cytopathologically positive for metastatic breast
carcinoma cells and also positive with MBr1. The results obtained
confirmed that the labeled cells were mammary epithelial tumor
cells. Mesothelial cells, as well as polymorphonuclear leukocytes,
lymphocytes and red blood cells were always negative by electronmicroscopy.

In conclusion, the use of MBr1 by IF in immunocytodiagnosis
allowed the detection of 37% false negative cases. Antibody MBr1
may not substitute conventional diagnostic procedures, due to its
failure to react with subsets of breast cancers, but may be
helpful in supporting current diagnostic techniques.

We believe that the development of "cocktails" of monoclonal
antibodies with complementary specificities will progressively
increase the role of immunodiagnostic techniques.

REFERENCES

1. Colcher D., Horan Hand P., Nuti M., Schlom J.: A spectrum of
    monoclonal antibodies reactive with human mammary tumor cells.
    Proc. Natl. Acad. Sci. U.S.A. 78: 3199 (1981).

2. Schlom J., Wunderlich D., Teramoto Y.A.: Generation of human
    monoclonal antibodies reactive with human mammary carcinoma
    cells. Proc. Natl. Acad. Sci. U.S.A. 77: 6841 (1980).

3. Taylor-Papadimitriou J., Peterson J.A., Arklie J., Burchell J.,
    Ceriani R.L., Bodmer W.F.: Monoclonal antibodies to epithelium-
    specific components of the human milk fat globule membrane:
    production and reaction with cells in culture. Int. J. Cancer,
    28: 17 (1981).

4. Canevari S., Fossati G., Balsari A., Sonnino S., Colnaghi M.I.:
    Immunochemical analysis of the determinant recognized by a
    monoclonal antibody (MBr1) which specifically binds to human
    mammary epithelial cells. Cancer Res., 43: 1301 (1983).

5. Mènard S., Tagliabue E., Canevari S., Fossati G., Colnaghi M.I.:
    Generation of monoclonal antibodies reacting with normal and
    cancer cells of human breast. Cancer Res., 43: 1295 (1983).

6. Nuti M., Teramoto Y.A., Mariani-Costantini R., Horan Hand P.,
    Colcher D., Schlom J.: A monoclonal antibody (B.72.3) defines
    patterns of distribution of a novel tumor associated antigen in
    human mammary carcinoma cell populations. Int. J. Cancer 29:
    539 (1982).

7. Horan-Hand P., Nuti M., Colcher D., Schlom J.: Definition of
    antigenic heterogeneity and modulation among human mammary
    carcinoma cell populations using monoclonal antibodies to
    tumor associated antigens. Cancer Res., 43: 728 (1983).

8. Colnaghi M.I., Clemente C., Della Porta G., Della Torre G.,
    Mariani-Costantini R., Mènard S., Rilke F., Tagliabue E.:
    Monoclonal antibodies to human breast cancer. In "Monoclonal
    Antibodies '82" - Elsevier Press, 1982.

GENERATION OF MONOCLONAL ANTIBODIES REACTIVE

WITH HUMAN COLON CARCINOMAS

Raffaella Muraro, David Wunderlich, and
Jeffrey Schlom
National Institutes of Health
National Cancer Institute
Bethesda, Maryland

ABSTRACT

Monoclonal antibodies have been generated that are reactive
with human colon carcinomas. The rationale for the studies was
to utilize extracts from patient biopsy material (and not colon
cancer cell lines) as immunogen to increase the probability
that any monoclonal antibody generated be reactive with colon
carcinomas in a clinical setting. Five immunization protocols
were used employing extracts and membrane enriched fractions
from both primary and metastatic colon carcinoma lesions.
Twenty nine monoclonal antibodies from double-cloned hybridoma
cultures have been characterized; all are of the IgG isotope.
Preliminary results indicate that the monoclonal antibodies
can be placed into 15 groups on the basis of their differential
reactivities to six colon carcinoma extracts, the surface of
three colon carcinoma cell lines and five partially purified
CEA preparations from bloods of colon cancer patients. Some of
the monoclonal antibodies were shown to bind from one to five
of the five CEA preparations, while others showed no anti-CEA
reactivity. None of the 29 monoclonal antibodies reacted
with extracts of 21 normal human tissues including livers,
spleens, kidneys, red blood cells, (of several blood groups),
or polymorphonuclear leucocytes. All the 29 monoclonal antibodies could be distinguished, on the basis of differential
reactivities to various tumors and normal human tissues, from
several monoclonal antibodies (B1.1, B6.2, B72.3) reactive with
colon carcinomas that have been previously generated in our
laboratory. Further immunohistochemical and radiolocalization
studies will further define the potential clinical utility of
the monoclonals described.

117

INTRODUCTION

Numerous investigators have reported the existence of
human colon carcinoma associated antigens (1,2). These anti
gens have been first detected with hyperimmune polyclonal sera
(3,4,5) and subsequently with monoclonal antibodies (MAbs)
which were generated using colon carcinoma cell lines as
immunogen (1,2,6). Some of these MAbs thus far generated have
shown some utility in blood tests and immunohistochemical
analysis of human colon cancers (1,2,6). However, no MAbs
have been generated thus far that are (a) reactive with all
neoplastic cells of all colon tumors, or (b) not reactive with
any normal human tissues (1,2,6,7).

Three monoclonal antibodies (B1.1,B6.2,B72.3) generated
in our laboratory using human mammary carcinoma tissues as
immunogens (8), have shown reactivities with the surfaces of
human colon adenocarcinomas (9,10). Of these, MAb B72.3 which
reacts with a 200,000–400,000d high–molecular weight glycoprotein complex, binds to approximately 85% of human colon
adenocarcinomas tested (10). Monoclonal B1.1, which reacts
with the 180,000d glycoprotein carcinoembryonic antigen (11,12)
(CEA) and MAb B6.2 which reacts with a 90,000d glycoprotein
show binding to 94 and 88% of human colon adenocarcinomas,
respectively (10). These two monoclonals (B1.1 and B6.2) have
shown a great deal of coordinate expression on the surface of
many tumor cell lines and tumor tissue sections; they also
have shown reactivities to extracts of polymorphonuclear leukocytes, and certain spleens (9).

Of the colon antigens thus far described, CEA has been
the most extensively studied. It has previously been shown
that most antisera raised against CEA react with many different types of carcinomas (13) as well as with antigenic
determinants present in some normal tissues such as spleen,
lung, and polymorphonuclear leukocytes of some individuals
(14,15,16). Many of these CEA–related determinants are on
molecules which are either coordinately expressed with or
cross–reactive with CEA (13-18). At this time, however, there
is a great deal of discrepancy in the literature as to the
degree of expression of both "CEA" and "CEA-related antigens"
in carcinomas as well as in normal tissues.

The production and use of monoclonal antibodies which
react with CEA and other colon carcinoma antigens, but do not
react or cross–react with "CEA-related antigens" present in
normal tissues, should help greatly in the phenotypic characterization of colon carcinoma cells.

The rationale of the studies reported here was to utilize
tissue extracts of both primary and metastatic human colon
carcinomas as immunogens in an attempt to generate monoclonal

antibodies reactive with antigenic determinants present in primary and/or metastatic colon carcinomas. The selective pressure in the establishment of a cell line may modify or eliminate some antigens present in the original tumor tissue. For this reason we chose to use extracts of tumor tissues from colon cancer patients (and not cell lines) as immunogen in our studies. Multiple assays using tumor and normal cell extracts, purified CEA, live cells in culture, and tissue sections have been employed to reveal the diversity of the monoclonal antibodies generated.

MATERIALS AND METHODS

Cell Extract and Membrane Preparation

Cell extracts were prepared from colon carcinoma metastasis to lymph nodes and spleens of two patients, from six primary colon carcinomas and from apparently normal human tissues including 4 spleens, 3 livers, 2 kidney, 1 granulocyte, as previously described (9). All the tumor specimens were obtained from biopsies of colon cancer patients. Tissues were minced finely and homogenized. The homogenate was subjected to nitrogen cavitation at 1000 lb/in^2 and clarified at 1000xg for 5 min. Cell membrane enriched fractions were prepared from one primary colon tumor extract by centrifugation of the 1000xg extract supernatant in a discontinuous 20-40% (w/w) sucrose-gradient for 17 h at 130,000xg. The 20-40% interface was diluted and pelleted at 130,000xg for one hour. The pellet was resuspended in PBS and sonicated for 1 min. The sonicate was centrifuged at 10,000xg for 10 min and the supernatant used as immunogen. Protein concentrations were determined by the method of Lowry (19).

Immunization

Four week old Balb/c mice were immunized by intraperitoneal inoculation of 100 ug of antigen emulsified with an equal volume of complete Freund's adjuvant. Seven days later mice were boosted with an intraperitoneal inoculation of 100 ug of immunogen mixed with an equal volume of incomplete Freund's adjuvant. On the fourteenth day, 10 ug of immunogen in saline was injected intravenously. The spleens were removed for cell fusion three days later.

Hybridoma Methodology

Somatic cell hybrids were prepared using the method of Herzenberg (20) with some modifications (21). Single cell suspension of spleens from immunized mice were prepared by passage through a stainless steel screen. Spleen cells and NS-1, a non-immunoglobulin secreting myeloma cell line, were

mixed at a ratio of 4:1 and fused with 50% polyethelene glycol
1500. After fusion, cells were seeded in 96-well microtiter
plates at a concentration of 1×10^6 total cells/0.1ml/well.
Fused cells were selected using RPMI 1640 medium containing 15%
heat-inactivated fetal calf serum, 2mM glutamine, 1mM sodium
pyruvate, 0.25 ug/ml Fungizone, 1×10^{-4} M hypoxanthine, 4×10^{-7} M
aminopterin, and 1.6×10^{-5} M thymidine (HAT media). The
hybridoma cell lines were cloned twice by limiting dilution in
96-well microtiter plates using mouse thymocytes from 4-week
old Balb/c mice as feeder cells. Cloning wells containing a
single hybridoma colony were chosen for further screening.

Solid Phase Radioimmunoassay

Hybridoma supernatant fluids were harvested and assayed
for specific antibody production using solid phase radioimmunoassays (sRIA) (8). 50 ul of cell extract (5 ug) or purified
CEA (50 ng) were added to each well of 96-well polyvinyl microtiter plate and allowed to dry overnight at 37°C in a non-
humidified incubator. In order to decrease the non-specific
binding, 100 ul of 5% bovine serum albumin (BSA) in phosphate-
buffered saline (PBS) containing calcium and magnesium were
added and incubated 1 hour at 37°C. The BSA was removed and 50
ul of hybridoma tissue culture supernatant was added. After
one hour of incubation, the unbound immunoglobulin was removed
by washing the plates with PBS 1% BSA. The wells were then
incubated with ^{125}I goat anti-mouse IgG (^{125}IGaMuIgG; 75,000
cpm/25 ul) for 1 hour. The unbound ^{125}IGaMuIgG was removed by
extensive washing with 1% BSA in PBS. The plates were then
subjected to autoradiography using Kodak XAR film and inten-
sifying screen. The films were developed after an exposure of
16 hours at -70°C. The bound ^{125}IGaMuIgG was also detected by
cutting the individual wells and measuring the radioactivity
in a gamma-counter.

Cell Surface Binding

Subconfluent established cell lines were detached from
75 cm^2 tissue culture flasks using 0.1% trypsin containing 0.5
mM EDTA. Cells were then seeded into 96-well flat-bottom
tissue culture plates at 5×10^4 cells/well and incubated 18-24
hours in an incubator. The diluting and washing buffer was
RPMI 1640 medium containing 10% (w/v) bovine serum albumin
(BSA) and 0.08% (w/v) sodium azide. The assay was performed
as described for the solid phase RIA. To determine bound cpm,
100 ul of 2 N NaOH were added to each well. Cotton swabs were
then used to absorb the fluid from each well and then counted
in a gamma-counter (9).

Immunoperoxidase Studies

Paraffin blocks of tissues were obtained from the Depart-

ment of Surgical Pathology of the George Washington University
Medical Center, Washington, D.C. A slight modification of the
avidin-biotin-peroxidase complex (Vecastain ABC Kit, Vector
Laboratory) method was used. This method has been described
in detail by others (22). Gelatinized slides were used to
collect 5 um sections and then heated for 60 min at 60°C.
The sections were deparaffinated in xylene and rinsed in
absolute ethanol. To block endogenous activity, the sections
were immersed in methanol with 0.3% H_2O_2 for 30 min at room
temperature. After rinsing in PBS, the sections were incubated
with 10% normal horse serum for 15 min at room temperature.
This and all subsequent reagents were diluted in PBS 1% BSA;
the experiment was performed at room temperature. The pretreatment serum was removed and hybridoma tissue culture supernatant containing the antibody were added at 200 ul/slide.
The slides were incubated 30 min, then the monoclonal was
removed and the slides rinsed in PBS. The sections were then
incubated with biotinylated horse anti-mouse antisera (Vector
Labs, Inc) at a 1:500 dilution for 30 min and then rinsed in
PBS. Avidin-biotinylated-horseradish peroxidase complex (ABC)
was added, incubated for 30 min, and then removed by rinsing
in PBS. The peroxidase reaction was initiated by the addition
of 0.06% diaminobenzidine (Sigma) and 0.01% H_2O_2; after 5 min
the slides were rinsed in PBS. The sections were counter-
stained with hematoxylin, dehydrated in ethanol, cleared in
xylene, mounted under a coverslip with Permount and examined
with a light microscope.

Cells and Antigens

The Balb/c myeloma cell line P3-NS1-1-Ag4-1 (NS-1), was
obtained from Dr. J. Kim, N.I.H., Bethesda, Maryland. The
WI-DR and LS-174T colon carcinoma cell lines, and the WI-38
normal fetal lung cell line were obtained from the American
Type Culture Collection, Rockville, Maryland. The HT 29 colon
carcinoma cell line was obtained from the Breast Cancer Task
Force, National Cancer Institute, N.I.H., Bethesda, Maryland.
Purified carcinoembryonic antigen (CEA) from five different
colon cancer patients was kindly provided by Dr. H. Hausen,
Hoffmann-LaRoche, Nutley, N.J.

RESULTS AND DISCUSSION

Mice were immunized with extracts of human metastatic
colon carcinoma from either a lymph node or spleen, and with an
extract and membrane enriched fraction of a primary human colon
carcinoma. Five immunization protocols were followed (Table I).
In addition to using either metastases or primary carcinomas as
single immunogens, sequential immunizations with three different
tumors were used in an attempt to induce the production of antibodies to common determinants shared by both metastatic and
primary colon lesions (Protocol No. 4, Table 1).

Table 1

Protocal No.	Immunogen	ug per immunization
1	Colon carcinoma metastasis to lymphnode, extract.	100-100-10
2	Colon carcinoma metastasis to spleen, extract.	100-100-10
3	Primary colon carcinoma, extract.	100-100-10
4	Sequential immunization with two colon carcinoma metastases and a primary colon carcinoma, extracts.	100-100-100-30
5	Partially purified membrane of primary colon carcinoma.	100-100-10

Splenocytes of immunized mice were fused with non Ig secreting NS-1 myeloma cells to generate 5,052 primary hybridoma cultures (Table II). Supernatant fluids from these cultures were harvested and tested in a solid phase RIA to detect the presence of immunoglobulins reactive with extracts of the immunogen and not with an extract of an apparently normal human spleen. The spleen used for initial screening was previously shown to be reactive with some MAbs reactive with CEA and CEA-related determinants. Whereas many cultures demonstrated reactivity with both extracts, 308 cultures contained immunoglobulins reactive only with the colon carcinoma used as immunogen (Table 1). To define the reactivities of these immunoglobulins, the culture supernatants were assayed for binding to the extracts of six colon carcinomas and several apparently normal human tissues, including 4 spleens, 2 kidneys and 3 livers. After passage and double cloning by limiting dilution, 29 MAbs were chosen which were shown to be non-reactive with any of the normal tissues. These MAbs were also shown to be non-reactive with 11 extracts of red blood cells from 11 different patients as well with granulocytes.

The 29 MAbs selected for non-reactivity to the 21 normal human tissues were then assayed for differential reactivities to human colon carcinomas. This was done by testing each of the MAbs for (a) binding to extracts of six colon carcinomas, (b) binding to the surface of three colon carcinoma cell line and (c) binding to partially purified CEA preparations from 5

Table 2. Logistics of Generation of MAb's Reactive With Human
          Colon Carcinomas

Colon Carcinomas		Normal Spleen
4,403 Cultures	Neg	Neg
341 Cultures	+	+
308 Cultures	+	Neg

different colon cancer patients. The colon carcinoma extracts
were prepared from 5 different primary carcinoma lesions and
one colon carcinoma metastasis to the lymph node, all from
different patients. The 29 MAbs could be divided into 6 groups
on the basis of their differential reactivities to the various
extracts (Table III). Twelve reacted with all 6 extracts, five
MAbs reacted with 5/6 extracts, eight MAbs reacted with 4/6
extracts, two MAbs reacted with 3/6 extracts and one MAb
reacted with 2/6 extracts. One MAb (see Group 15, Table III)
did not react with any of the tumor extracts but did react with
an extract of the LS 174 colon carcinoma cell line and was thus
taken for further study.

Table 3. Monoclonal Antibody Grouping

Group	Tumor Extracts[a]	Tumor Cell Surface[b]	CEA[c]	No. MAb's	Isotype
1	6/6	3/3	5/5	7	IgG_1, IgG_{2a}
2	6/6	2/3	5/5	5	IgG_1
3	5/6	3/3	5/5	1	IgG_{2b}
4	5/6	3/3	1/5	1	IgG_{2a}
5	5/6	2/3	5/5	2	IgG_1, IgG_{2b}
6	5/6	0/3	0/5	1	IgG_{2a}
7	4/6	3/3	5/5	3	IgG_1, IgG_{2b}
8	4/6	3/3	1/5	1	IgG_1
9	4/6	3/3	0/5	1	IgG_1
10	4/6	2/3	5/5	2	IgG_1
11	4/6	1/3	2/5	1	IgG_1
12	3/6	3/3	1/5	1	IgG_1
13	3/6	2/3	1/5	1	IgG_{2a}
14	2/6	0/3	5/5	1	IgG_{2b}
15	0/6 (1/7)[d]	0/3	5/5	1	IgG_3

[a] Extracts of 6 colon carcinomas.
[b] Live cell assay on 3 colon carcinoma cell lines.
[c] 5 different preparations.
[d] Positive to extract of LS174T cell line.

To further define the reactivities of the 29 MAbs, each
antibody was tested for binding to the surface of three established colon carcinoma cell lines in culture, LS174T, WiDr, and
HT29 (Table III). Fifteen MAbs bound to the surface of all
three lines, ten MAbs bound the LS174 and WiDr but not the HT29
cell line, one MAb bound only to the surface of the LS174T cell
line and three MAbs did not bind the surface of any of the
three lines tested. All 29 MAbs did not bind the WI38 normal
embryonic lung cell line. The 29 MAb could thus be divided
into 4 groups on the basis of their binding to the surface of
colon carcinoma cells, and 12 groups on the basis of differential reactivities to tumor extracts and cell surface binding.

The 29 MAbs were then tested for their binding to 5
partially purified CEA preparations from 5 colon carcinoma
patients (Table III). One MAb bound to 2/5 CEAs, four bound to
1/5 CEAs and two MAbs did not bind to any of the 5 CEA preparations. It is unclear at this time whether the five MAbs which
bound to 2/5 or 1/5 CEA preparations are reacting with "CEA"
or another colon tumor associated antigens in the "CEA" preparations. On the basis of differential reactivities to the tumor
extracts, line cells, and CEA preparations, the 29 MAbs could
be placed into 15 groups (Table III).

All the antibodies from the fifteen groups were of the IgG
isotype, of varying subclasses (Table III). This was not
unexpected since affinity purified goat anti-murine IgG was
used as the linker in all immunoassays (see Materials and
Methods). In most cases the immunization protocol used did not
seem to influence the placement of the antibodies in any particular group. However, four of the six antibodies generated
after sequential immunization with three different colon
tumors (Protocol 4, Table 1) could be placed in group number
1, i.e. they were reactive with six of six colon tumor extracts,
with the surface of three of three carcinoma cell lines, and
with five of five CEA preparations. It would appear that the
sequential immunization protocol gave rise to antibodies that
react to determinants shared by different colon carcinoma
cells.

As mentioned above, some antisera and monoclonal antibodies reactive with CEA also show reactivities to some normal
human tissues. In fact, monoclonal antibody B1.1, generated
against human mammary carcinoma (8), while reactive with CEA,
also binds to certain normal spleen extracts and with polymorphonuclear leukocytes. Table IV displays a comparison of
the reactivities of B1.1 and 22 of the antibodies generated in
this study. The anti-CEA antibodies generated in this study do
not react with any of the normal tissues tested, indicating
that these MAbs may recognize a determinant on CEA that is not
present on normal tissues.

Table 4. Differential Reactivities of MAb's to CEA

Extracts	B1.1	22 MAb's
CEA	5/5	5/5
Liver	0/3	0/3
Kidney	0/2	0/2
Spleen	2/4	0/4
Polymorphonuclear Leukocytes	1/1	0/1

Some of the antibodies are also reactive with formalin fixed sections of human colon carcinomas using the immuno-peroxidase technique. None of the 29 MAb generated in this study were derived from immunization protocol number 2 (Table 1), in which a colon carcinoma metastasis to spleen was used as immunogen. The hybrid cultures derived from these fusions produced immunoglobulin equally reactive with both the spleen metastasis and the normal spleen extract. Also worthy of note is the fact that the majority of the 29 MAbs were derived from the fusion in which the membrane fraction of a primary colon tumor was used as immunogen (Protocol No. 5, Table 1). A comparison of the number of MAbs generated when membranes or extract from the same primary carcinoma were used as immunogens is shown in Table 5. These results suggest that the use of partially purified membranes from human tumors as immunogen may be the most efficient method to produce anti-tumor monoclonal antibodies.

Studies are now in progress to further define the range of reactivities of the 29 MAb described here. Those with the more restricted range of reactivities for tumor vs. normal tissues will be assayed for their ability to detect antigens in bloods of colon cancer patients and their ability to radio-localize human tumor transplants in experimental models.

Table 5. Comparison of Colon Carcinoma Cell Extracts Versus Cell Membranes for Immunogen

Immunization Protocol	No. 3	No. 5
Immunogen	extract	Membranes
No. Mice	5	4
No. Cultures Planted	885	1,377
No. MAb's	1	16
No. MAb's Groups	1 (Group No. 3)	11 (Groups No. 1,2, 4,7,8,9,10,11, 12,13,15)
Percent Efficiency[*]	0.11%	1.16%

[*]Number of Specific Antibodies Generated Divided By The Total Number Of Wells Planted X100.

REFERENCES

1. Heryln, M., Steplewsky, Z., Herlyn, D. and H. Koprowsky,
   1973, Colorectal carcinoma - specific antigen: Detection by
   means of monoclonal antibodies, Proc. Natl. Sci. USA 76:
   1438-1442.
2. Koprowsky, H., Steplewsky, Z., Mitchel, K., Herlyn, M.,
   Herlyn, D. and P. Fuhrer, 1979, Colorectal carcinoma antigens detected by hybridoma antibodies, Somatic Cell Genet.
   5:957-971.
3. Sell, S., 1978, in Water, H. (Ed.): The Handbook of Cancer
   Immunology, vol. 3, New York, Garland STP M, p.1.
4. Lewis, M.G., Phillips, T.M., Rowden, G., 1978, in Water, H.
   (Ed.): The Handbook of Cancer Immunology, vol. 3, New York,
   Garland STP M, p. 159.
5. Ferrone, S., Pellegrino, M.A., 1978, in Walter H. (Ed.): The
   Handbook of Cancer Immunology, vol. 3, New York, Garland STP
   M, p. 291.
6. Leibovitz, A., Stinson, J.C., McCombs, W.B., McCoy, C.E.,
   Masur, C. and Malony, N.D., 1976, Classification of human
   colorectal adenocarcinoma cell lines, Cancer Res. 36: 4562-
   4563.
7. Brockhaus, M., Magnani, J.L., Blaszczy, K.M., Steplousky,
   Z., Kopvowski, H., Karlsson, K.A., Larson, G. and V.
   Ginsburg, 1981, Monoclonal antibody directed against
   the human Le^b blood group antigen, J. Biol. Chem. 256:13223-13225.
8. Colcher, D., Hand, P., Nuti, M. and J. Schlom, 1981, A spectrum of monoclonal antibodies reactive with human mammary
   tumor cells. Proc. Natl. Acad. Sci. USA 78:3199-3203.
9. Colcher, D., Hand, P., Nuti, M. and J. Schlom, 1983,
   Differential binding to human mammary and non-mammary
   tumors of monoclonal antibodies reactive with carcinoembryonic antigen, Cancer Invest. 1:127-138.
10. Stramignani, D., Bowen, R., Atkinson, B. and J. Schlom,
    1983, Differential reactivity of monoclonal antibodies
    with human colon adenocarcinomas and adenomas, Int. J.
    Cancer 31:543-552.
11. Krupey, J.T., Wilson, S., Freedman, O. and P. Gold, 1972,
    The preparation of purified carcinoembryonic antigen of
    the human digestive system from large quantities of tumor
    tissues, Immunochemistry 9:617-
12. Coligan, J.E., Lautenschleger, J.T., Egan, M.L. and C.W.
    Todd, 1972, Isolation and characterization of carcino-
    embryonic antigen, Immunochemistry 9:377-
13. Goldenberg, D.M., Sharkey, R.M. and J. Primus, 1976,
    Carcinoembryonic antigen in histopathology: immunoperoxi-
    dase staining of conventional tissue section, JNCI 57:
    11-22.
14. von Kleist, S., Charanel, G. and P. Butin, 1972, Identi-
    fication of an antigen from normal human tissue that cross
    reacts with CEA, Proc. Natl. Acad. Sci. USA 9:2492-2501.

15. Mach, J.P. and G. Pusztaszeri, 1972, CEA: demonstration of
    a partial identity between CEA and a normal glycoprotein,
    Immunochemistry 9:1031-1038.
16. Burtin, P., Quan, P.C. and M.C. Sabine, 1975, Non specific
    cross reacting antigen as a marker for human polymorphs,
    macrophages and monocytes, Nature 255:714-716.
17. Ahnen, D.J., Nokane, P.K. and W.R. Brown, 1982, Vetro-
    structural localization of carcinoembryonic antigen in
    normal intestine and colon cancer, Cancer 49:2077-2090.
18. O'Brien, M.J., Zamcheck, N., Burke, B., Kirkham, S.E.,
    Saravis, C.A. and L.S. Gottlieb, 1981, Immunocytochemical
    localization of CEA in benign and malignant colonrectal
    tissues, Amer. J. Clin. Path. 75:283-290.
19. Lowry, O.H., Rosenbrough, N.J. and A.L. Farr, 1951, Protein
    measurement with the Folin phenol reagent, J. Biol. Chem.
    193:265-275.
20. Herzenberg, L.A., Herzenberg, L.A. and C. Milstein, 1978,
    Cell hybrids of myelomas with antibody forming cells and T
    lymphocytes with T cells, in Weir, D.M. (Ed.): Handbook of
    Experimental Immunology, London, Blackwell Scientific Pub-
    lications, pp. 25.1-25.7.
21. Colcher, D., Hand, P., Teramoto, Y.A., Wunderlich, D. and
    J. Schlom, 1981, Use of monoclonal antibodies to define the
    diversity of mammary tumor vital gene products in virions
    and mammary tumors of the gene Mus, Cancer Res. 41:1451-59.
22. Hsu, S.M., Raine, L. and H. Fanger, 1981, Use of avidin-
    biotinperoxidase complex (ABC) in immunoperoxidase tech-
    niques: A comparison between ABC and unlabeled antibody
    (PA) procedures, J. Histochem. Cytochem. 29:577-580.

REACTIVITY OF CULTURED MOUSE NATURAL KILLER (NK) CELLS

AGAINST NORMAL NON-NEOPLASTIC CELLS

C.Riccardi*, G.Migliorati*, L.Frati**, F.Guadagni*,
E.Bonmassar**, and R.B.Herberman***

*Inst.of Pharmacology, Univ.of Perugia, Italy
**Inst.of General Pathology Univ.of Rome, Italy
***Frederik Cancer Center, NCI, NIH, BRM
Frederik, USA

INTRODUCTION

In the last few years much interest has evolved in the
study of natural reactivity (1). Studies from many laboratories have demonstrated that cells from different lymphoid
tissues, including spleen and peripheral blood, show a spontaneous reactivity against neoplastic cells (2). This spontaneous reactivity, mediated by NK lymphocytes, has been
shown to play a major role in the rapid elimination in vivo
of neoplastic as well as of normal non-neoplastic targets
including syngeneic bone marrow, thymocytes and fibroblasts
(3-4). This reactivity directed against normal cells suggest
an autocytotoxic function of NK effectors which could be
involved in the homeostatic control of growth and differentiation of normal tissues (5-6). Also in vitro experiments
showed some spontaneous reactivity against ^{51}Cr-labelled
non-neoplastic cells, but in this case it was not possible
to obtain high cytotoxic levels of reactivity, comparable
to those found against neoplastic targets (7-8). This
fact is probably due to the low frequency of NK cells
able to recognize "self" structures as targets. More
recently it has been shown that it is possible to culti-
vate in vitro splenocytes of normal mice in the presence of T-cell-growth-factor (TCGF) and that these cultures
generate lymphocytes with NK cell-like activity (9-10).
In all cultures showing this activity, the frequency of cytotoxic cells correlates well with the frequency of proliferating cells in that the growth and development of NK effectors is dependent on the levels of

cell proliferation (11). Based on the assumption that
in these cultures we could find a frequency of NK cells
higher than that detectable in uncultured splenocytes
as a result of NK cell growth, we analyzed the possible
cytotoxic activity of cultured NK cells against normal
non-neoplastic targets. The results show that cultured
NK cells are cytotoxic against syngeneic Con-A-induced
blasts as well as against syngeneic peritoneal macrophages. In addition to that we also tested the possible
cytotoxic activity of cultured splenocytes of F1 hybrid
mice against syngeneic or parental non-neoplastic cells.
The results here reported demonstrate that these effector NK cells are able to lyse F1 and parental peritoneal
macrophages in a fashion comparable to that reported for
the in vitro hybrid resistance (12).

MATERIALS AND METHODS

Mice - Six to 8 week old inbred BALB/c, C57Bl/6 (B6),
SJL/J and C3H/HeN mice were obtained from inbred lines
maintained in our laboratory.

Target cells - A variety of target cells were used:
1) Peritoneal exudate cells (PEC) were obtained by injecting mice i.p. with 2 ml of thioglicolate medium. Three
days later, PEC were collected from the peritoneal cavity. 2) Con-A-induced target cells: $10x10^6$ viable lymphocytes were incubated with 2 ug/ml Con-A in complete medium. 3) YAC-1 tumor cells were passaged in RPMI supplemented with 10% fetal calf serum and antibiotics.

Culture conditions - 10^5 spleen cells/well were cultured
for 7-8 days in a 96 well microtiter plates, together
with 10^5 irradiated (3000 R) spleen cells as feeder and
20 U/ml TCGF. RPMI was used as medium supplemented with
10% FCS, 1% Sodium pyruvate, 1% Glutamine, $2x10^{-5}$ M 2-ME,
1% Gentamycin, 25mM Hepes buffer, penicillin 1000 U/ml,
streptomycin (100 mg/ml).

Assay for cell-mediate cytotoxicity - The cytotoxicity
assay was performed as previously described (3-5). Standard errors were consistently below 5% of the mean values and for clarity have been omitted from the results.

TABLE 1
Natural Cytotoxic Activity of C3H/HeN Cultured Spleen
Cells against NK-sensitive YAC-1 Tumor Cells

Effector cells	% Cytotoxicity			
	100:1	50:1	25:1[a]	LU[b]
Uncultured	30.5	23.8	17.6	2
Cultured	65.0	58.3	56.0	392

a) Effector: Target ratios.
b) Lytic units/10^6 spleen cells.

Cytotoxic activity of uncultured and cultured NK cells
In Table 1 are reported the data obtained in a representative experiment in which the spontaneous cytotoxic activity against YAC-1 target cells of uncultured and cultured mouse spleen cells was measured in a 4-hr ^{51}Cr-re-
lease assay. As shown in the table, a significant increase
of the lytic capability was found with cultured splenocytes as comparated to uncultured effector cells at all
the effector-to-target ratios tested. The difference appears more evident when the lytic units/10^6 spleen cells
were calculated.

Target specificity of cultured NK cells - We compared
the target selectivity of uncultured and cultured mouse
splenocytes as tested against NK-sensitive and NK-insensitive tumor target as well as against Con-A induced blasts.
Data reported in Table 2 confirm the results of Table 1
showing that cultured cells are significantly more cytoxicity
was found when uncultured spleen cells were used as attackers
against the NK- insensitive EL-4 and P-388 tumor targets.
Similary, very limited cytotoxicity was found when cultured
cells were tested against the same NK-insensitive tumor
targets. However, when effector cells were tested against
Con-A blasts, while the uncultured splenocytes did not
show any cytotoxic activity, marked cytotoxicity was
found when cultured cells were used as effectors.

TABLE 2

Cytotoxic Activity of Fresh and Cultured Spleen Cells
Against Neoplastic and Non-Neoplastic Cells

Effector	Target	% Cytotoxicity[a]		
		100:1	50:1	25:1
Fresh BALB/c	YAC-1	32.0	21.2	11.3
	P-388	5.0	4.1	2.0
	EL-4	1.7	1.9	0.5
	BALB/c blasts	0.8	0.9	0.5
Cultured BALB/c	YAC-1	78.0	75.6	65.7
	P-388	6.5	3.8	2.5
	EL-4	12.4	10.8	9.1
	BALB/c blasts	42.7	38.5	30.9

a) As measured in a 4-hr ^{51}Cr-release assay.

Cytotoxic activity of cultured NK cells against syngeneic and allogeneic non-neoplastic cells - Based on the
observation reported in Table 2 we performed experiments
to analyze the possible cytotoxic activity of cultured NK
cells against syngeneic as well as allogeneic Con-A induced
blasts. Table 3 shows the results of a representative experiment
in which the cytotoxic activity of cultured spleen cells
of 2 different strains of mice was tested against syngeneic
and allogeneic Con-A induced blasts.
As shown in the Table, cultured cells were cytotoxic for
syngeneic as well as allogeneic targets. Interestingly
enough, the cytotoxic activity directed against syngeneic
cells was significantly higher than that obtained against
allogeneic targets.

TABLE 3

Spontaneous Cytotoxic Activity of Culture NK Cells Against
Syngeneic and Allogeneic Con-A-induced Blasts

Effector	Target	% Cytotoxicity[a]
BALB/c	BALB/c	35.8
	SJL/J	5.0
	B6	18.5
B6	B6	30.0
	BALB/c	10.0

a) Effector: Target ratio 50:1

Cytotoxic activity of cultured B6D2F1 spleen cells against
neoplastic and non-neoplastic targets - It has been previously
reported that F1 hybrid spleen cells cultured in vitro in the
presence of irradiated parental splenocytes are able to develop cytotoxic activity against parental as well as F1
non-neoplastic cells (12-13). In the attempt to obtain preliminary
information on the possible relevance of cultured NK cells
in the in vitro hybrid reactivity, we performed experiments
in wich spleen cells of normal B6D2F1 mice were cultured
in vitro in the presence of TCGF and irradiated syngeneic
splenocytes as feeder cells. Table 4 illustrates the results
obtained in a representative experiment in which the reactivity
of cultured B6D2F1 spleen cells was tested against YAC-1
tumor cells, syngeneic F1 and parental (B6 and DBA/2) normal
peritoneal macrophages. As shown in the Table, cultured cells
showed cytotoxic activity against YAC-1 tumor cells (line
1, Table 4). More interestingly, high cytotoxic activity
was also found against DBA/2 parental macrophages while a
significantly lower cytotoxicity was obtained parental B6
macrophages (line 3, Table 4). When the F1 syngeneic macrophages
were used as targets again appreciable levels of reactivity
were measured (line 2).

TABLE 4

Cytotoxic Activity of Cultured B6D2F1 Spleen Cells
Against Neoplastic and Non-neoplastic Targets.

Target cells	% Cytotoxicity		
	100:1	50:1	25:1[a]
YAC-1	35.3	27.9	16.9
BD2F1 Per.Macroph.	40.4	36.7	27.2
DBA/2 Per.Macroph.	54.5	50.8	47.7
B6 Per.Macroph.	27.8	23.0	19.5

a) Effector: Target ratios.

DISCUSSION

In this paper we show the spontaneous cytotoxic activity
of cultured mouse NK cells against normal non-neoplastic
targets. The results are in line with previous data obtained in our and other laboratories suggesting an autoreactive activity of mouse NK cells (4-8). We have previously shown that cultured NK lymphocytes have characteristics similar to those of uncultured NK effector cells
by different criteria, including strain distribution, target selectivity and phenotypic characteristics (9-11, 14).
The data reported here add new information to our previous work demonstrating the functional similarity between these cultured cells and fresh mouse NK lymphocytes,
i.e. the capability of killing neoplastic as well as non-
neoplastic targets (3-5). Very recently it has been reported in the human NK system that interferon (IFN)-ac-
tivated Large Granular Lymphocytes are able to kill autologous and allogeneic non-neoplastic targets without
preference (15). In the human system, fresh NK cells
were enriched by percoll density gradient centrifugation
and then boosted by human leucocyte IFN. In our culture

system enrichment of NK effector cells occurred as a result of in vitro proliferation in the presence of TCGF.
The fact that TCGF is also able to boost NK cells suggests that the above cited human system and our culture
system may have common characteristics (16). In any case,
it is evident from aur and other authors' data that NK
cells are able to kill syngeneic as well as allogeneic
targets. The question of the possible target preference
between the human and the murine system remains open.
Our data (Table 3) suggest for a self-preference so that
one is tempted to propose an autoreactive role of NK
cells (5). As previously described, another in vitro system was found to be able to generate autocytotoxic cells,
which can kill in a 4-hr ^{51}Cr-release assay Con-A induced
blasts as well as peritoneal macrophages (12-13, 17). In
this case F1 lymphocytes cocultured in vitro with irradiated parental cells for 5 days were able to kill parental as well as syngeneic non-neoplastic targets (17). In
the attempt to further analyze the possible function of
in vitro growing NK cells obtained in our culture system
without irradiated parental cells, we tested the possible
cytotoxic activity of cultured F1 NK cells against
F1 and parental macrophages (Table 4). The data obtained
clearly resemble those described in the experiments on
the in vitro hybrid resistance system (12-13, 17). These
observations are in line with data previously described,
suggesting some similarities between NK activity and hybrid resistance (18). These results are strongly in favour of an autocytotoxic function of these natural reactivities, i.e. NK and hybrid resistance. These observations must be taken into proper consideration and could
be helpful to a better understanding of the actual role
of spontaneous cytotoxicity previously described against
some tumor cell lines. A pool of autocytotoxic lymphocytes
normally present in the spleen and peripheral blood of
mice and humans can be evidenced in vitro as a spontaneous cytotoxicity against some neoplastic cell and
against normal non-neoplastic syngeneic targets. It is
possible that cytolytic effects of NK cells could be mainly directed against self components as a homeostatic
mechanism. Similar cytotoxic activities against selected
tumor lines could be merely a component of a general control system not directed specifically against cancer
cells.

ACKNOWLEDGEMENT
    This work was supported by contract n. 83.00927.96
within "Progetto Finalizzato Controllo della Crescita
Neoplastica" C.N.R., Rome, Italy.

REFERENCES

1. Natural Resistance System Against Foreign Cell,
   Tumors and Microbes, eds. Cudkowicz G., Landy M.,
   and Shearer G.M., Academic Press, New York, 1982.
2. NK Cells and Other Natural Effector Cells, ed. R.B.
   Herbermann, Academic Press, New York, 1982.
3. C.Riccardi, A.Santoni, T.Barlozzari and R.B. Herberman:
   Role of NK cells in rapid in vivo clearance of radiolabeled tumor cells. In "Natural Cell-Mediated Immunity Against Tumors" ed. R.B. Herberman, Academic
   Press, New York, p.1121, 1980.
4. C.Riccardi, A.Santoni, T.Barlozzari, C.Cesarini and
   R.B.Herberman: In vivo role of NK cells against neoplastic or non-neoplastic cells. In "Human Cancer
   Immunology", North-Holland Press, vol.4 p.57, 1982.
5. C.Riccardi, A.Santoni, T.Barlozzari and R.B.Herberman:
   In vivo Reactivity of mouse Natural Killer (NK) cells
   against Normal Bone Marrow Cells. Cell.Immunol., 60,
   136, 1981.
6. G.Cudkowicz and P.S.Hochman: Do Natural Killer Cells
   Engage in Regulater Reactions Against Self to Ensure
   Homeostasis. Immunol. Rev., 44, 13, 1979.
7. M.E.Nunn, R.B.Herberman and H.T.Holden: Natural cell-
   mediated cytotoxicity in mice against nonlymphoid
   tumor cells and some normal cells. Int. J. Cancer, 20,
   381, 1977.
8. M.Hansson, R.Kiessling, B.Andersson, K.Kärre and J.
   Roder: Natural Killer (NK) cell sensitive T-cell subpopulation in the thymus: inverse correlation to NK
   activity of the host. Nature, 278, 174, 1979.
9. C.Riccardi, B.M.Vose and R.B.Herberman: Regulation by
   Interferon and T cells of IL-2-dependent growth of NK
   progenitor cells: a limiting dilution analysis. In
   "NK Celles and Other Natural Effector Cells" ed. R.B.
   Herberman, Academic Press, New York, pag. 909, 1982.

10. C.Riccardi, B.M.Vose and R.B.Herberman: Modulation of
    IL-2-dependent growth of mouse NK celles by interferon
    and T lymphocites. J. Immunol., 130, 228, 1983.
11. C.Riccardi, G.Migliorati and R.B.Herberman: Partially
    Restorative Role of T Cells for Low IL-2-Dependent
    Growth of NK Cell Progenitors from Nude Mice. Submitted
    for publication.
12. K.Nakano, I.Nakamura and G.Cudkowicz: Generation of F1
    hybrid cytotoxic T lymphocytes specific for self H-2.
    Nature, 289, 559, 1981.
13. G.M. Shearer and G.Cudkowicz: Induction of F1 hybrid
    antiparental cytotoxic effector cells: an in vitro
    model for hemopoietic Histoincompatibility. Science
    190, 890, 1975.
14. C.Riccardi, G.Migliorati and L.Frati: Induction of
    Naturally Cytotoxic Cells by T-Cell-Growth-Factor:
    Auto-Cytotoxic Activity Against Syngenic Non-Neoplastic
    Cells. Proc. 13th International Congress of Chemotherapy,
    in press, 1983.
15. J.Tarkkanen: Interferon-evidenced autologous reactivity
    of human natural killer cells. Scand. J. Immunol., 17,
    513, 1983.
16. C.S.Henney, K.Kuribayashi, P.E. Kern and S.Gillis:
    Interleukin 2 augments natural killer cell activity.
    Nature, 291, 335, 1981.
17. H.Ishikawa and R.W. Dutton: Characterization of the
    target antigen of F1 antiparent cytotoxic lympholysis:
    analysis of the spontaneous in vitro F1 cytotoxic T
    lymphocytes. J.Immunol., 125, 656, 1980.
18. R.Kiessling, P.S.Hochman, O.Haller, G.M.Shearer, H.
    Wigzell and G.Cudkowicz: Evidence for a similar or
    common mechanism for natural killer cell activity and
    resistance to hemopoietic grafts.
    Eur. J. Immunol., 7, 655, 1977.

MODULATING EFFECTS OF THYMIC FACTORS ON NATURAL CELL-MEDIATED

REACTIVITIES OF NATURAL AND CYCLOPHOSPHAMIDE-TREATED MICE

Francesco Bistoni[1], Manuela Baccarini[1], Lucia Scaringi[1], Rosanna Mazzolla[1], Paolo Puccetti[2], Pierfrancesco Marconi[1]

[1]Institute of Medical Microbiology - University of Perugia - 06100 Perugia - Italy
[2]Institute of Pharmacology - University of Perugia - 06100 Perugia - Italy

INTRODUCTION

Our laboratory has been concerned for some time with the problem of the effects of in vivo administration of thymic extracts to mice on the expression of natural cell-mediated cytotoxicity against both fungal (1) and neoplastic cells (2) in intact as well as immunode- pressed hosts. This seems particularly important because of the recent interest in the possible therapeutic use of thymus extracts (3, 4) and in consideration of the possible role of natural immuni- ty in resistance mechanisms against neoplasia and microbial infect- ions (5, 6). The issue is even more relevant when dealing with com- promised hosts that are known to experience an increased suscepti- bility to infections and development of malignancies. In the present paper we report on the effects of thymus extract administrations in intact or cyclophosphamide treated mice on in vitro cell-mediated cytotoxicity against radiolabelled YAC-1 cells (7) and C. albicans particles (8).

MATERIALS AND METHODS

Mice

Six to 8 week old hybrid (BALB/c Cr x DBA/2 Cr) F1 (CD2F1) mice were obtained from Charles River Breeding Laboratories, Calco, Milan, and from our colony.

Drugs

Cyclophosphamide (Cy, Endoxan-Asta, Asta Werke, West Germany) was
injected i.p. in a volume of 0.1 ml/10 gr body weight. The polypeptide α_1 (α_1) (RO 21-9199/5) was a kind gift from dr. Armin Ramael
(Hoffman-LaRoche, Nutley, N.J., U.S.A.). The lyophilized drug was
dissolved in 1.4% sterile solution of sodium bicarbonate, and injected s.c. within 20 minutes in a volume of 0.1 ml/10 gr body weight.
Thymostimulin (TS) was obtained from the Istituto Farmacologico
Serono, Rome, Italy. The lyophilized drug was dissolved in sterile
saline and injected by s.c. route within 20 min in a volume of 0.1
ml/10 gr body weight.

Preparation of effector cells

Spleen cells (SC) were obtained by standard techniques. Peritoneal
polymorphonuclear neutrophils (PMN) were induced by i.p. injection
of 1 ml of 10% thioglycolate broth (Bacto brewer thioglycolate
medium, Difco Labs., Mich., U.S.A.), 18 hrs before testing. The elicited cells were harvested by peritoneal washing.

In vitro microcytotoxicity assays against ^{51}Cr labelled C. albicans
and YAC-1 tumor cells

The microcytotoxicity assays against both yeasts and tumor cells and
the culture conditions of target cells have been described in detail
elsewhere (7, 8).

Statistical analysis

Differences between groups have been evaluated according to Student's
"t" test.

RESULTS

As a preliminary approach to the problem we tested the effect of multiple exposure to α_1 (100 µg/Kg s.c. each) of CD2F1 mice of which
spleen cells and polymorphonuclear neutrophils were reacted in vitro
against radiolabelled YAC-1 and C. albicans cells. It is indeed
known that splenocytes are potent anti-YAC effectors (9) whereas PMN
exhibit the highest levels of reactivity against C. albicans particles (8,10). Table 1 shows that thymosin α_1 had a considerable impac

Table 1 - Effect of thymosin α_1 administration on natural killer
and candidacidal activity of murine SC and PMN

α_1 [a] treatment (days)	Effector cell population	% ^{51}Cr specific release from					
		YAC-1 cells			C. albicans cells		
		100:1 [b]	50:1	25:1	10:1	5:1	2.5:1
-	SC	20.78 [c]	12.6	9.98	18.64	13.42	8.91
-	PMN	5.4	5.6	3.2	40.32	34.7	23.9
-10-8-6-4-2	SC	32.47*	26.7*	19.42*	20.33	12.65	10.2
-10-8-6-4-2	PMN	6.75	4.32	0.77	54.6*	45.6*	36.75*

a) Mice were given 5 repeated administrations of thymosin α_1 (100
   µg/Kg each, by s.c. route) on the days reported in the column,
   with respect to the test on day 0.
b) Effector : target ratios.
c) Percentage of ^{51}Cr specific release; standard errors, always
   below 2%, have been omitted.
* P < 0.01 (α_1-treated vs. untreated mice) according to Student's
   "t" test.

on the two reactivities when spleen cells were assayed for anti-YAC
cytotoxic potential and PMN were reacted against C. albicans. On the
other hand, no major effects could be observed on the cytotoxic activity of PMN against YAC-1 tumor cells and on the candidacidal reactivity of splenocytes against C. albicans. Data not reported in
the present study, however, indicate that other treatment schedule
of thymosin α_1 administration can modulate these apparently unaffected reactivities. In further experiments we studied the effects of
TS administration on the anti-YAC and anti-Candida activities of
splenocytes from Cy-treated mice subjected to 2 different immunotherapeutic regimes. Table 2 shows that the splenic anti-YAC cell-
mediated cytotoxicity of mice given Cy (150 mg/Kg, i.p., 12 days
before the test on day 0) was depressed by 5 subsequent exposures
to TS (100 µg/Kg s.c. each) on days -8, -7, -6, -5 and -4 before
testing. The same regimen, however, failed to affect the activity
of splenocytes against radiolabelled C. albicans particles. The same

Table 2 - Effect of TS administration on the natural killer and
candidacidal activity of splenocytes from Cy-treated
mice

Cy[a] treatment (day)	TS[b] treatment (days)	% ^{51}Cr specific release from					
		YAC-1 cells			C. albicans cells		
		100:1	50:1	25:1[c]	10:1	5:1	2.5:1
-12	-	36.65[d]	30.32	23.7	29.9	24.6	20.2
-12	-8-7-6-5-4	25.4*	19.96*	14.3*	30.3	23.7	20.6
-9	-	33.4	24.3	18.84	34.45	30.6	19.11
-9	-5-4-3-2-1	29.6	20.4	19.6	41.9*	39.75*	27.03*

a) Mice were given a single Cy injection (150 mg/Kg, i.p.) on
the day reported in the column, with respect to the test on
day 0.
b) Mice received 5 repeated administration of TS (50 µg/Kg, s.
c.) on the days reported in the column, with respect to the
test on day 0.
c) Effector : target ratios.
d) Percentage of ^{51}Cr specific release (mean of quadruplicate
samples); standard errors, always below 2%, have been omitted.
* P < 0.01 (TS treated vs. TS untreated mice) according to Student's "t" test.

table shows that, by administering TS on days -5, -4, -3, -2 and -1
it was possible to augment the fungicidal activity whereas lysis of
YAC-1 target remained unaffected.

DISCUSSION

In the present study we investigated the combined effects of Cy +
thymus extract treatment on two natural cell-mediated functions,
i.e. in vitro lysis of YAC-1 tumor cells by NK lymphocytes and in
vitro killing of radiolabelled C. albicans particles. In selected
experiments we also studied the effect of thymosin α_1 administration
on the natural reactivities of splenocytes and polymorphonuclear
neutrophils of intact mice. It was found that the administration of
thymosin α_1 to intact mice resulted in augmentation of NK cell acti-

vity in the spleen against YAC-1 leaving reactivity of PMN unaffected. The same regime affected anti-Candida activity of PMN, but lacked
major impacts on the candidacidal functions of spleen cells. It is
to be noted, however, that, in studies not reported in present paper,
we also defined immunotherapeutic regimes that were able to modulate
the activity of splenocytes against Candida, a finding in line with
the notion that the biological activity of immunoactive substances
given in vitro may considerably vary according to multiple conditions
including treatment schedules and route of administration (11, 12,
13). When the study was extended to Cy-treated mice, it was found
that the TS regime capable of affecting anti-YAC reactivity was different from that able to enhance candidacidal functions. This finding
is important for at least two different reasons. Firstly, the concept
is reinforced that no unitary effect can be ascribed to thymus extracts in modulating natural cell-mediated functions. Secondary, further evidence is provided that the anti-YAC-1 effectors are distinct
from the candidacidal effectors, a notion in line with previous data
from our laboratory. In conclusion, our study points out that thymus
extracts can modulate in vitro natural cell-mediated cytotoxicity in
intact as well as Cy-conditioned host. No unitary pattern, however,
can be defined and even in a given system, with rigorously defined
conditions, the overall effect of thymus extract administration can
be considerably affected by the multiple parameters concerning the
administration regime.

REFERENCES

1. F. Bistoni, M. Baccarini, E. Blasi, C. Riccardi, P. Marconi, E.
   Garaci, Modulation of polymorphonucleate-mediated cytotoxicity
   against Candida albicans by thymosin α_1, Thymus, in press.
2. F. Bistoni, M. Baccarini, P. Puccetti, P. Marconi, E. Garaci, Enhancement of natural killer cell activity in mice by treatment
   with a thymic factor, Cancer Immunol. Immunother., submitted for
   publication.
3. M. H. Cohen, P. B. Chretien, D. C. Ihde, B. E. Fossieck, R. Mazuch,
   P. A. Bunn, A. V. Johnston, S. E. Shackney, M. J. Matthews, S. D.
   Lipson, D. E. Kenady, J. D. Mirna, Thymosin fraction V and intensive combination chemotherapy prolonging the survival of patients
   with small-cell lung cancer, J. Am. Med. Assoc. 241: 1813 (1979).
4. J. Shoham, E. Theodor, H.J. Brenner, B. Goldman, A. Lusky, S.
   Chaitchick, Enhancement of the immune system of chemotherapy-
   treated cancer patients by simultaneous treatment with thymic extract TP-1, Cancer Immunol. Immunother. 9: 173 (1980).

5. G. Cudckowicz, M. Landy, G. M. Shearer, Natural resistance systems against foreign cells, tumours and microbes, Academic Press, N. Y. (1978).

6. R. B. Herberman, H. T. Holden, Natural cell-mediated immunity, in: "Advances in Cancer Research", G. Klein, S. Weinhouse, eds., Academic Press, N. Y., vol. 27, p. 305 (1978).

7. R. K. Oldham, J. R. Ortaldo, H. T. Holden, R. B. Herberman, Direct comparison of three isotopic release microassay as measures of cell-mediated immunity to virus-induced lymphoma in rats, J. Natl. Cancer Inst. 58: 1061 (1977).

8. F. Bistoni, M. Baccarini, E. Blasi, P. Puccetti, P. Marconi, A radiolabel release microassay for phagocytic killing of Candida albicans, J. Immunol.Methods 52: 369 (1982).

9. R. B. Herberman, M. E. Nunn, D. H. Lavrin, Natural cytotoxic reactivity of mouse lymphoid cells. I. Distribution of reactivity and specificity, Int. J. Cancer 16: 216 (1975).

10. M. Baccarini, E. Blasi, P. Puccetti, F. Bistoni, Phagocytic killing of Candida albicans by different murine effectors, Sabouraudia in press.

11. A. S. Klein, J. Shoham, Effect of the thymic factor thymostimulin (TP-1) on the survival of tumor-bearing mice, Cancer Res. 41: 3217 (1981).

12. C. Y. Lau, G. Goldstein, Functional effect of thymopoietin$_{32-36}$ (TP-5) on cytotoxic lymphocytes precursors units (CLP-U). I. Enhancement of splenic CLP-U in vitro and in vivo after suboptimal antigenic stimulation, J. Immunol. 124: 1861 (1980).

13. P. Puccetti, A. Santoni, C. Riccardi, H. T. Holden, R. B. Herberman, Activation of mouse macrophages by pyran copolymer and role in augmentation of natural killer activity, Int. J. Cancer 24: 819 (1979).

This work was supported by contract n. 83.00628.52 within Progetto Finalizzato per il controllo delle Malattie da Infezione, from The Consiglio Nazionale delle Ricerche, Italy.

EFFECT OF INACTIVATED C. ALBICANS ON NATURAL KILLER (NK)

CELL ACTIVITY AND BLASTOGENESIS IN MICE

Pierfrancesco Marconi[1], Lucia Scaringi[1], Antonio Cassone[2], Luciana Tissi[1]
[1]Institute of Medical Microbiology, University of Perugia, 06100 Perugia, Italy.
[2]Laboratory of Bacteriology and Medical Mycology, Istituto Superiore di Sanità, 00100 Rome, Italy

INTRODUCTION

The Candida albicans (CA) is an important example of microbial cell with antitumor adjuvant activity (1). Our previous in vivo data are compatible with the hypothesis that CA antitumor activity could be strictly dependent on an intact T-cell compartment since this antitumor effect is not obtained in congenitally athymic mice or in animals treated by total-body irradiation (3). On the other hand, CA does not seem to be able to augment the in vitro expression of splenic natural killer (NK) cell activity which could exclude a possible role of NK lymphocytes in the CA-induced antitumor activity (3). However, since induction of NK cells with cytotoxic activity against tumor cells, as has been shown in the peritoneal cavity of mice treated with BCG (8) or C. parvum (5), we examined in the present study possible effect of CA administration on peritoneal NK cell activity. We also examined the in vitro response to mitogens of spleen cells from CA-treated mice.

MATERIALS AND METHODS

Mice. Eight to ten week-old hybrid (BALB/c Cr x DBA/2 Cr)F1 mice were obtained from Charles River Breeding Laboratories (Calco, Milan), and from our colony.

145

Biological agents. The origin and growth conditions of CA have
been described elsewhere (2). Vials containing 1×10^9 CA orga-
nisms/ml inactivated with sodium merthiolate (0.01 wt/vol, 24 h) were
diluted in sterile 0.85% NaCl solution to yield 1×10^8 organisms/ml.
All injections were given intraperitoneally in a total volume of
0.2 ml/mouse. Pyran copolymer (NSC 46015, Hercules Research Center,
Wilmington, Del., 50 mg/Kg) was administered intraperitoneally.

Mitogens. Concanavalin A (Con A, Difco Laboratories, Detroit,
Michigan), phytohemagglutinin (PHA-P, Difco Laboratories) and lipo-
polysaccharide (LPS, from E. coli, Difco Laboratories) were obtained
in a lyophilized form and were reconstituted with RPMI 1640 medium.

Preparation of effector cells. Spleen cell suspensions were
obtained by standard techniques. Peritoneal exudate cells (PEC) were
collected by washing the peritoneal cavity with 10 ml of RPMI 1640
medium. Effector cells from the spleen and the peritoneal cavity
were resuspended at the desired concentrations in RPMI 1640 medium
supplemented with 10% fetal calf serum, 25 mM Hepes buffer and
0.1% gentamycin sulphate.

^{51}Chromium release assay (CRA). YAC-1 tumor cells resuspended
in 1 ml of complete medium were incubated for 30 min at 37°C with
200 μCi of Na$_2$^{51}CrO$_4$ (spec. act. 1 mCi/ml; Radiochemical Center).
The cells were washed twice, counted and resuspended. Various numbers of effector cells in 0.1 ml were mixed in U-shaped 96-well
microtiter plates (Sterilin, Teddington, Middx., England) with
1×10^4 labelled target cells in 0.1 ml and then incubated at 37°C
in a 5% CO$_2$ incubator. At the end of the incubation period, the
plates were centrifuged (800 g, 10 min) and the radioactivity of
0.1 ml of the supernatant was measured in a γ-scintillation counter.
All groups were tested in quadruplicate. Baseline ^{51}Cr release was
determined by means of an autologous control with equal numbers of
unlabelled target cells in place of lymphoid cells. This baseline
was less than 10% of the total ^{51}Cr incorporated by target cells.
The percentage of the specific lysis was calculated as follows:

$$\text{Percentage cytotoxicity} = \frac{\text{test cpm} - \text{autologous control cpm}}{\text{total cpm incorporated}} \times 100$$

where test cpm is the mean cpm released in the presence of effector cells, autologous control cpm is the mean cpm released by targets incubated with autologous cells, and total cpm is the total amount of ^{51}Cr incorporated by target cells.

Blastogenesis assay. A total of 4×10^5 spleen cells were dispensed (in quadruplicate) in a volume of 0.1 ml into flat-bottom wells (Falcon, Catalog No. 3040). Wells containing cells alone had 0.1 ml incubation medium added in addition. Wells to contain mitogen were added with 0.1 ml of mitogen solution to obtain final concentration of 0.1, 0.5 and 1 μg/well of Con A, 0.1, 0.5 and 10 μg/well of PHA and 0.1, 0.5 and 1 μg/well of LPS. The cell cultures were incubated at 37°C in a humidified atmosphere of 5% CO_2 in air, for 48 h. Twenty hours before harvesting 0.01 γ of 5-fluoro-2'-deoxyuridine in a volume of 0.05 ml of RPMI plus 0.1 μCi of $^{125}IdUrd$ in a volume of 0.05 ml of RPMI (spec. act. 8.5 mCi/mg; Amersham/Searle Corp. Ardington Heights, Ill.) were added to each well. After reincubation the cultures were harvested with a Mash II sampler. Radioactivity was measured in a γ-scintillation counter (Packard Autogamma 500 C, Packard Instruments, Downers Grove, Ill., U.S.A.).

Stimulation index calculation and statistical analysis. The stimulation index (SI) was calculated according to following equation:

$$SI = \frac{\text{Mean counts per minute of stimulated cultures}}{\text{Mean counts per minute of unstimulated cultures}}$$

The variation among the cultures was consistently less than 10%. The SI was not used to assess the statistical significance of a given stimulation. Student's "t" test was used to compare the statistical significance of the mean count per minute for one group versus another group (after correction for incorporation by non-stimulated control cultures).

RESULTS

CD2F1 mice (10 week-old) were immunized intraperitoneally with 2×10^7 CA cells. Peritoneal exudate cells and splenocytes were harvested 3 days after immunization and lytic activity was assessed in a short-term (4-h) ^{51}Cr release assay against YAC-1 tumor target. The results reported in Table 1 show that exudates from unimmunized

Table 1 - Effect of CA and Py copolymer treatment on peritoneal or splenic NK activity.

| Treatment i.p. | % SPECIFIC CYTOLYSIS[a] | | | | | |
| | Peritoneal exudate cells | | | Spleen cells | | |
	100:1[c]	50:1	25:1	100:1	50:1	25:1
None	3.5	2.7	1.8	18.6	13.1	9.4
CA[b]	40.1*	34.6	24.8	10.7*	6.1	3.0
Py[b]	66.2*	46.2	34.7	43.8*	35.4	27.9

a) Chromium release assay.
b) Peritoneal exudate cells or spleen cells from 10 week-old
   CD2F1 mice untreated or injected 3 days previously with
   2×10^7 CA cells or with Py (50 mg/Kg) were assayed with
   ^{51}Cr YAC-1 tumor target cells.
c) Effector : target ratios.
d) *, P< 0.01 (CA or Py-treated versus untreated mice) according to Student's "t" test. Standard errors, always
   below 2%, have been omitted.

animals were not cytotoxic under these assay conditions.
     In contrast, peritoneal cells obtained from CA-treated mice
caused target cells destruction similar to that obtained when pyran
treatment (50 mg/Kg i.p.) was given to mice 3 days before the in
vitro assay. The amount of lysis occurring with effector cells from
CA or pyran-treated mice was proportional to the number of exudate
cells added in the assay. This lytic activity was not confined to
CD2F1 mice, similar results have been observed with CA induced
exudates of C57B1/6 or DBA/2 mice (data not shown). CA administration, on the other hand, significantly decreased splenic NK reactivity, while pyran treatment resulted in an augmentation of splenic
NK activity. Further experiments were carried out to evaluate the
effect of CA administration (given 3 days before assay) on in vitro
blastogenic responses of spleen cells to Con A, PHA or LPS mitogens.
The results show that a significant decrease in responsiveness to
stimulation by Con A or PHA-P occurred in the spleen of CA-treated

Table 2 – Effect of CA treatment on the _in vitro_ mitogenic response
of spleen cells to different mitogens.

Dose of[a] mitogen	STIMULATION INDEX								
	Con A-induced blastogenesis			PHA-P-induced blastogenesis			LPS-induced blastogenesis		
	None[b]	CA[c]	%[d]	None	CA	%	None	CA	%
0.1	20.7	10.5*	(50.7)	ND	ND	–	4.3	3.2	(74.4)
0.5	67.5	38.9*	(57.6)	3.8	2.0*	(52.6)	13.8	10.5	(76.0)
1	55.4	33.0*	(59.5)	13.8	6.4*	(46.3)	16.9	13.8	(81.6)
10	ND	ND	–	7.9	4.6*	(58.2)	ND	ND	–

a) μg/well.
b) Spleen cells from untreated control mice.
c) Spleen cells from mice injected i.p. 3 days previously with
   2×10^7 CA cells.
d) The values represent the percentage of blastogenesis of CA-treated
   mice calculated with respect to untreated control mice.
*, $P < 0.01$ (CA-treated versus untreated mice) according to Student's
   "t" test.

mice. This suppression was evident at all the lectin concentrations
tested. The response of spleen cells from CA-treated mice to LPS
was only slightly suppressed (Table 2).

DISCUSSION

The data here reported follow our previous observations on the
cellular mechanisms underlying the immunoadjuvant activity of
inactivated CA cells (3). Previous results showed that CA administration to 16-week-old mice did not affect splenic NK activity.
However, in the present study, when we used a different approach to
the problem and the NK activity of peritoneal exudate cells from
CA-treated mice was tested, we found a significant augmentation of
NK cell cytotoxicity comparable to that obtained with pyran copoly-

mer treatment (6). On the contrary, treatment with CA (3 days before
the in vitro test) significantly depressed NK cell activity of spleen
cells (Table 1). The evaluation of blastogenic response of spleen
cells from CA-treated mice also revealed that responses to Con A or
PHA (T-cell dependent) were markedly depressed (Table 2). The finding that CA administration depressed blastogenic responses to mitogens could suggest the possible induction by CA treatment of suppressor cells responsible for such suppression, as previously reported in other experimental systems (4). Moreover, the existence of
suppressor cells able to inhibit the lytic phase of NK cells has
been previously reported (7). Based on the data here reported showing that both mitogenic response and splenic NK activity are depressed by CA treatment, one is tempted to suggest the possibility that
the decrease of NK cell activity is also due to the induction of
splenic suppressor cells able to inhibit the lytic phase during the
4-hr cytotoxicity assay. Further experiments are necessary to clarify this point and in particular the cellular nature of these suppressor cells and the mechanisms responsible for their induction
following CA administration.

REFERENCES

1. Bistoni F., Marconi P., Pitzurra M., Frati L., Spreafico F.,
   Goldin A., Bonmassar E., 1979. Combined effects of BCG or Candida
   albicans (CA) with antitumor agents against a virus-induced
   lymphoma in mice. Europ. J. Cancer, 15: 1305-1314.
2. Cassone A., Marconi P., Bistoni F., Mattia E., Sbaraglia G.,
   Garaci E., Bonmassar E., 1981. Immunoadjuvant effects of Candida
   albicans and its cell wall fraction in a mouse lymphoma model.
   Cancer Immunol. Immunother., 10: 181-190.
3. Marconi P., Cassone A., Tissi L., Baccarini M., Puccetti P.,
   Garaci E., Bonmassar E., Bistoni F., 1982. Cellular mechanisms
   underlying the adjuvant activity of Candida albicans in a mouse
   lymphoma model, Int. J. Cancer, 29: 483-488.
4. Noar D., 1979. Suppressor cells: Permetters and promoters of
   malignancy. Adv. Cancer Res., 29: 45-125.
5. Ojo E., Haller O., Kimura A., Wigzell H., 1978. An analysis of
   conditions allowing Corynebacterium parvum to cause either augmentation or inhibition of natural killer activity against
   tumor cells in mice. Int. J. Cancer, 21: 444-452.
6. Puccetti P., Santoni A., Riccardi C., Holden H., Herberman R.,

1979. Activation of mouse macrophages by pyran copolymer and role in augmentation of natural killer activity. Int. J. Cancer, 24: 819-825.

7. Riccardi C., Santoni A., Barlozzari T., Cesarini C., Herberman R. 1981. Suppression of natural killer (NK) activity by splenic adherent cells of low NK-reactive mice. Int. J. Cancer, 28: 811-818.

8. Wolfe S., Tracey D., Henney C. 1978. Induction of "natural killer" cells by BCG. Nature, 262: 584-586.

ACKNOWLEDGEMENT

This work was supported by Contract n. 81.01322.96 within the "Progetto finalizzato Controllo della crescita neoplastica" - C.N.R. - Italy.

ANTITUMOR ADJUVANTS FROM CANDIDA ALBICANS : EFFECTS ON HUMAN

ALLOGENIC T-CELL RESPONSES "IN VITRO"

Clara Ausiello[1,2], Giulio Spagnoli[1], Francesca Mondello[2],
Pierfrancesco Marconi, Francesco Bistoni, and
Antonio Cassone[2]

1. Ist.Tipizzazione Tissutale, CNR, L'Aquila
2. Lab.Batteriol.Micol.Medica, ISS, Roma, Italia

INTRODUCTION

Candida albicans (CA) and other yeasts have recently been shown to act as strong, non-specific immunoadjuvants in combined chemo-immunotherapy in a mouse lymphoma model (1,2). Several cell wall fractions of distinct antigenicity and chemical composition have been used in "in vivo" experiments and showed a differential capacity of stimulating both anticancer effects and immunoresponsiveness (2). Other pieces of experimental evidence strongly suggest that the overall immunostimulating activity of yeast adjuvants depend on the potentiation of classical T-cell responses against products of minor histocompatibility loci or tumor-associated transplantation antigens of experimental, virus-induced tumors (2,3).

Because of the importance of T-cell responses in the immuno-surveillance against tumors, as opposed to or integrated with, the natural immunity system (4,5), attempts were done to explore the effect of yeast adjuvants in human T-cell systems which can be characterized by well-established "in vitro" responses. We report here that a mannan-protein (MP) component of CA cell wall inhibits the mixed lymphocyte culture. Both MP and, to a greater extent, the insoluble cell wall glucan ghosts (GG) are also able to reduce T-cell cytotoxic activity of human peripheral blood lymphocytes.

MATERIALS AND METHODS

Candida albicans and cell wall preparations. The origin and growth conditions of the yeast have been reported previously (2). In all

153

reported experiments, CA was used after glutaraldehyde inactivation (2% v/v,1h). Chemical extraction of glucan ghosts (GG) and mannan-protein (MP) and their preparation for experimental purposes have been reported in detail elsewhere (2). All biological reagents were diluted in culture medium.

Cells. Peripheral blood mononuclear cells (PBL) of healthy volunteers were isolated by centrifugation on density gradient as described by Böyum (6) and resuspended in RPMI medium supplemented with 15% pooled AB serum and antibiotics.

Mixed lymphocyte cultures (MLC). PBL of one donor were cocultured with irradiated (4200 rad) allogenic PBL (10^6/ml) in 0.2ml for six days in 96 flat bottomed wells, microtiter trays, under 5% CO_2, at 37°C. 18 hours before harvesting, radiolabeled thymidine (methyl-^{3}H-thymidine, 25 Ci/mmol, 1 mCi/ml) was added and its uptake was evaluated by standard methods. All tests were performed in triplicate and the associated radioactivity was measured by the two channel ratio using the external standard method, at a Beckman LS 9100 liquid scintillator.

Cytotoxic T-limphocytes (CTL) and natural killer (NK)-like activities. CTL were generated from bulk MLC, cultured in 24 wells trays in CO_2 with or without the considered CA materials. After washing, cells were seeded in 0.1 ml in 96 wells round bottom trays at three different effector:target ratios with target lymphocytes of the original stimulator (transformed with PHA for 72 hours) and labeled with 150 microCi sodium chromate (^{51}Cr). After 4 hours, supernatants were collected by Titertek system and counted at LKB 1282 compugamma. NK-like effectors, generated as for CTL, were tested against ^{51}Cr-labeled K562 target. Culture conditions and evaluation of specific killing by this assay were as reported elsewhere (7).

RESULTS

Table 1 shows the chemical composition of yeast materials used throughout this study. MP is representative of yeast surface cell wall components as also shown by its strong response in ELISA test using a CA-whole cells rabbit antiserum. GG represent the internal cell wall materials, essentially made up of insoluble beta-glucan free of surface MP. GG did not react with anti-CA serum.As shown in Table 2, CA whole cells, MP and GG had differential effects on human MLC response. While whole cells (in the range of 0.1-10 micrograms/ml) led to a dose-dependent increase of thymidine incorporation, no effect at all was observed in presence of comparable amount of GG. On the other hand, MP (0.5-50 micrograms/ml)determined a marked dose-dependent inhibition of the uptake. At a dose of

50 micrograms/ml a complete block of MLC was observed.

Table 1. Chemical compositions[a] of whole cells and fractions of C. albicans used as immunomodulators.

Material	Protein	Polysaccharide	Mannan
Whole cells	27.3	23.0	8.1
Glucan ghosts	- -	94.3	1.2
Mannanprotein	13.0	85.0	83.7

a) values expressed as % cell dry weight for whole cells and glucan ghosts. For the mannanprotein, the values are expressed in % of purified, lyophilized material.

CTL effectors were generated in presence of CA cell wall preparations. Mean values of three independent experiments are shown in Table 3. A slight inhibition of CTL activity could be detected both with GG and MP at a dose of 10 micrograms/ml and 5 micrograms /ml, respectively. No inhibition of NK-like activity was observed using similar amounts of the same materials.

Table 2. Effect of whole Candida cells (CA), insoluble glucan (GG) and mannanprotein (MP) on MLC:results of a typical experiment.

Component	Dose[a]	Thymidine uptake[b]		%Control
None	--	$83,242 \pm 8490$		--
CA	10	$119,782 \pm 11728$	P 0.05	143
CA	1	$108,694 \pm 3433$		130
CA	0.1	$103,954 \pm 7042$		124
GG	10	$77,093 \pm 5492$		92
GG	1	$93,783 \pm 4746$		112
GG	0.1	$89,672 \pm 3475$		107
MP	50	381 ± 15	P 0.001	0.45
MP	5	$62,334 \pm 7136$		74
MP	0.5	$74,680 \pm 3923$		89

a)in micrograms/ml; b)dpm + MSE; final amount of radiolabeled thymidine was 1 microCi/20 microliters/well. P less than 0.05 or 0.0
01, respectively.

Table 3. Effect of MP and GG on CTL and NK-like activities.

Component	Dose[a]	CTL-activity[b]	NK-like activity[b]
None	--	33 + 7.3	25.5 + 1.4
MP	5	20 + 7.7	26.0 + 1.1
MP	0.5	20 + 7.5	26.0 + 1.7
MP	0.05	31 + 2.3	27.0 + 2.3
GG	10	13.3 + 2.6	25.5 + 4.3
GG	1	15.3 + 4.2	20.0 + 4.0
GG	0.1	23.5 + 3.1	23.5 + 4.3

a) in micrograms/ml; b)Mean values + MSE of three independent
experiments. The values of both CTL and NK-like activities are
expressed as %specific killing using an effector target ratio of
30:1. Comparable results were obtained using different ratios.

DISCUSSION

Previous studies showed differences in the antitumor effects
of various CA cell wall components. Briefly, it was found that the
minimal immunoadjuvant structure capable of synergizing with chemotherapy was the insoluble GG. No effect was shown by soluble fractions even if they retained full antigenicity (2). The present "in
vitro" study with human PBL indicate that yeast cells induce a little
enhancement of thymidine uptake in MLC. Such an increase of a classical T-dependent response is consistent with the results obtained
in the mouse lymphoma model where the adjuvant activity of CA was
found to rely upon the integrity of T cell compartement (8).It should
be noted, however, that CA cells are also able to induce a moderate
degree of blastogenesis in a three day culture (data not shown).

The insoluble GG did not affect MLC reactivity but MP preparations, essentially consisting of phosphorylated mannan polysaccharide, had a strong, dose-dependent, inhibitory effect on MLC response
with a total block at 50 micrograms/ml. This inhibition is not due
to a direct cytotoxiceffect of the substance as no inhibition of

thymidine uptake was observed either in spontaneous or in PHA-induced blastogenesis. This material is not endowed with endotoxin-like property but a long-term toxic effect cannot be excluded.

Both MP and GG exerted an inhibitory effect on CTL activity but no effect on NK-like activity suggesting they may influence some specific aspect or mechanism of CTL reactivity. We have, however, no data to attribute the reduction in CTL to an actual decrease in the effector generation or to an inhibition of target cell killing.

REFERENCES

1) F.Bistoni,P.Marconi,M.Pitzurra,L.Frati,F.Spreafico,A.Goldin and E.Bonmassar. Combined effects of BCG or Candida albicans (CA) with antitumor agents against a virus-induced lymphoma in mice. Eur.J. Cancer 15:1305 (1979).

2) A.Cassone,P.Marconi,F.Bistoni,E.Mattia,G.Sbaraglia,E.Garaci and E.Bonmassar. Immunoadjuvant effects of Candida albicans and its cell wall farctions in a mouse lymphoma model. Cancer Immunol.Immunother. 10:101 (1981).

3) P.Marconi,A.Cassone,M.Baccarini,L.Tissi,E.Garaci,E.Bonmassar,L. Frati and F.Bistoni. Relationship among tumor load, route of tumor inoculation and response to immunochemotherapy in a murine lymphoma model. J.Natl Cancer Inst.71:299 (1983).

4) R.B.Herberman and J.R.Hortaldo. Natural killer cells:their role in defenses against disease. Science 214:24 (1981).

5) J.L.Collins,P.Q.Patek and M.Cohn. Tumorigenicity and lysis by natural killers. J.Exptl Med.153:89 (1981).

6) A.Böyum. Isolation of mononuclrar cells and granulocytes from human blood. Scand.J.Clin.Lab.Invest.21:77 (1968).

7) C.Ausiello,P.Hokland and I.Heron. Interferon induced augmentation of cytotoxic killer cell generation in mixed lymphocyte cultures. Analysis of the effector cell product. Scand.J.Immunol.13:268 (1981).

8) P.Marconi,A.Cassone,L.Tissi,M.Baccarini,P.Puccetti,E.Garaci,E. Bonmassar and F.Bistoni. Cellular mechanisms underlying the adjuvant activity of Candida albicans in a mouse lymphoma model. Int.J.Cancer 29:483 (1982).

ACKNOWLEDGMENT

This work was supported in part by Contract N° 82.00262.96 within the Progetto Finalizzato Controllo della Crescita Neoplastica, CNR, Italy.

IL-2 AND LYMPHOCYTES FROM TUMOR BEARING MICE: A COMBINATORY

IMMUNOTHERAPY OF TUMORS

Guido Forni*, Mirella Giovarelli*, Susanna Cerruti Sola+
and Angela Santoni§

*Department of Microbiology, University of Turin
 Via Santena 9, 10126 - Turin, Italy
+Department of Animal Pathology, University of Turin
 Via Nizza 52, 10126 - Turin, Italy
§Department of General Pathology, University of Rome
 Viale Regina Elena 324, 00161 - Rome, Italy

INTRODUCTION

The way a membrane antigen enters the immune system is a feature of critical importance on which the efficient induction of distinct reaction patterns depends (Mitchison, 1979). This is especially true when we are dealing with proliferating tumor cells (Forni et al., 1983).

Natural cell-mediated immunity potentially plays an important immunosurveillance role against incipient tumors and metastases (Herberman, 1984). It rests on NK cells and macrophages and does not require specific antigen recognition (Herberman, 1982). Tumors may escape natural resistance because of their proliferative kinetics and because natural mechanisms are often operative only marginally (Herberman, 1984). In several cases, however, unspecific recognition of some tumor associated structures triggers the release of soluble mediators which lead to an amplification of natural reactivity (Trinchieri et al., 1978; Djeu et al., 1980; Sarzotti et al., 1982). Such mediators can be released by the same cells as are responsible for natural resistance or by T lymphocytes (Domzig and Stadler, 1982; Djeu et al., 1982; Kasahara et al., 1983).

159

T lymphocytes play pivotal roles in resistance to tumors, since following specific recognition of tumor associated membrane antigens, they regulate both specific and non-specific immune reactivity. However, activation of T lymphocyte responses efficient enough to overcome tumor proliferative capacity and hinder tumor growth requires the recognition of tumor associated surface antigens in the framework of the glycoproteins coded by the major histocompatibility complex (MHC). The absence or rarefactions of class II or class I MHC glycoproteins hampers the physiological cell-cell interactions required by T lymphocytes to recognize (Forni et al., 1976; Forni et al., 1982) and to react (Schrier et al., 1983).

Tumor growth can even lead to the induction of negative responses that actively suppress both natural and adaptative host resistance (Varesio et al., 1979; Gerson et al.,1981; Berendt and North, 1980). Several lines of evidence indicate that, while the immune system potentially recognizes syngeneic or autochthonous tumors (Herberman, 1977), its actual reaction is marginal and vanishes as tumor size increases (Forni et al., 1979).

Previous studies have shown that efficient anti-tumor reactivity can be elicited from lymphocytes that have already lost their primary war against the tumor (Forni and Giovarelli, 1984). Spleen cells (Spc) from mice harboring small but clinically evident tumors, stimulated in vitro by tumor cells and expanded in the presence of interleukin 2 (IL-2) and tumor cells, displayed efficient reactivity both in vitro and in vivo. In the present study, we show that efficient activation of lymphocytes from tumor bearing mice can also be achieved directly in vivo by multiple local injections of IL-2. The experiments to be reported show various characteristics of this phenomenon, which we have called lymphokine-activated tumor inhibition (LATI).

MATERIALS AND METHODS

Mice and tumors. Female BALB/c mice (H-2^d) 8-10 weeks of age used in these experiments were bred in our animal facilities from breeders obtained from Dr. G. Parmiani, Ist. Naz. Tumori, Milan, Italy. Age and sex matched nu/nu BALB/c mice were bred from pairs obtained from Dr. C. Riccardi, Univ. Perugia, Perugia, Italy. The CE-2 and CA-2 tumors are two antigenically non cross-reacting methylcholanthrene-induced sarcomas of BALB/c mice induced by Dr. Parmiani (Carbone et al, 1983). Their earlier transplant generations were preserved by slow freezing and storage at -80°C. TSA is a non-immunogenic adenocarcinoma that arose spontaneously in BALB/c mice and was kindly provided by Dr. P. Nanni, Inst. Cancerol., Bologna, Italy (Nanni et al, 1983). A tissue culture cell line of YAC-1, a Moloney virus induced lymphoma of A/Sn mice, was used as the target for NK activity (Herberman, 1982). Mice were challenged sc in the inguinal region with 0.2 ml of a single cell suspension containing the minimal 100% tumor inducing dose (4 x 10^4 trypan blue dye excluding cells for CE-2, 10^5 for CA-2, and 2 x 10^4 for TSA). Mice were palpated twice weekly to pinpoint the moment of tumor appearence, after which neoplastic mass was measured with calipers in the two perpendicular diameters (Forni and Giovarelli, 1984). Survival time was defined as the period (in days) between challenge and the growth of a neoplastic mass of 15 mm mean diameter when mice were killed for humane reasons.

Winn assay. Inhibition of tumor growth was assessed by the Winn-type neutralization assay as previously described (Forni and Giovarelli, 1984). Various numbers of lymphoid cells were mixed with tumor cells and 0.2 ml of the mixture were immediately injected sc. The lymphoid cell to tumor cell ratio, referred as the effector-to-target (E:T) ratio was specified in each experiment. Normal and mice bearing already clinically evident 5 mm mean diameter tumors (TB-mice) were used as spleen cell donors.

Lymphocytes. Single cell suspensions from normal and TB-mice spleens were fractionated on nylon wool columns as previously described in detail (Forni and Giovarelli, 1984). The column emerging cells, consisting of more than 85-90% Thy 1.2^+ lymphocytes as determined by immunofluorescence, were used in the experiments. Those obtained from TB-mice are hereafter referred as TB-lymphocytes. In a few instances, they were also fractionated by centrifugation on discontinuous density gradients of Percoll (Pharmacia, Uppsala, Sweden) as previously described (Santoni et al, 1984). Seven concentrations of Percoll were prepared, with the top having 38.6% Percoll, the next (F1) 47.6%, followed by 4.5% graded increases to 70.1% (F. 6). After centrifugation at 300 G for 40 min the fractions were collected. The lymphocyte recovery was about 80% of the original input, and the viability was greater than 95%. Antibody treatments plus non toxic rabbit C of TB-lymphocytes were performed by using monoclonal antibody to Thy

1.2, Lyt 1.2, Lyt 2.2, (NEN, Boston, Ma.), or rabbit antiserum to
Asialo GM1 (kindly supplied by Dr. R.B. Herberman, BRMP,
Frederick, Md.) as previously described (Forni and Giovarelli,
1984). Proliferative response, interferon (IFN) titration, and 4
and 18 h cytotoxicity assays were performed as previously described
(Giovarelli et al, 1982a; Forni and Giovarelli, 1984).

    IL-2.   IL-2 containing supernatants were prepared from clone
16 of the EL-4 thymoma (kindly provided by Dr. H. Engers, Swiss
Inst.Cancer Res., Epalinges, Switzerland) stimulated by 10 ng/ml of
phorbol-12-myristate-13-acetate as described by Farrar et al.,1980.
IL-2 in the supernatants was quantified by determining the ability
to maintain the growth of an IL-2 dependent murine T cell line
(CTLL) kindly provided by Dr. F. Manca, Univ. of Genova, Italy.
The IL-2 unit of activity is defined as the amount required to
give 50% of the maximal proliferative response of CTLL cultured at
10^5/ml for 24 h. Typically, crude EL 4 supernatant has an IL-2
activity of about 700 and 1,000 U/ml. Purification of IL-2 was done
by precipitation of the supernatant with 85% saturated $(NH_4)_2SO_4$.
The precipitate was dissolved in a small volume of phosphate
buffered saline, dialyzed for 48 h and cromatographed on Sephacryl
S-200 (Pharmacia). Active fractions between 25,000 and 30,000 m.w.
were pooled. Their titer was similar to that of the starting
material and were devoid of macrophage activating factor and IFN
activity.   0.4 ml were injected sc daily for ten days where the
tumoral challenge was made (Fig.1).

RESULTS

    Normal and CE-2 TB-lymphocytes were tested for their ability
to react towards CE-2 tumor cells both in vitro and in vivo, and
for NK cytotoxicity against YAC-1 target cells (Table 1). For in
vitro reactivity to CE-2, we chose three independent lymphocyte
functions, namely IFN release, proliferation and cytotoxicity since
they have different activation requirements (Giovarelli et al.,
1982b). IFN release and proliferation were evaluated for a period
of 20 - 120 h by using a wide range of responder to stimulator cell
ratios. For the sake of simplicity, only the data obtained after
96 h of culture at responder to stimulator ratio of 1:0.17, where
both sets of values culminated, are reported. Cytotoxicity against
CE-2 and YAC-1 target was assayed respectively for 18 and 4 h in
^{51}Cr release assay at E:T cell ratio of 50:1. A very marginal,
even if consistently positive response to CE-2 was found. NK

Table 1. Reactivity of lymphocytes from normal and CE-2 TB-mice
          against CE-2 tumor cells.

Lymphocytes from:	Target cells	Tested activity		
		IFN release	Proliferation	Cytotoxicity[a]
Normal mice	–	3	1.0^b (1.0)^c	–
	B6 Spc	80	12.4 (11.4)	–
	CE-2	9	1.6 (1.2)	7.0
	YAC-1	–	– –	7.9
TB-mice	–	6	1.0 (1.0)	–
	B6 Spc	70	16.4 (8.8)	–
	CE-2	18	2.0 (1.1)	4.0
	YAC-1	–	– –	13.0

[a] E:T ratio 50:1.
[b] Total cpm x 10^{-3}.
[c] Stimulation index.

activity was not depressed in CE-2 TB-lymphocytes but slightly
enhanced.   In vivo lymphocytes from both normal and TB-mice were
assayed for tumor inhibitory activity in a Winn-type neutralization
assay by mixing 4 x 10^4 CE-2 cells with various numbers of
lymphocytes at E:T ratios from 5:1 to 500:1. No inhibition of tumor
growth was observed (data not shown).

     The in vitro data indicate that the reactivity of normal and
CE-2 TB-lymphocytes to CE-2 cells is very poor. In vivo, too, it
was not enough to affect tumor growth rate and takes.   The
following studies examined the possibility of enhancing in vivo
the reactivity of TB-lymphocytes by the local injection of IL-2
rich preparations. Almost complete inhibition of tumor takes was
found when the protocol outlined in Fig.1 was adopted. When IL-2
was omitted, or injected only once at the moment of tumor
challenge, or for the following 1 or 2 days, there was no
significant inhibition in tumor growth and takes. After 5 and 10
days' injections, however, 40% and 100% rejection was observed
(Table 2). The latter period was therefore used in all subsequent
experiments.

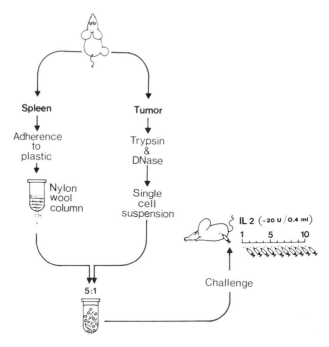

Fig. 1   Schematic drawing of the basic protocol adopted   for the   study   of   tumor   inhibition by CE-2   TB-lymphocytes   in   the presence of exogenous IL-2.

Since   CE-2 TB-lymphocytes inhibit tumor growth in presence of IL-2,   we compared their activity with that of normal   lymphocytes. As shown in Table 3, both can be activated by IL-2 in vivo to block CE-2   tumor   growth.   However, CE-2 TB-lymphocytes are always   more effective.   In addition, there is a direct relationship between the degree   of tumor inhibition and the number of lymphocytes added   up to   8   x 10^5.   Decrease in efficiency when this number is   exceeded may   reflect   an   overcrowding   effect   and a   mutual   hindering   of activity, or competition for the injected IL-2.

We   next   assessed   the   role   of   the   immune   system   of   the recipient mice.   As shown in Table 4, the combination of IL-2   and TB-lymphocytes was effective in normal and nu/nu mice but not in

Table 2. Effect of the period of IL-2 injection on the tumor
          inhibitory activity of CE-2 TB-lymphocytes.

TB-lymphocytes[a]	Days of IL-2 treatment	Surviving/total challenged mice	
−	0	0/20	(0%)[b]
+	0	0/20	(0%)
+	1	0/18	(0%)
+	2	0/20	(0%)
+	3	0/20	(0%)
+	5	8/20	(40%)
+	10	20/20	(100%)
−	10	0/24	(0%)

[a] E:T ratio 5:1.
[b] Percentage survival in brackets.

sublethally irradiated recipients, showing that a radiosensitive
mechanism of the host immune system plays a crucial role in this
very local reaction to tumor. To determine which lymphocyte
subpopulations are responsible for   the   induction of tumor
inhibition in the presence of IL-2, TB-lymphocytes were both
treated with antibody and C and fractionated on Percoll density
gradients. As shown in Table 5, pretreatment with anti Thy 1.2,
anti Lyt 1.2 or anti Asialo GM1 antibody decreased their capacity
to inhibit tumor growth but never abolished it. Anti-Lyt 2.2
antibody had no effect, whereas anti Lyt 1.2 followed by anti
Asialo GM1 antibody resulted in total abolition.

These findings are most compatible with the hypothesis that
Lyt 1.2^+ and Asialo $GM1^+$ lymphocytes independently elicit tumor
rejection in the presence of exogenous IL-2. This possibility is
further supported by the data obtained by fractionation on Percoll
density gradient, since both Fraction 1-2   and 4-5-6 pools
triggered similar tumor rejection in the presence of IL-2 (Table
6).   Considerable enrichment of NK activity and large granular
lymphocytes (LGL) takes place in low density Percoll fractions
(1-2), while both are lost in high density fractions (4-5-6)
containing predominantly small lymphocytes (Santoni et al., 1984).

Table 3.   Tumor inhibitory capacity of normal and CE-2
TB-lymphocytes in the presence of IL-2.

		Lymphocytes added		
IL-2	E:T ratio[a]	None	Normal	TB
+	0.0 : 1	0/12[b](0%)[c]	–	–
+	0.5 : 1		0/10 (0%)	2/10 (20%)
+	1.0 : 1		0/10 (0%)	2/10 (20%)
+	5.0 : 1		1/ 9 (11%)	16/18 (89%)*
+	10.0 : 1		6/10 (60%)	10/10 (100%)*
+	20.0 : 1		9/12 (75%)	9/ 9 (100%)*
+	40.0 : 1		4/12 (33%)	6/20 (30%)
–	40.0 : 1		0/10 (0%)	0/10 (0%)

[a]Mice challenged with 4×10^4 CE-2 cells
[b]Surviving/total challenged mice.
[c]Percentage of survival in brackets.
*Values significantly different ($P < 0.05$) from those observed with
normal lymphocytes as determined by chi square method with Yate's
modification for small sample sizes.

Table 4.   Role of the host immune system in tumor inhibition by
combination of CE-2 TB-lymphocytes and IL-2.

		Surviving/total challenged mice.		
TB-lymphocytes[a]	IL-2	Normal	Irradiated (450 rad)	Nude
+	+	24/26 (86%)[b]*	3/30 (10%)	5/6 (90%)*
+	–	0/10 (0%)	0/10 (0%)	0/6 (0%)
–	+	0/16 (0%)	1/21 (5%)	0/5 (0%)
–	–	0/10 (0%)	0/10 (0%)	0/5 (0%)

[a]E:T ratio 5:1.
[b]Percentage of survival in brackets.
*Significantly different from the corresponding values in
irradiated mice ($P < 0.05$).

Table 5.   Effect of antibody   and C on the capacity of
           CE-2 TB-lymphocytes to inhibit CE-2 growth.[a]

Treatment	% lymphocytes recovered	Surviving/total challenged mice
None	100	23/25 (92%)[b]
C only	85	17/20 (85%)
a-Thy 1.2	11	7/24 (29%)*
a-Lyt 1.2	20	7/15 (47%)*
a-Lyt 2.2	52	14/15 (93%)
a-Asialo GM1	40	6/15 (40%)*
a-Lyt 1.2 + Asialo GM1	18	2/15 (13%)*

[a] E:T ratio 5:1.
[b] Percentage survival in brackets.
*Significantly different from   corresponding values displayed   by
 untreated TB-lymphocytes.

    Next,   we   evaluated the specificity of tumor inhibition in   a
criss-cross   experiment   by using TB-lymphocytes from mice   bearing
apparently   non cross-reacting tumors (Table 7).   Lymphocytes   from
CE-2   and   CA-2   bearing mice blocked the growth of both   CE-2   and
CA-2, but had virtually no effect on the non immunogenic TSA tumor.
Lymphocytes   from   TSA   TB-mice failed to inhibit   CE-2   and   CA-2
growth,   and had no effect upon TSA tumor growth pattern.   Neither
of   these   distinct   TB-lymphocyte   populations   inhibited   various
BALB/c lymphoid tumors (data not shown).

DISCUSSION

    The   LATI   phenomenon   described in this paper   is   an   unique
immunotherapeutic   approach based on the activation of   lymphocytes
by   interleukins   in   vivo.   The experiments   reported   show   that
combination of TB-leukocytes and IL-2 triggers such a strong immune
reaction   that tumors are very efficiently rejected.   In vitro   and
in   vivo   tests   show that CE-2 TB-lymphocytes   by   themselves   are
apparently   unable   to   react   against CE-tumor   cells.   Repeated
injections   of   IL-2   at   the challenge site do   not   affect   tumor
growth.   Their   local   combination with   CE-2   TB-lymphocytes   is
required for tumor inhibition.

Table 6. Effect of Percoll fractionation on the capacity of
          CE-2 TB-lymphocytes to inhibit tumor growth.

TB-lymphocytes[a]	IL-2	% LGL	NK activity[b] (50:1 E:T)	Surviving/total challenged mice
Unfractionated	−	5	7.5	1/20 (5%)[c]
	+			18/23 (78%)
Percoll F. 1-2	−	25	15.8	2/22 (10%)
	+			21/31 (68%)
Percoll F.4-5-6	−	0	0.0	2/21 (10%)
	+			25/36 (69%)

[a] E:T ratio 5:1.
[b] Expressed as % ^{51}Cr specific release.
[c] Percentage survival in brackets.

Table 7. Specificity of tumor inhibition by combination of
          TB-lymphocytes and IL-2.

Lymphocytes from mice bearing:	IL-2	Target tumor[a]		
		CE-2	CA-2	TSA
No tumor	−	0/5[b] (0%)[c]	ND[d]	0/10 (0%)
	+	1/5 (20%)	ND	0/ 5 (0%)
CE-2	−	0/5 (0%)	0/ 8 (0%)	0/ 5 (0%)
	+	5/5 (100%)	8/ 8 (100%)	1/ 5 (20%)
CA-2	−	0/5 (0%)	0/10 (0%)	0/ 5 (0%)
	+	5/5 (100%)	10/10 (100%)	0/ 5 (0%)
TSA	−	0/5 (0%)	0/ 5 (0%)	0/ 5 (0%)
	+	0/5 (0%)	ND	0/10 (0%)

[a], [b], [c] As specified in Table 3.
[d] Not done.

IL-2 is well known for its ability to support T and NK cell proliferation in vitro (Dennert and De Rose, 1976; Dennert et al., 1981, Riccardi et al., 1983). In vivo it may restore immune functions in nude mice (Wagner et al., 1980). However, when injected iv, IL-2 is rapidly inactivated by serum inhibitors (Donohue and Rosenberg, 1983) that restrict its physiological activity to a very short range. In these studies, IL-2 was therefore used as a local mediator, and administered where TB-lymphocytes contacting neoplastic cells express IL-2 receptor and are selectively triggered by exogenous IL-2.

Precursor CE-2 TB-lymphocytes responsible for LATI in vivo are a dishomogeneous cell population. They sediment in both high and low density Percoll fractions. Moreover, depletion with antibody and C shows that Lyt 1.2 and Asialo GM1 positive cells are independently involved in LATI. It is thus possible that all lymphocytes expressing IL-2 receptors through specific or non-specific recognition of tumor cell surface structures are activated by exogenous IL-2. When unfractionated CE-2 TB-lymphocytes are injected, the simultaneous activation of various cells may also lead to significant cooperation between distinct cell populations. It is worth noting that CE-2 TB-lymphocytes mediate LATI more efficiently than lymphocytes from normal mice on a per cell basis. They contain slightly more LGL and display a slightly enhanced NK activity. In addition, they may contain an expanded cell population potentially able to recognize tumor associated membrane structures. These cells are inactive or suppressed, as shown by in vitro and in vivo tests, but can be quickly activated by IL-2.

The LATI phenomenon described here could be the in vivo counterpart of the in vitro lymphokine-activated killer (LAK) activity described by Grimm et al. (1983). LAK activity becomes evident on day 3 of culture in the presence of IL-2, and reaches maximum between day 3 and 5. LAK cells lyse a broad spectrum of fresh tumor cells . Their precursors are serologically distinct from NK cells and specifically cytotoxic T-lymphocytes. Unfortunately, no reports are yet available on the capacity of LAK cells to release lymphokines or sustain delayed type hypersensitivity in vivo.

Immune mechanisms of the recipient host are directly involved in LATI in vivo. This apparently very local reaction based on the combination of lymphocytes and IL-2 is, in fact, fully ineffective in 450 rad irradiated mice. This may be a key point in elucidating the mechanisms leading to tumor rejection. Activation of the cytotoxic function of TB-lymphocytes does not appear to be the mechanism on which LATI depends, since local cytotoxicity is also fully operative in irradiated hosts (Engers et al, 1983). Furthermore, depletion of Lyt 2.2$^+$ cells does not affect the ability of residual TB-lymphocytes to reject the tumor. Cytotoxicity is not the only function activated by exogenous IL-2. In vitro studies have shown that CE-2 TB-lymphocytes are triggered by IL-2 to release various lymphokines in the presence of CE-2 tumor cells (Forni and Giovarelli, 1984). In this way, they recruit several host lymphocyte populations and initiate a delayed type hypersensitivity reaction. By continuous release of IFN-γ and other lymphokines, they may boost NK and natural cytotoxic (NC) cells, activate macrophages, and induce the generation and expansion of specifically cytotoxic T-lymphocytes. The inductive phase of all these functions is radiation-sensitive. Germane to this interpretation are the findings we have obtained in parallel in vivo and in vitro with CE-2 TB-lymphocytes restimulated by CE-2 cells in vitro, showing that the most important function in the local tumor inhibition in vivo is the ability to recruit specific and non-specific host immune mechanisms, rather than direct lysis of tumor cells (Forni and Giovarelli, 1984). The broad spectrum of specificity of LATI observed could be fully explained by the dynamic integration of specific and less specific effector mechanisms that is an hallmark of the cellular reaction in vivo (Varesio et al., 1980).

Finally, the LATI system, based on a combinatory use of quite low levels of IL-2 and TB-lymphocytes, is a new way of looking at lymphokine mediated immunotherapy which may have interesting applications.

ACKNOWLEDGMENTS

We wish to thank John Iliffe for careful review of the manuscript. This work was supported by grants from CNR-PFCCN, Italy, No. 83.00820.96 and the Italian Department of Education (MPI 40% to GF).

REFERENCES

Berendt, M. T., and North, R. J., 1980, T-cell mediated suppres-
    sion of anti-tumor immunity. An explanation for progressive
    growth of an immunogenic tumor. J. Exp. Med., 151:169.
Carbone, G., Colombo, M., P., Sensi, M. L., Cernuschi, A., and
    Parmiani, 1983, G., In vitro detection of cell mediated
    immunity to individual tumor specific antigens of chemically
    induced BALB/c fibrosarcomas, Int. J. Cancer, 31:483.
Dennert, G., and DeRose, M., 1976, Continuously proliferating T
    killer cells specific for H-2^b targets: selection and
    characterization, J. Immunol., 116:1601.
Dennert, G., Yogeeswaran, G., and Yamagata, S., 1981, Cloned cell
    lines with natural killer activity. J. Exp. Med., 153:545.
Djeu, J. Y., Huang, K. Y., and Herberman, R. B., 1980,
    Augmentation of mouse natural killer activity and induction
    of interferon by tumor cells in vivo. J. Exp. Med., 151:781.
Djeu, J. Y., Timonen, T., and Herberman, R. B., 1982,Production of
    interferon by human natural killer cells in response to
    mitogens, viruses, and bacteria, in "NK Cells and Other
    Natural Effector Cells", R. B. Herberman, ed., Academic
    Press, New York.
Domzig, W., and Stadler, B. M., 1982, The relation between human
    natural cells and interleukin 2, in "NK Cells and Other
    Natural Effector Cells", R. B. Herberman, ed., Academic Press,
    New York.
Donohue, J. H., and Rosenberg, S.A., 1983, The fate of IL 2 after
    in vivo administration, J. Immunol., 130:2203.
Engers, H. D., Sorenson, G. D., Terres, G., Howath, C., and
    Brunner, K.T., 1982, Functional activity in vivo of effector
    cell populations. I. Anti-tumor activity exhibited by
    allogeneic mixed leukocyte culture cells. J. Immunol.,
    129: 1292.
Farrar, J. J., Fuller-Farrar, J., Simon, P. L., Hilfiker, M.,
    Stadler, B. M., and Farrar W. L., 1980, Thymoma production of
    T cell growth factor (interleukin 2) , J. Immunol., 125:2555.
Forni, G., and Giovarelli, M., 1984, In vitro reeducated T helper
    cells from sarcoma-bearing mice inhibit sarcoma growth in
    vivo, J. Immunol., 132:156.
Forni, G., Shevach, E. M., and Green, I., 1976, Mutant lines of
    guinea pig L2C leukemia. I. Deletion of Ia alloantigens is
    associated with a loss in immunogenicity of tumor associated
    transplantation antigens, J. Exp. Med., 143:1067.

REFERENCES

Forni, G., Varesio, L., Giovarelli, M., and Cavallo, G., 1979, Dynamic state of spontaneous immune reactivity towards a mammary adenocarcinoma, in: "Current Trends in Tumor Immunology", S. Ferrone, S. Gorini, R. B. Herberman and R. A. Reisfeld, eds., Garland STPM Press, New York.

Forni, G., Landolfo, S., Giovarelli, M., Whitmore, A. C., and R. B. Herberman, 1982, Immune recognition of tumor cells in vivo. I. Role of H-2 gene products in T lymphocyte activation against minor histocompatibility antigens displayed by adenocarcinoma cells, Eur. J. Immunol., 12:664.

Forni, G., Giovarelli, M., Sarzotti, M., and Whitmore, A. C., 1983, RSV-induced tumors in mice. II. Contribution of H-2 and non-H-2 alloantigen barriers to tumor immunogenicity in vivo, J. Immunogenetics, 10:209.

Gerson, J. M., Varesio, L., and Herberman,R.B., 1981, Systemic and in situ natural killer activity and suppressor cell activities in mice bearing progressively growing murine sarcoma virus induced tumors, Int.J. Cancer, 27:243.

Giovarelli, M., Landolfo, S., Whitmore, A. C., and Forni, G., 1982a, Rous sarcoma virus-induced tumors in mice. I. Macrophage mediated natural cytotoxicity, Eur. J. Cancer Clin. Oncol., 18:307.

Giovarelli, M., Landolfo, S., Scher, I., and Forni, G., 1982b, Distinct alloantigens trigger proliferative and non proliferative T lymphocyte activation in CBA/N, CBA/J, and C3H mice, Transplantation, 33: 260.

Grimm, E. A., and Rosenberg, S. A., 1983, The human lymphokine activated killer cell phenomenon, The lymphokines, 9:435

Herberman, R. B., 1977, Existence of tumor immunity in man, in "Mechanisms of Tumor Immunity", I.Green, S. Cohen, R. T. McCluskey, eds., J. Wiley & Sons, New York.

Herberman, R. B., ed., 1982, "NK Cells and Other Natural Effector Cells", Academic Press, New York.

Herberman, R. B., 1984, Immune surveillance hypothesis: Updated formulation and possible effector mechanisms, in "Immunology 1983", T. Tada, ed., Academic Press, New York, (1984).

Kasahara, K., Djeu, J. Y., Dougherty, S. F., and Oppenheim, J. J., 1983,Capacity of human large granular lymphocytes to produce multiple lymphokines: Interleukin 2, interferon, and colony stimulating factor, J. Immunol., 131:2379.

Mitchison, N. A., Regulation of the response to cell surface
    antigens, in: "Current Trends in Tumor Immunology", S.
    Ferrone, S. Gorini, R. B. Herberman and R. A. Reisfeld, eds.,
    Garland STPM Press, New York (1979).

Nanni, P., De Giovanni, C., Lollini, P. L., Nicoletti, G., and
    Prodi, G., 1983, TS/A: a new metastatizating cell line
    originated from a BALB/c spontaneous mammary adenocarcinoma,
    Clin. Expl. Metastasis, 1:373.

Santoni, A., Piccoli, M., Ortaldo, J. R., and Herberman, R. B.,
    1984, Changes in number and density of large granular
    lymphocytes upon in vivo augmentation of mouse natural killer
    activity, J. Immunol., in press.

Sarzotti, M., Giovarelli, M., and Forni, G., 1982, Interferon
    production in mixed cultures of murine leukocytes and
    syngeneic L1210 leukemia cells, Boll. Ist. Sieroter. Mil.,
    147:1314.

Schrier, P.I., Bernards, R., Vaessen, R. T. M. J., Houweling, A.,
    and van der Eb, A.J., 1983, Expression of class I major
    histocompatibility antigen switched off by highly oncogenic
    adenovirus 12 in transformed rat cells, Nature, 305:771.

Trinchieri, G., and Santoli, D., 1978, Anti viral activity induced
    by culturing lymphocytes with tumor derived or virus
    transformed cells. Enhancement of human natural killer cell
    activity by interferon and antagonistic inhibition of
    susceptibility of target cells to lysis, J. Exp. Med.,
    147:1314.

Varesio, L., Giovarelli, M., Landolfo, S., and Forni, G., 1979,
    Suppression of proliferative response and lymphokine release
    during the progression of a spontaneous tumor, Cancer Res.,
    39:4983.

Varesio, L., Landolfo, S., Giovarelli, M., and Forni, G., 1980,
    The macrophage as the social interconnection within the
    immune system, Dev. Comp. Immunol., 4:11.

Wagner, H., Hard, C., Heeg, K, Rollinghoff, M., and Pfizenmaier,
    K., 1980, T cell derived helper factor allows in vivo
    induction of cytotoxic T cells in nu/nu mice, Nature,
    284:278.

HYPORESPONSIVENESS OF NATURAL KILLER ACTIVITY INDUCED IN VIVO BY

MULTIPLE TREATMENT WITH MALEIC ACID ANHYDRIDE DIVINYL ETHER (MVE-2)

Mario Piccoli, Angela Santoni, Francesca Velotti,
M. Cristina Galli, Luigi Frati and Michael A. Chirigos[o]

Istituto di Patologia Generale, Università di Roma,
viale Regina Elena, 324 00161 Roma - Italy
[o] Immunopharmacology Section, BTB, BRMP, NCI, FCRF
Frederick MD - USA

INTRODUCTION

The immunomodulators include a variety of biological and chemical compounds whose mechanisms of action involve the individual's own biological responses. A modifier of the immune response should possess the following requirements:
-lack of carcinogenicity or tumor enhancing influence;
-no antigenicity;
-defined effects on the components of the immune system;
-known pharmacology;
-low experimental and clinical toxicity.

Interest in immunomodulators has gained popularity such as immunotherapeutic treatment for a large number of diseases as cancer, viral and bacterial infections, as well as immunodeficiencies etc.. Although the ability of specific stimulation of immune response with antigen bearing tumor cells or non specific stimulation with viruses, bacteria and adjuvant type compounds has been demonstrated in many experimental and human systems (Mathe' 1978, Rosenberg et al. 1977), clear to investigators should be some problems related to the relative purity of the biological and chemical agents and to the specificity of the reactions that are being stimulated.

175

A main role of the immune system in host defence against neoplasia is widely demonstrated. However, in tumor-bearing hosts immunosurveillance is impaired by the disease itself and by cytoreductive therapy. In the last years a large body of evidence has described the attempts of cancer therapists to reconstitute the depressed humoral and cellular immune responses by treatment with several biological response modifiers (BRMs). The restoration of immune response may be crucial for the successful control of neoplasia and for the prevention of secondary infectious diseases. However the mechanisms by which the immunomodulating agents interact with the several components of immune response are still largely unknown.

In the last years we have been particularly interested in one of these immunomodulators: maleic anhydride divinyl ether (MVE-2),previously known also as pyran copolymer (Chirigos et al. 1982), a powerful interferon inducer and stimulator of Reticulo Endothelial System (RES). A series of synthesized maleic anhydride divinyl ether polyanions, of molecular weights ranging from 12,500 to 52,600 has been reported to be able to enhance macrophage tumoricidal function and natural killer activity (Chirigos et al.1983). Treatment with pyran copolymer, a mixture of MVEs with an average molecular weight of 18,000 resulted both in augmentation and in inhibition of NK activity depending on timing, route of inoculation (Santoni et al.1980). Results of phase I studies in which MVE-2 was administered on a weekly basis for 4 or more courses demonstrated an increase of NK and K cell function (Reinhart J.J. et al.1982, Rios et al.1982). Recently, testing the efficacy of a single versus multiple treatments with MVE-2, we have found that repeated injections of this agent led to an hyporesponsiveness of NK cells whereas macrophage activity remains high (Piccoli et al.1984).

We undertake the present study to better understand the mechanisms underlying the hyporesponsiveness of NK cells induced by multiple treatment with MVE-2. In particular we tested: 1. the possibility to reverse the low NK reactivity by in vivo or in vitro treatment with NK augmenting agents such as interferon (IFN) or IFN-inducers or interleukin-2 (IL-2); 2. the effect of a single versus multiple treatment on large granular lymphocytes (LGLs), a subpopulation of lymphoid cells recently associated with natural killer activity with a characteristic morphology: large lymphocytes with an indented nucleus and azurophilic granules in the cytoplasm (Timonen et al.1981).

MATERIALS AND METHODS

Mice

Specific pathogen-free (SPF) inbred BALB/C and (C57BL/6xC3H)-F1 (B6C3F1) hybrid mice were obtained from the Animal Production Area, NCI-Frederick Cancer Research Facility, Frederick, MD, and mantained in SPF conditions.

Reagents

C. parvum (CN 6134) was kindly provided by Dr. R. Tuttle, Burroughs Wellcome Inc., Research Triangle Park, NC. Maleic vinyl ether-2 (MVE-2) and poly inosinic-poly cytidylic acid complexed with poly-L-lysine and carboxymethyl cellulose (Poly ICLC) were kindly provided by Dr. M.A.Chirigos, NCI FCRF Frederick MD., IFN, purchased from Enzo Biochem. Inc., New York, was a mixture of both alpha and beta IFN produced following infection of mouse fibroblasts by Newcastle disease virus partially purified, with a specific activity of 2.3×10^{7} U/mg protein); IL-2 was obtained by Collaborative Research Inc.. This IL-2 was prepared from conditioned medium of cultures of Concanavalin A-stimulated rat splenocytes and was partially purified by ammonium sulfate precipitation and ion-exchange chromatography.

"In vivo" augmentation of NK activity

Appropriate concentrations of C. parvum, MVE-2, Poly ICLC or IFN were administrated i.p. in Hanks' balanced salt solution (BSS). Mice from each group were killed at various times after treatment and their spleens were pooled before separation procedures or testing for NK activity.

"In vitro" augmentation of NK activity

   1-2 x 10^6 spleen cells were incubated at 37°C for 18 hrs with 10^3 U/ml of IFN or 6 U/ml of IL-2.

Effector cell preparations

   Spleen cells were prepared as described by De Landazuri et al.(1973). Removal of adherent cells was performed by passage through a nylon column according to the method of Julius et al.(1973).

Discontinuous Percoll density gradient centrifugation

   Spleen cells depleted of adherent cells were fractionated by centrifugation on a discontinuous density gradient of Percoll (Pharmacia Chemicals, Uppsala, Sweden), by a modification (Kumagai et al.1982, Luini et al.1981) of the original method of Timonen and Saksela (1981). Growth medium and Percoll were adjusted to 290 mOsmol/kg H_2O with sterile distilled water and 10x concentrated phosphate-buffered saline (PBS) (pH 7.4), respectively. Seven different concentrations of Percoll in medium were prepared, with the top fraction having 38.6% Percoll, the next having 47.6% (F.1) and the subsequent fractions having graded increases of 4.5% until the last fraction (F.6) of 70.1%. After a careful layering of the gradient into 15 ml conical test tubes, 5×10^7 nonadherent spleen cells were placed on the top of gradient and the tube was centrifuged at 300xg for 40 min at room temperature. The fractions were collected with a Pasteur pipette from the top and were washed once with RPMI 1640 medium plus 5% fetal bovine serum. Recovery of the cells was $\simeq$ 80% of the original input, and the viability was greater than 95%.

Cytochemical staining

   For the morphologic analysis of the effector cell population, 2×10^5 lymphocytes on 0.2 ml of medium were centrifuged for 7 min at 900 rpm on to microscope slides by using a Cytospin (Shandon Instruments Co., Bewickley, PA) centrifuge. Air-dried preparations were fixed for 10 min in methanol and stained for 25 min with 10% Giemsa (Fisher Scientific Company, Fairlawn, N.J.) diluted in pH 7.4 phosphate-buffered distilled water. Morphologic differential count were obtained by inspection of the slides by oil immersion microscopy. At last 200 cells were analyzed on each slide.

Cytotoxicity assay (Cromium Release Assay - CRA)

Various concentrations of effector cells were incubated with 5×10^3 ^{51}Cr-labeled target cells ($100 \mu Ci/5 \times 10^6$ cells, 37 °C water bath, 1hr) for 4 hr at 37 °C in round-bottomed 96-well plastic microtiter plates. After incubation the supernatant was removed by the Titertek automatic harvesting system and counted in a Y-scintillation counter. All combinations were performed in quadruplicate. YAC-1, a tissue culture cell line of YAC, a Moloney-virus induced lymphoma of A/Sn origin, was used as the target for NK activity. Baseline ^{51}Cr-release was determined by use of unlabeled autologous target cells in place of lymphoid cells. Standard errors were less than 2% and are not included in the tables. The percent cytotoxicity was calculated as follows:

$$\frac{\text{cpm released from exp. group-cpm released from autol. control}}{\text{total cpm incorporated}} \times 100$$

Tests were always performed with multiple ratios of effector: target (E:T) cells and the differences in results shown in the Figure at one E:T ratio were paralleled by those at other ratios.

RESULTS

We have previously reported the lack of NK boosting following repeated injections with MVE-2 (Piccoli et al. 1984). In an attempt to understand the mechanisms underlying the development of NK hyporesponsiveness to MVE-2, we tested the possibility to reconstitute the low levels of cytotoxic activity observed in the

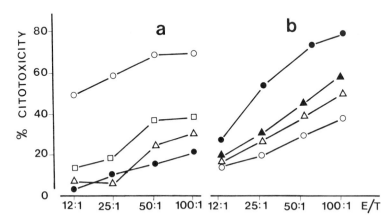

Fig. 1.   Susceptibility of spleen cells from mice repeatedly trea-
          ted with MVE-2 to in vivo augmentation by Poly ICLC or C.
          parvum.

Panel a. NK activity of spleen cells from normal 7 - 9 week-old
BALB/c mice (●) or BALB/c mice which have received one (day -3)(○)
two (day -17,-10)(□) or three (day -17,-10,-3)(▲) injections of
MVE-2 (25 mg/Kg,ip) was tested in a 4 hrs CRA against YAC-1 targets
at various E/T ratios.

Panel b. NK activity of spleen cells from BAL/c mice treated with
C. parvum (0.7 mg/muose, ip, day -3)(●) or MVE-2 (day -17,-10) and
C. parvum (day -3)(○) or Poly ICLC (4 mg/Kg, ip, day -1)(▲) or
MVE-2 (day -17,-10) and Poly ICLC (day -1)(▲) was tested in a 4 hrs
CRA against YAC-1 targets at various E/T ratios.

spleen of mice repeatedly treated with MVE-2, by in vivo treatment
with other NK boosting agents such as C. parvum or Poly ICLC
(Fig.1). C. parvum was not effective in increasing the low levels
of NK augmentation in mice which had received 2 weekly treatments
with MVE-2. In contrast, the additional treatment with Poly ICLC
to   these   mice   resulted in higher NK cell cytotoxicity,
significantly higher than in those which had received 3 treatments
with MVE-2. These results prompted us to examine whether a similar
response could be achieved by in vitro treatment of spleen cells
from mice which have received two inoculations of MVE-2, with
either alpha/beta -IFN or IL-2 (Fig.2). Both IFN and IL-2 failed
to augment in vitro the NK activity of spleen cells from mice
repeatedly injected with MVE-2, suggesting that overstimulation by
MVE-2 can exhaust the precursor pool of NK cells inhibiting their
maturation.

   To consider the possibility that multiple treatment with
MVE-2 could exert inhibitory effects directly on NK cells or their
precursors, we studied the association of cytotoxic activity with
the presence of LGLs in the spleen of mice treated with a single
or multiple injections of this agent (Fig.3). Augmentation of
cytotoxic activity 3 days after a single MVE-2 treatment was
accompanied by a marked increase of LGLs number. However, repeated
injections of the drug resulted in a lower number of LGL as
compared to that observed following a single treatment.

DISCUSSION

   In the present study we have attempted to explain the
development of hyporesponsiveness of NK cells following multiple
injections with MVE-2. Mice which had received 2 treatments with
MVE-2 did not show NK boosting, not only to a subsequent injection
of this drug, but also of C. parvum, a potent NK cell augmenting
agent (Ojo et al.1978). Moreover spleen cells from mice repeatedly
treated with MVE-2 were not susceptible to in vitro treatment with
NK activating factors such as IFN or IL-2. However, Poly ICLC,
another known NK boosting agent (Djeu et al.1979), was capable of
augmenting NK activity in hyporesponsive mice.

   At last three possibilities may be considered to explain the
lack of NK boosting: 1. induction of suppressor cells in the

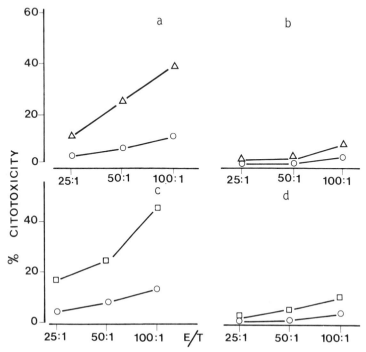

Fig. 2.   Susceptibility of spleen cells from mice repeatedly
treated with MVE-2 to in vitro augmentation by IL-2
or $\alpha - \beta -$ IFN.

NK activity of spleen cells from normal 7-9 week old B6C3F$_1$ mice
(panel a) or from B6C3F$_1$ treated with MVE-2 (25mg/kg ip, day-
17,-10) (panel b) after overnight incubation at 37°C with medium
(O) or with IL-2 (△) was tested in a 4hrs CRA against YAC-1 targets at various E/T ratios.

NK activity of spleen cells from normal 7-9 week-old B6C3F$_1$ mice
(panel c) or from B6C3F$_1$ treated with MVE-2 (25mg/Kg, ip, day-17
-10) (panel d) after overnight incubation at 37°C with medium
(O) or with IFN (□) was tested in a 4hrs CRA against YAC-1 targets
at various E/T ratios.

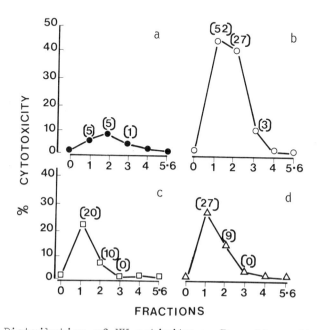

Fig. 3.   Distribution of NK activity on Percoll gradient after
           single or multiple treatment with MVE-2.

Spleen cells from normal 7-9 week old BALB/c mice (●) or from
BALB/c which have received one (day-3), (O), two (day-17 -10)
(■) or three injections (day-17,-10, -3) (△) with MVE-2 (25mg/Kg
ip) were separated and then tested for NK activity (E/T ratio 50:1)
and for the percentage of LGL (numbers in parenthesis).

spleen of repeatedly treated mice; 2. production of prostaglandins
E (PGE), which are known to inhibit NK cytotoxicity (Droller et
al.1978); 3. inhibition of NK cell maturation with exhaustion of
NK cells or their precursors.

We tend to rule out the first possibility since preliminary
results obtained in mixture experiments demonstrated that adherent
spleen cells from repeatedly treated mice were not capable of
inhibiting NK lysis of normal effector cells.

Prostaglandins E are reported to be produced and secreted by
peritoneal macrophages incubated in the presence of MVE-2
(Chirigos et al.1983). However, it is still unclear whether this
mechanism of inhibition is operative in vivo. Moreover, recent
findings by Leung and Koren (1982) have shown that "activated" NK
cells are quite resistant to inhibition by PGE2. To better explore
the role of PGE in the establishment of NK cell
hyporesponsiveness, experiments in which inhibitors of PGE
synthesis, such as aspirin or indomethacin are administered in
vivo, should be performed to analyze whether this treatment is
effective in recovering NK activity.

Consistent with the third possibility is the observation that
reduced levels of cytotoxic activity by spleen cells from
repeatedly treated mice were associated with a reduced number of
LGLs compared to that observed in the spleen of mice treated with
a single injection of MVE-2 (Fig.3). However, these results are in
contrast with the boosting of NK activity seen in hyporesponsive
mice following in vivo treatment with Poly ICLC. This indicates
that a variety of mechanisms might be responsible for the
augmentation of NK activity in vivo and the phenomenon is quite
complex and needs further investigation.

The lack of a sustained or cyclic augmentation of NK activity
by multiple treatment with MVE-2 are consistent with the previous
results of clinical trials with IFN where the treatment did not
induce NK boosting, but was rather associated with a depression of
NK activity in a substantial proportion of patients (Maluish et
al. 1983). Recent results from mouse experiments also show that
multiple injections with IFN do not augment NK cytotoxicity, but
rather reduce this activity as compared to the effect obtained
with a single treatment (Bruley-Rosset et al. 1983).

The overall findings emphasize the necessity to determine the pharmacokinetics of Biological Response Modifiers to establish the most effective treatment protocols which sustains augmented NK activity. Such a protocol would be expected to be most effective for the treatment of neoplasia and immunodeficiency diseases.

REFERENCES

Bruley-Rosset M., Rappaport H. (1983)
Natural killer cell activity and spontaneous lymphoma development.
Effects of single and multiple injections of interferon in young
and aged C57Bl/6 mice. Int. J. Cancer 31, 381.

Chirigos M.A., Mastrangelo M.J. (1982)
Immunorestoration by chemicals. In Immunological Approaches to
Cancer Therapeutics, E. Mihich Ed, J. Wiley & Sons, New York, 191.

Chirigos M.A., Schlick E., Piccoli M., Read E., Hartung K.,
Bartocci A. (1983)
Characterization of Agents. In Advances in Immunopharmacology, J.
Hadden et al. Eds. Pergamon Press, 669.

De Landazuri M.O. and R.B. Herberman (1973)
Immune response to Gross virus-induced lymphoma. III.
Characterization of the cellular immune response. J. Natl. Cancer
Inst. 49, 147.

Djeu J.Y., Heinbaugh J.A., Holden H.T. and R.B. Herberman (1979)
Augmentation of mouse natural killer cell activity by interferon
and interferon inducers. J. Immunol. 122, 175.

Droller M.J., Schneider M.V. and P. Perlman (1978)
A possible role of prostaglandins in natural and
antibody-dependent lymphocyte mediated cytotoxicity against tumor
cells. Cell. Immunol. 37, 165.

Julius M.H., Simpson E., Herzenberg L.A. (1973)
A rapid method for the isolation of functional thymus derived
murine lymphocytes. Eur. J. Immunol. 3, 645.

Kumagai K., Itoh K., Suzuki R., Hiruma S. and F. Saitoh (1982)
Studies of murine large granular lymphocytes. I. Identification as
effector cell in NK and K cytotoxicities. J. Immunol. 129, 2788.

Leung K.H., Koren H.S. (1982)
Regulation of human natural killing. II. Protective effect of
interferon on NK cells from suppression of PGE . J. Immunol. 129,
1742.

Luini W., Boraschi D., Alberti S., Aleotti A. and A. Tagliabue
(1981)
Morphological characterization of a cell population responsible
for natural killer activity. Immunology 127, 282.

Maluish A.E., Coulon J., Ortaldo J.R., Sherwin S.A., Seavitt R.,
Fein S., Weirnick P., Oldham R.K. and R.B. Herberman (1982)
Modulation of NK and monocyte activity in advanced cancer patients
receiving interferon. In Interferons, T.C. Merigan &R.M. Friedman
Eds. Academic Press, New York, 377.

Mathe' G. (1978)
Immunotherapy: experimental and rational basis. In Immunotherapy
of human cancer, M.D. Anderson Ed, Raven Press New York, 5.

Ojo E., Haller O., Kimura A. and H. Wigzell (1978)
An analysis of conditions allowing corynebacterium parvum to cause
either augmentation or inhibition of natural cell activity against
tumor cells in mice. Int. J. Cancer 21, 444.

Piccoli M., Saito T., and M.A. Chirigos (1984)
Bimodal effects of MVE-2 on cytotoxic activity of Natural Killer

cell and macrophage tumoricidal activity. Int. J. Immunopharmacol. in press.

Reinhart J.J., Wilson H.F., Neidhart J.A. (1982)
Phase I evaluation of MVE-2 in man. Proc. Am. Soc. Clin. Oncol. 1, 37 (C-145)

Rios A., Rosenblum M.L., Powell M. and E. Hersh (1982)
Phase I. Study with MVE-2 therapy in human cancer. Proc. Am. Soc. Clin. Oncol. 1, 37 (c-146).

Rosenberg S.A., Terry W.D. (1977)
Passive immunotherapy of cancer in animals and in man. Adv. Cancer Res. 25, 323

Santoni A., Riccardi C., Barlozzari T. and R.B. Herberman (1980)
Suppression of activity of mouse natural killer (NK) cells by activated macrophages from mice treated with pyran copolymer. Int. J. Cancer 26, 837.

Timonen T., Saksela E., Ranki A. and P. Hayry (1981)
Characteristics of human large granular lymphocytes and relationship to natural killer and K cells. J. Exp. Med. 153, 569.

EPSTEIN-BARR VIRUS MARKERS IN NASOPHARYNGEAL CARCINOMA

Alberto Faggioni, Giuseppe Barile, Mario Piccoli and
Luigi Frati

Istituto di Patologia Generale, Università degli Studi
di Roma "La Sapienza"

Nasopharyngeal carcinoma (NPC) is, along with Burkitt's lymphoma (BL), one of the two human cancers which are thought to be associated with the Epstein-Barr virus (EBV), the etiological agent of infectious mononucleosis. The EBV was first discovered by M.A. Epstein in a Burkitt's lymphoma (Epstein et al., 1964), and its association with NPC was casual, when testing for anti-EBV antibodies sera of BL patients and using nasopharyngeal carcinoma sera as controls, it was seen that both series of sera contained high levels of EBV antibodies (Old et al., 1966). Now the constant presence of EBV DNA in the tumor tissue strenghtens this association of EBV with NPC.

NPC represents a leading cause of death for large populations in south-east Asia. It is one of the three most common tumors in southern chinese males and it is not uncommon in northern Africa. Worldwide there are areas with a strong incidence of the disease and areas in which it is almost unknown; this fact suggests that EBV, which is an ubiquitous virus, could be only one of the etiologic agents, along with genetic and environmental factors. One of the unsolved questions is how the EBV genome become associated with the carcinoma cells. There may exist epithelial cells in the nasopharynx which have EBV receptors and therefore are infectible or transformable. Recently, evidence has been obtained which suggests that salivary glands may be a habitat, aside of B lymphocytes, in which EBV persists permanently after the primary infec-

tion. Another possibility is that viral genomes may be introduced into nasopharyngeal epithelial cells by fusion. Enveloped virus particles of EBV genome-carrying lymphocytes, that are inter-
mittently present in the nasopharynx of viral carriers, might be
merged with nasopharyngeal epithelial cells during infection by
parainfluenza or other viruses known to cause cellular fusion.
Glaser et al. (1975, 1977) obtained in this manner somatic cell
hybrids of lymphoid cells and human and murine epithelial cells;
Bayliss and Wolf (1980) have shown that even EBV alone might be
able to enter epithelial cells by such a process, since at high
multiplicity it causes cell fusion of various cells independent
of virus-receptors.

It is most likely that, in addition to EBV, various other
factors play important roles in the emergence of NPC. A strict
genetic disposition among the Chinese has been shown by Ho et al.
(1972) and Simons et al. (1975) demonstrated the frequent association of a particular HLA type (Singapore-2) with the disease in
Malaysian patients. That environmental carcinogens may play a role in NPC development is suggested by the fact that Chinese born
in the United States have a lower risk for the disease than those
who have migrated there (King and Haenszel, 1972). Traces of di-
methylnitrosamines were found in salted fish, and this could play
a role in NPC etiology, as Huang and associates (1978) succeeded
in inducing carcinomas in the nasal and paranasal regions of rats
fed with extracts of salted fish. Extracts derived from Croton ti-
glium, Euphorbia lathyris, Croton megalocarpus and Jatropa curcas,
compounds present in high-NPC areas and used as herbal medicines,
have been found to increase the transforming efficiency of EBV by
10-fold, and to induce the EBV cycle and bind to the same receptor as did the 12-0-tetradecanoylphorbol-13-acetate, perhaps triggering the event that leads to EBV induction (Ito et al., 1981).
Similarly, Faggioni et al. (in press) have shown that the alkylat-
ing agent N-methyl-N-nitro-N-nitrosoguanidine (MNNG) is able to
enhance EBV transformation and antigen expression. Based on these
findings a closer review of the association of environmental carcinogens or tumor promoters in affected geographical areas should
be recommended. Attempts should be made to remove the carcinogen
from one geographical portion of that territory and to monitor
the population of the entire area for any changes in NPC incidence.

The EBV association with NPC is based on EBV serology and on

Table 1. Compilation of the most important specific and unspecific
         immunologic methods for describing the immune defense of
         the tumor carrier against the tumor.

Specific Testing	Unspecific Testing
- antibody dependent cellular cytotoxicity test (ADCC)	- T and B lymphocytes in the peripheral blood and tumor tissue
- EBV serology	- Intracellular immunoglobins in the tumor tissue
- macrophage inhibition test (MIT)	- granulocyte phagocytosis test (NBT)
- specific intracutaneous tests (NPC-membrane antigen)	- unspecific intracutaneous testing of the delayed type immune reaction.

the presence of EBV DNA in the tumor tissue. The initial immunofluorescence test was shown to detect viral capsid antigen (VCA).
Subsequently it was noted by Henle et al. (1971) that virus from
a producer culture of BL cells induced in cells from a nonproducer
culture an abortive cycle of viral replication in which two early
antigens, the diffuse (D) and restricted (R) components, were synthesized but not VCA. Antibodies to VCA, D and R are titrated by
the indirect immunofluorescence technique which also serves to i-
dentify the immunoglobulin class (IgG, IgM or IgA) of the reactive
antibodies. Reedman and Klein (1973) discovered the EBV-associated nuclear antigen (EBNA), which is present in every EBV transformed cell and can be detected only by the highly sensitive anti-
complement immunofluorescence technique. In addition, there are
early and late EBV determined cell membrane antigens (EMA and LMA)
which are detected on live cells by immunofluorescence tests. Antibodies to MA are partly identical with EBV neutralizing antibodies and antibodies reactive in the antibody dependent cellular
cytotoxicity (ADCC) reaction. The most important of these appears
to be the antibody response to the diffuse (D) component of the

EBV induced early antigen (EA) complex and the IgA antibody titers
to viral capsid antigens (VCA) and to a lesser extent to D (Henle
and Henle, 1978; Pearson et al., 1980). Studies primarily on Chinese patients with NPC have established the potential clinical
importance of these antibody response patterns to EBV-associated
antigens (Henle et al., 1977).

    The IgA antibodies to EBV have been useful to detect NPC pat-
ients before the onset of the disease. Lanier et al. (1980) found
IgA to VCA in a serum sample taken 22 months before the clinical
diagnosis of NPC was made. In two serological surveys involving a
total of 148.000 individuals, aged 30 or more, were detected by
means of an immunoenzymatic test, 1267 IgA/VCA positive individuals who were clinically examined. Of these, 230 were biopsied;
NPC diagnosis was established early in 46 cases, and 18 months
later in 12 more cases (Zeng et al., 1980). Desgranges et al.
(1982) found 64 Chinese individuals exhibiting IgA antibodies to
EBV for 18 months and presenting nasopharyngeal abnormalities. At
biopsy, 4 nasopharyngeal carcinomas, two at a very early stage,
were detected. In 14 further individuals, without clinical or his-
topathologica evidence of tumor, EBV/DNA internal repeats and/or
EBNA were detected in the biopsied mucosae. This fact suggests
that the presence of IgA/EBV antibodies and EBV markers in the nasopharyngeal mucosa may characterize pre-cancerous contitions.

    There have been few studies directed primarily in the role
of cell-mediated immunity (CMI) to EBV-associated antigens in NPC.
Although the role of CMI in the control of viral infections (Notkins, 1974) and malignancy (Hellstrom and Hellstrom, 1969) has
been considered to be of great importance, there are relatively
few studies specifically related to EBV CMI in NPC patients due
to the difficulty and the high cost in producing large amounts of
virus and for the characterization of standardized antigens. An
additional difficulty has been the concentration of NPC patients
in areas where there has been a relative scarcity of reserach laboratories interested in developing studies of CMI. While most
studies have been of a pilot nature involving less than twenty
patients, there have been some that provided intriguing suggestions as to areas needing further investigation. Based on the early
studies of Pearson et al. (1976), who showed that humoral antibody could trigger lymphocytes to kill EBV infected cells specifically, a series of reports indicated that the presence of ADCC

correlated with long-term survival to NPC (Levine et al., 1978; Pearson et al., 1978; Chan et al., 1979). These observations have now been extended to several population groups and the predictive value of ADCC has been observed in Chinese, East African, Algerian (Ablashi et al., 1981), German and North American (Pearson et al., 1981) NPC patients.

In contrast to the apparent beneficial effect of certain sera on the CMI response, another serum factor has been identified which appears to abrogate the immune response of lymphocytes to EBV associated antigens. Designated lymphocyte stimulation inhibitor (LSI) and apparently associated with the IgA fraction (Sundar et al., 1982) this factor has been found thus far only in NPC patients with active disease (Kamaraju et al., 1982). A comparison of LSI activity with IgA antibodies to EBV VCA and IgG antibodies to VCA, EA, EBNA and MA (as measured in the ADCC assay) indicate that LSI is the most sensitive indicator of local/regional disease activity thus far reported, but may not be useful in detection of metastatic dissemination. A correlation of LSI and ADCC in 11 sera reported by Kamaraju et al. (1982) indicated the the two assays were measuring independent phenomena, and therefore although IgA has been associated with both the presence of LSI and the inhibition of ADCC, either there are additional factors influencing the assay or more than one IgA function is involved in these assays.

As international cooperation in the establishment of assays for CMI has developed, several groups have adapted more widely used in vitro assays to the direct study of lymphocyte response to EBV-related antigens in NPC. The assays used most consistently have been the lymphocyte stimulation assay (LS) and the leukocyte migration inhibition assay using as antigen either extracts from tumor cells (Ng et al., 1977), or relatively specific EBV antigens (Sundar et al., 1982). Because of the different antigens used, direct comparison of results between laboratories is not possible. There are general conclusions, however, that can be reached from these limited studies: a) while LMI and LS frequently correlate, they can also be discordant both in NPC patients and controls (Ng et al., 1977; Levine et al., 1981). The evidence thus far indicates that these assays are measuring different aspects of the cellular immune response to EBV, and is consistent with data obtained in other immunologic studies; and b) NPC patients appear to have

cellular immunity to EBV, and in the one study correlating disease
stage with LS response, a more pronounced reactivity to extracts
of tumor biopsies was suggested in patients with more advanced disease, a finding that was compatible with the longitudinal study
of skin test reactivity in NPC patients (Ho et al., 1978). One
other EBV CMI assay that was reported in a pilot study in NPC patients investigated the presence of T-cells with activity against
EBV (Chan and Chew, 1981) based on an assay developed by Moss et
al. (1978). Unlike the normal controls, NPC patients were unable
to generate EBV-specific cytotoxic T-cells.

In conclusion, it can be said that there is a bulk of evidence for the involvement of EBV in the development of NPC. Further
studies aimed to find animal models for NPC, which are still lacking, on the development of an EBV vaccine, in an attempt to prevent NPC in the high-risk areas, on the understanding how EBV can
enter in the epithelial nasopharyngeal cell, and on the possible
involvement of some onc-gene, are particularly needed.

REFERENCES

Ablashi, D., Allal, L., Armstrong, G., Bouguermou, A., Pearson,
    G., Levine, P., Bengali, Z., Easton, J., Zaghouani, S., Chou-
    ter, A. and Ghoudali, R., 1981, Some characteristics of Naso-
    pharyngeal carcinoma in Algeria, in: "Nasopharyngeal carcino-
    ma, Grundman et al. eds., Gustav Fischer Verlag, Stuttgart,
    New York, 157.
Bayliss, G.J. and Wolf, H., 1980, Epstein-Barr virus induced cell
    fusion. Nature, 287, 164.
Chan, S.H., Levine, P.H., DeThe', G., Mulroney, S., Lavoue, M.,
    Glen, S., Goh, E., Connelly, R., 1979, A comparison of the
    prognostic value of antibody dependent cellular cytotoxicity
    and other EBV antibodies in Chinese patients with nasopharyn-
    geal carcinoma. Int. J. Cancer, 23, 181
Chan, S.H. and Chew, T.S., 1981, Lack of regression in Epstein-
    Barr virus infected leukocyte cultures of nasopharyngeal car-
    cinoma patients. Lancet, 2, 1353.
Desgranges, C., Bornkamm, G., Zeng, Y., Wang, P., Zhu, J., Shang,
    M. and DeThe', G., 1982, Detection of Epstein-Barr viral DNA
    internal repeats in the nasopharyngeal mucosa of Chinese with
    IgA/EBV specific antibodies. Int. J. Cancer, 29, 87.
Epstein, M.A., Achong, B.G. and Barr, Y.M., 1964, Virus particles

in cultured lymphoblasts from Burkitt's lymphoma. Lancet, 1,7.

Faggioni, A., Ablashi, D., Armstrong, G., Dahlberg, J., Sundar, S., Rice, J. and Donovan, P., Enhancing effect of N-methyl-N-nitro -N-nitrosoguanidine (MNNG) on Epstein-Barr virus (EBV) replication and comparison of short term and continuous TPA treatment of producer and nonproducer cells for EBV antigen induction and/or stimulation. In: "Nasopharyngeal carcinoma: current concepts", Prasad et al. eds., in press.

Glaser, R., Nonoyama, M., Shows, T.B., Henle, G., Henle, W., 1975 Epstein-Barr virus: Studies on the association of virus genome with human chromosomes in hybrid cells. In: "Oncogenesis and Herpesviruses II, DeThe' et al. eds., IARC, Lyon, 457.

Glaser, R., Ablashi, D., Nonoyama, M., Henle, W., Easton, J., Fellows, C., Armstrong, G., 1977, Enhanced oncogenic behaviour of human and mouse cells following cellular hybridization with Burkitt's tumor cells. Proc.Natl.Acad.Sci. USA, 74, 2574.

Hellstrom, K.E., and Hellstrom, I., 1969, Cellular immunity against tumor antigens. Adv. Cancer Research, 12, 167.

Henle, G. and Henle, W., 1966, Immunofluorescence in cells derived from Burkitt's lymphoma. J. Bact., 91, 1248.

Henle, G., Henle, W., and Klein, G., 1971, Demonstration of two distinct components in the early antigen complex of Epstein-Barr virus infected cells. Int. J. Cancer, 8, 272.

Henle, W., Ho, H., Henle, G., Chan, J, Kwan, H., 1977, Nasopharyngeal carcinoma: significance of changes in Epstein-Barr virus related antibody patterns following therapy. Int. J. Cancer, 20, 663.

Henle, W., Henle, G., 1978, The immunological approach to study of possible virus-induced human malignancies using the Epstein-Barr virus as an example. Prog. Expt. Tumor Res., 21, 19.

Ho, J.H.C., 1972, Nasopharyngeal carcinoma. Adv. Cancer Res. 15, 7.

Ho, J.H.C., Chau, J., Tse, K.C., Levine, P.H., 1978, In vivo cell mediated immunity in Chinese patients with nasopharyngeal carcinoma. In: "Nasopharyngeal carcinoma: etiology and control" DeThe' et al. eds., IARC, Lyon, 545.

Huang, D.P., Ho, J.H.C., Saw, D., and Teoh, T.B., 1978, Carcinoma of the nasal and paranasal regions in rats fed with Cantonese salted marine fish. In: "Nasopharyngeal carcinoma: etiology and control", DeThe' et al. eds., IARC, Lyon, 315.

Ito, Y., Yanase, S., Fujita, J., Harayama, T., Takashima, M., and Imanaka, H., 1981, A short term in vitro assay for promoter substances using human lymphoblastoid cells latently infected with Epstein-Barr virus. Cancer Lett., 13, 29.

Lanier, A.P., Henle, W., Bender, T.R., Henle, G. and Talbot, M.L., 1980, Epstein-Barr virus specific antibody titers in seven A-laskan natives before and after diagnosis of nasopharyngeal carcinoma. Int. J. Cancer, 26, 133.

Levine, P.H., DeThe', G., Brugere, J., Schwabb, G., Mourali, N., Herbermann, R., Ambrosioni, J., Revol, P., 1978, Delayed hypersensitivity reactions of cancer patients to antigens of lymphoid cell lines. Int. J. Cancer, 22, 400.

Levine, P.H., Pizza, G., Cannon, G., Ablashi, D., Armstrong, G., Viza, D., 1981, Cell-Mediated immunity to Epstein-Barr virus associated membrane antigens in patients with nasopharyngeal carcinoma. In: "Nasopharyngeal carcinoma", Grundmann et al., eds., Springer Fischer Verlag, Stuttgrart, New York, 137.

Kamaraju, L., Levine, P., Sundar, S., Ablashi, D., Faggioni, A., Armstrong, G., Bertram, G. and Krueger, G., 1983, Epstein-Barr virus related lymphocyte stimulation inhibitor. A possible prognostic tool for nasopharyngeal carcinoma. JNCI, 70, 643.

King, H. and Heinszel, K., 1972, Cancer mortality among foreign and native born Chinese in the United States. J. Chronic. Dis. 26, 623.

Moss, D.J., Rickinson, A.B. and Pope, J.H., 1978, Long term T-cell mediated immunity to EBV in man. I. Complete regression of virus induced transformation in cultures of seropositive donor leukocytes. Int. J. Cancer, 22, 662.

Ng, W.S., Ng, M.H., Ho, H.C., Lamelin, P., 1977, In vitro immune response to PPD extracts from Raji cells and nasopharyngeal carcinoma biopsies in nascpharyngeal carcinoma leukocytes. Br. J. Cancer, 36, 713.

Notkins, A.L., 1974, Immune mechanisms by which the spread of viral infections is stopped. Cell. Immunol., 11, 478.

Old, J.L, Boyse, E.A., Oettgen, H.F., Geering, G., Williamson, B., Clifford, P., 1966, Precipitating antibody in human serum to an antigen present in cultured Burkitt's lymphoma cells. Proc. Natl.Acad.Sci. USA, 56, 1699.

Pearson, G. and Orr, T.W., 1976, Antibody dependent cellular cytotoxicity against cells expressing Epstein-Barr virus antigens. JNCI, 56, 485.

Pearson, G., Johanson, B. and Klein, G., 1978, Antibody dependent cellular cytotoxicity against Epstein-Barr virus associated antigens in African patients with nasopharyngeal carcinoma. Int. J. Cancer, 22, 120.

Pearson, G., Weiland, L., Neel, H.B., 1981, Evaluation of antibodies to EBV in the diagnosis of American nasopharyngeal carcinoma. In: "Nasopharyngeal Carcinoma", Grundmann et al, eds., Gustav Fischer Verlag, Stuttgart, New York, 231.

Reedman, B.M. and Klein, G., 1973, Cellular localization of an EBV associated complement fixing antigen in producer and non producer lymphoblastoid cell lines. Int. J. Cancer, 11, 499.

Simons, M.J., Wee, G.B., Chan, S., Shanmugaratnam, K., Day, N., DeThe', G., 1975, Probable identification on an HLA second-locus antigen associated with an high risk of a nasopharyngeal carcinoma, Lancet, 1, 142.

Sundar, S., Ablashi, D., Kamaraju, L., Levine, P.H., Faggioni, A., Armstrong, G., Pearson, G., Krueger, G., Hewetson, J., Bertram, G., Sestherhenn, K. and Menezes, J., 1982, Sera from patients with undifferentiated nasopharyngeal carcinoma contain a factor which abrogates specific Epstein-Barr virus antigen induced lymphocyte response. Int. J. Cancer, 29, 407.

Zeng, Yi., Liu, Yuxi., Liu, Chunren, Chen, S., Wei, J., Zhu, J., Zai, H., 1980, Application of an immunoenzymatic and an immunoradiographic method for a mass survey of nasopharyngeal carcinoma. Intervirology, 13, 162.

INTERFERON-MEDIATED REGULATION OF THE NK TARGET STRUCTURES OF NORMAL OR LYMPHOMA CELLS

G. Graziani, C. Grandori, B. Macchi, S. Pastore,
E. Bonmassar, and A. Giuliani Bonmassar

Department of Experimental Medicine and Biochemical
Sciences, Second University of Rome, Rome, Italy
Institute of General Pathology, Viale Regina Elena 324
Rome 00161 Italy

It is well know that Interferon (IF) has antitumor activity presumably based on different mechanisms of action. This class of compounds is capable of inhibiting the growth of neoplastic cells (1), and of enhancing the cytotoxic activity mediated by natural killer (NK) lymphocytes (2,3) and by activated macrophages (4). However, additional studies have shown that a decrease of the susceptibility of normal or neoplastic cells to NK attack occurs after in vitro pretreatment with IF (5,9). These findings indicate that IF interacts in some way with NK target structures (NKTS) on the cell membrane, modifying their expression, or affinity, for effector lymphocytes. A number of studies pointed out that IF pretreatment of the target produces a profound influence on the antigenic makeup of tumor cells, increasing the expression of histocompatibility antigens specified by the major histocompatibility complex (MHC) both in mice (10) and in humans (11, 13). More detailed studies showed that two subsets of class II Molecules specified by DR and DC loci of human MHC, are differentially susceptible to IF-mediated modulation. DC products were found to be increased more than DR products under the influence of gamma-IF (14). These observations prompted us to investigate whether IF would also be able to produce differential effects on distinct subsets of NKTS. Actually, the results of the present paper support this hypothesis and suggest that different cell lines contain non-cross reacting NKTS susceptible to IF-mediated modulation.

MATERIAL AND METHODS

Animals

Six-to ten-week old congenitally athymic mice of the strain
BALB/c/A/BOM Cr, nude strain of BALB/c background (hereafter
referred to as BALB/c-nu/nu) originally obtained from the NCI were
bred in a closed but not strictly inbred colony at the Institute
of Pharmacology, University of Perugia, Perugia, Italy, in a
pathogenfree environment.

Tumor

A tissue-culture cell line of YAC, a Moloney virus-induced
lymphoma of A/Sn origin, YAC-1(15)(hereafter referred to as YAC)
was used as the target for NK activity. Tumor cells were maintained
as stationary suspension cultures in medium RPM1 1640 supplemented
with 10% fetal calf serum (FCS) and 2mM glutamine from Grand
Island Biological Co., Grand Island, N.Y., USA, and 1% gentamycin
sulphate reagent solution (Schering Corp., Kenilworth, N.J., USA).
L929 cells a continous mouse liver fibroblast line, were propagated
on monolayers in the culture medium previously described.

Chemicals

Purified mouse fibroblast interferon (IF) (Type 1), purchased
from Calbiochem. Inch. La Jolla, Ca, USA, was used for these
studies. Interferon titers were assayed measuring its ability to
inhibit the cytopathic effect of Vesicular Stomatitis Virus on
L929 cultures(16). Poly-L-Lysine (PLL, mol wt 90, 000) was
purchased from Sigma Chemical Co., St. Louis, Mo, USA.

Treatment of target cells with IF

YAC cells were suspended in culture medium at the concentration of 10^6 cells/ml, distributed in 25 cm^2 flasks, 5-10ml/
flask, and incubated at 37° C in 5% CO_2 atmosphere for 18 hrs,
with medium alone or with IF at the final concentration of 10^3
units/ml, if not otherwise stated. Non treated control tumor cells
or IF-treated cells (YAC/IF) were washed 2 times with culture
medium and resuspended at the desired concentration in the same
medium. L929 monolayers were also pretreated with 10^3 units/ml of
IF for 18 hrs. Then control and IF-pretreated cells were dispersed
with trypsin, washed and resuspended at the required concentration.

Preparation of effector cells nonadherent to nylon-wool column

Spleen cells were passed over nylon fiber columns as previously

described (17). Briefly, the sterile nylon columns were rinsed
with 20ml RPM1 1640 supplemented with 5%FCS. The columns were
drained of the excess medium and placed in a CO_2 incubator at
37° C for 1 hr. Then 10^8 cells in a volume of 1 ml were added
to the column and washed into the nylon wool with 0.5-1 ml of
warm (37°) medium. The columns were kept for 45 min. at 37° C
and the washed slowly with warm medium. The first 25 ml of
effluent were collected in 50 ml tubes, washed once and
resuspended in RPM1 1640 supplemented with 10% FCS, 25 mM Hepes
buffer and 50 μg/ml gentamycin, (hereafter referred to as Complete Medium, CM). Cell recovery was about 30%.

Monolayers of target cells for immunoabsorption of NK lymphocytes

Monolayers were prepared by some modification of previously
described methods (18,19). Briefly, 1 ml of PLL (500 μg/ml in
M 199 supplemented with 10 mM Hepes buffer), was added to each
35x10 mm Petri dishes (Nunc Denmark)for 1 hr at room temperature.
The plates were then washed three times in M199 + Hepes (ph 7,2)
to remove unbound PLL. The tumor-cells suspension (1 ml) was
washed three times in M 199 to deplete FCS, was plated on the
dishes at room temperature for 45 min. Non-attached tumor cells
were then poured off and the Petri dishes were rinsed three times
with M 199 + Hepes. One milliliter of spleen cells suspended in
medium RPM1 1640 containing FCS 10% and 25 mM Hepes was
immediately added. After gentle agitation, the plates were
incubated at 37°C for 45 min. At the end of the incubation period
the non-adherent spleen cells were removed by careful pipetting,
1 ml of warm RPM1 1640 + Hepes + FCS was added for two times to
wash the plates and recover all the non-absorbed cells. Cell recovery was about 30%. The immunoadherent assay for L929 was
almost the same, except that effector splenocytes were added
to freshly confluent monolayers of L929 adherent cells, obtained
without using PLL- coated Petri dishes.

Cytotoxicity assay

The activity of NK cells was determined in a ^{51}Cr-release
assay, as previously described (20). Briefly, graded concentration
of effector spleen cells (E) were suspended in cell culture medium
(see "Tumors") containing 25 mM Hepes buffer, mixed with 10^4 ^{51}Cr-
labeled target cells (T) in U-shaped 96-well microtiter plates
(Greiner C.A. and Söhone, Nürtingen, West Germany) (final volume
0,2 ml) and incubated for 4 hrs at 37° C in a 5% CO_2 incubator.
At the end of the incubation period the plates were centrifuged
(800 x g for 10') and the radioactivity in 0,1 ml of the supernatant
was measured in a γ-scintillation counter (Packard Instrument Co.,
Downers Grove, IL, USA). The baseline ^{51}Cr release was that released spontaneously from target cells and in no case did it exceed

10% of the total radioactivity incorporated by target cells. Experimental results were expressed as the percentage of specific lysis over spontaneous release and were calculated as follows:

$$\% \text{ specific lysis} = \frac{\text{cpmt} - \text{cpms}}{\text{cpmT}} \times 100$$

where cpmt is the mean cpm released in the presence of effector cells, cpms is the mean cpm released spontaneously by target cells, cpmT is the total amount of ^{51}Cr incorporated into target cells. Cold competition experiments were performed by fixing the E:T ratio at 100:1 and by adding graded numbers of cold cells to the E+T mixture in the microwells, containing 10^4 target cells/well.

Calculation of the lytic units

Dose-response curves were obtained by plotting the percentage of specific ^{51}Cr-release and the effector-target (E/T) ratios. The best fit curve for this function was found to be logarithmic (Hewelett-Packard Calculator HP- 97; program, "Standard Pac"03-01) in accordance with previous reports (21-22). A lytic unit, LU_n, was defined as the number of effector cells, extrapolated from the dose-response curve, which was required to achieve n% specific target cell lysis. The amount of $LU_n/10^6$ effector spleen cells was calcutated dividing 10^6 by the number of splenocytes corresponding to 1 LU_n.

Calculation of the inhibitory units

Dose-response curves were obtained by plotting the percentage of specific ^{51}Cr-release and the number of cold cells added. The best fit curve for this function was found to be linear when inhibition values ranged approximately between 0 and 70%. An inhibitory unit, IU_n, was defined as the number of cold cells, extrapolated from the dose-response curve, which was capable of producing n% inhibition of specific target cell lysis. Values indicating $IU_n/10^6$ cells were obtained dividing 10^6 by the number of cold cells corresponding to 1 IU_n.

Statistical analysis

Differences in cytolytic effects produced by NK effector in various experimental conditions were evaluated taking into account the percent of specific cytotoxicity at all E/T ratios. Therefore P values were calculated using covariance analysis performed on the regression of the number of effector cells over the logs of the percentage of specific ^{51}Cr-release. A similar covariance analysis was applied for cold-inhibition tests, using the regression

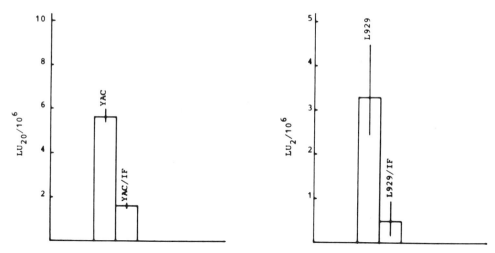

Fig. 1. Cytotoxic activity of BALB/c-nu/nu splenocytes against
         YAC-1 or L929 target cells, non treated or preincubated
         with IF(1000 u/ml for 18 hrs at 37°C).

of the number of cold cells over the percentage values of specific
^{51}Cr-release. All parameters of regression lines (RL) of either LU_n
or IU_n were calculated in order to provide the standard deviation
(SD) values for the lines. In particular, SD for each point of LU_n
was calculated on the SD lines, i.e. the lines parallel to the
original RL and intercepting the y-axis at a + SD and a-SD
respectively, "a" being the intercept of the RL. The SD values for
each point of IU_n were calculated on the SD lines having the slopes
b +SD_b and b -SD_b respectively, "b" being the slopes of the RL and
SD_b the standard deviation of b.

Results
_____

     Effector splenocytes obtained from BALB/c-nu/nu mice were
tested against IF-treated and untreated YAC cells in a 4 hr ^{51}Cr-
release assay. The results (Fig. 1A) show that IF-pretreatment of
tumor cells resulted in a net impairment of target-susceptibility
to NK attack. The same phenomenon was observed using untreated or
IF-treated L929 fibroblasts as target cells. (Fig. 1B). Using
different amounts of IF, it was found that 10^3 units/ml was the IF
concentration capable of the maximal negative modulation of target
cell susceptibility (data not shown). Cold competition experiments
were performed by adding unlabeled YAC or YAC/IF cells to the
mixture of effector splenocytes and ^{51}Cr-labeled YAC or YAC/IF
targets at the ratio of 100:1, during the 4 hr assay. The results
of these experiments, illustrated in fig. 2, are expressed in

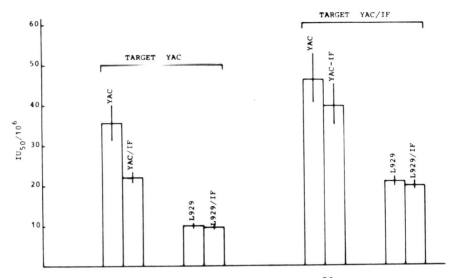

Fig. 2. Cold-inhibition assay performed with ^{51}Cr-labeled YAC or
YAC/IF target cells, in the presence of non-radioactive
competitor cells, and BALB.c-nu/nu effector splenocytes.
Results are expressed in terms of inhibitory units 50%
(IU_{50}) per 10^6 cold cells, being 1 IU_{50} the number of
competitor cells capable of inhibiting the cytolytic reaction by 50%.

"inhibitory units 50" (IU 50) present in 10^6 cells. Cold YAC-1
cells inhibit cytolysis more efficiently than YAC/IF when YAC is
used as target. Conversely YAC cold cells compete as well as cold
YAC/IF cells when labeled YAC/IF is used as target. Similar results
were obtained using effector splenocytes collected from euthymic
donors, untreated or stimulated with an IF-inducing agent such as
Poly- I:C or using splenocytes treated with IF in vitro (data not
shown). These results favour the hypothesis of the existence of
distinct subset of NKTS on the cell membrane, distinguishable on
the basis of their susceptibility to the effect of IF, i.e.
IF-susceptible (IFS) or IF-resistant (IFR) target structures (TS).
Therefore YAC cells showing both IFR-TS and IFS-TS compete more
efficiently than YAC/IF cells, bearing only IFR-TS for the effector
lymphocytes, when YAC is used as target lymphoma. On the other hand
when YAC/IF target is used, unlabeled YAC and YAC/IF cells provide
comparable competition for cytolysis, since IFS-TS subset associated
with YAC cells shoud be irrelevant, being absent on target YAC/IF
lymphoma. In order to confirm the existence of the two subsets of
NKTS, immunoadherence experiments were carried out, using monolayers
respective of YAC and YAC/IF lymphoma obtained stratifying the tumor
cells on PLL-coated Petri dishes as described in Material and

Methods. The results (Table 1) show that the effector splenocytes passed through nylon-wool column, not-adherent to YAC monolayers lose the capability of lysing either YAC or YAC/IF targets. In contrast, effector splenocytes not-adherent to YAC/IF cells, are still cytotoxic against YAC but not against YAC/IF targets. This could mean that splenocytes unbound to YAC/IF are depleted of effectors against IFS-TS present on YAC targets.

In order to test the cross-reactivity between the NKTS of lymphoma YAC cells and those of L929 fibroblasts, cold competition experiments were performed using unlabeled L929 and L929/IF cells and ^{51}Cr-labeled target YAC or YAC/IF cells. The results illustrated in Fig. 2 show that no difference can be found between cold competition afforded by L929 and L929/IF when either YAC or YAC/IF are used as target cells. Further experiments were performed stratifying effector cells on confluent monolayers of L929 or L929/IF cells on plastic flasks, and testing non-adherent lymphocytes against labeled YAC or YAC/IF targets. The results illustrated in Fig. 3 show that effector cells lose part of their cytolytic activity against YAC or YAC/IF cells, following adherence on both L929 or L929/IF monolayers. However no significant difference was found between L929 and L929/IF cells in their capacity to remove the NK activity of effector splenocytes.

DISCUSSION

The results illustrated in the present paper point out that IF-mediated negative modulation of target susceptibility to NK attack is presumably not due to a simple decrease in the density of NKTS or to a masking of their expression according to a model 1 of fig.4. In fact, if this hypothesis would hold true, YAC should compete more efficiently than YAC/IF cells in the cold-inhibition assay when either YAC or YAC/IF are used as labeled targets. Since this is in contrast to the results of the present studies, it seems more likely that IF mediates a partial or total disappearance (or masking) of an IF-susceptible subset of NKTS (i.e. IFS-TS), leaving relatively unaffected a separate subset of target structures, the IFR-TS, present on both YAC and YAC/IF cells. This hypothesis could explain the reason why:

a) "cold" YAC lymphoma competes more efficiently than YAC/IF cells when YAC target is used: in this case YAC/IF is not able to compete for IFS-TS subset of NKTS present on YAC cells.

b) "cold" YAC and YAC/IF cells produce comparable inhibitory effects when target YAC/IF is used, being the presence of IFS-TS on unlabeled YAC lymphoma, but not on labeled YAC/IF cells, not relevant for antigen competition.

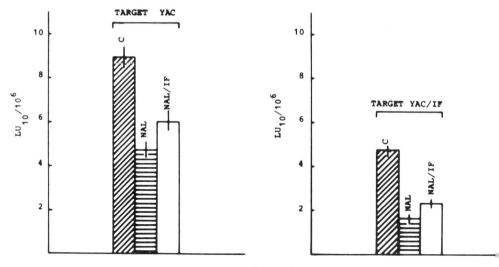

Fig. 3. Cytolytic activity of BALB/c-nu/nu splenocytes against
        labeled YAC or YAC/IF target cells, following absorption
        on confluent L929 or L929/IF monolayers. NAL, spleen cells
        non-adherent to L929 monolayer; NAL/IF, spleen cells non-
        adherent to L929/IF monolayer.

This hypothesis is illustrated in models 2 and 3 of Fig.4: the
duality of the model depends on the fact that it has not yet been
clarified whether IFS-TS and IFR-TS are contemporary present on
YAC cells or if distinct YAC clones bear IFS-TS or IFR-TS
respectively.

    The immunoabsorption experiments add further support to the
hypothesis of the existence of two subsets of NKTS. The results
(Table 1) indicate that effector lymphocytes not adherent to YAC/IF,
are capable of lysing YAC but not YAC/IF target cells. This is
compatible with the hypothesis that YAC expresses additional NKTS
(i.e. IFS-TS) not detectable on YAC/IF cell membrane.

    Two alternative models have been proposed for NK effector
cells, i.e. distinct NK lymphocytes capable of recognizing IFS-TS
or IFR-TS respectively (model 2A, 3A), or lymphocytes containing
membrane receptors for either IFS-TS and IFR-TS (model 2B, 3B).
Both models would be compatible with the results of cold
inhibition experiments. In particular, model B could be acceptable
if NK effector cells carrying both recognition sites for IFS-TS and
bound to cold YAC cells through IFS-TS only, would be still capable
of lysing YAC/IF lymphoma, as a result of their interaction with
IFR-TS expressed on the membrane of labeled target YAC/IF cells.
In this case, competitir YAC cells would possess inhibitory effects
similar to those obtainable with YAC/IF lymphoma. The results of

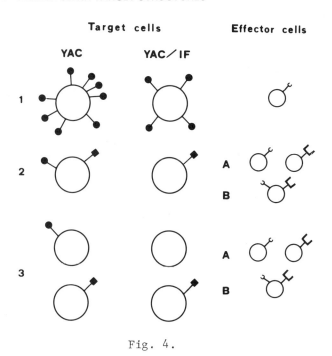

Fig. 4.

Table. 1 however seem to favour model A, although they could not exclude that clones of NK lymphocytes contain <u>predominantly but not exclusively</u> membrane structures capable of recognizing IFS-TS or IFR-TS. The overall picture appears to be more complicated when NKTS of YAC and L929 are comparatively analyzed. In both lines of IF produces negative modulation of the target structures (Fig. 1). However "cold" L929 and L929/IF compete equally well when target YAC or YAC/IF are used (Fig. 2).

TABLE 1. Differential NK activity afforded by BALB-c/nu-nu effector splenocytes non-adherent (NA) to YAC or YAC/IF monolayers.

Effector cells a)	Specific Lysis ($LU_{20}/10^6$) b) mean (M+SD,M-SD)	
	YAC	YAC/IF
Control	16.5(17.6-15.5)	5.5(5.8-5.2)
NA to YAC	0.3(0.6-0.2)	0.005(0.2-0.0001)
NA to YAC/IF	8.6(9.1-8.2)	0.2(0.3-0.1)

a) effector splenocytes passed through nylon-wool column.
b) Mean of $LU_{20}/10^6$, in parentheses mean + standard deviation, mean - standard deviation (see statistical analysis in Material and Methods)

This would suggest that: a) NKTS of L929 or of L929/IF fibroblasts cross-react with NKTS of YAC/IF cells. It follows that most of the cross-reactive structures of YAC lymphoma can be identified with the IFR-TS component of YAC NKTS, being present on YAC as well as on YAC/IF cells. This is also confirmed by the results of the immunoabsorption experiments illustrated in   . Fig. 4: (b) a subset of IFS-TS irrelevant for "cold" competition (Fig. 2), or immunoabsorption (Fig. 3) with respect to YAC or YAC/IF targets, would be expressed on L929 membrane. It follows that these IFS/TS do not cross-react with any NKTS associated with YAC cells.

In conclusion, the results of the present investigation provide evidence of a rather complex pattern of IF activity on NKTS of mouse lymphoma cells of fibroblasts. The available data are compatible with the hypothesis that IFR-TS and IFS-TS are present on both cell lines and that IF suppresses IFS-TS of L929 fibroblasts, distinct from those of YAC lymphoma cells.

REFERENCES

1. Gresser I., Brouty-Boye D., Thomas M.T., and Marcieira Coelho A., 1970, Interferon and cell division. I. Inhibition of the multiplication of mouse Leukemia L1210 cells in vitro by interferon preparation. Proc. Natl. Acad., 66, 1052.
2. Riccardi C., Santoni A., Barlozzari T., Puccetti P., and Herbermann R.B., 1980, in vivo natural reactivity of mice against tumor cells. Int. J. Cancer, 25, 475.
3. Roder J.C., Karre K., and Kiessling R., 1981, Natural killer cells, Prog. Allerg. 28, 66.
4. Gresser I., Interferon and the immune-system. Immunology 80M Fourgereau J., Dausset (ed.), 1980, Progress in immunology, Ac. Press. IV, 710.
5. Trinchieri G., and Santoli D., 1978, Anti-viral activity induced by culturing lymphocytes with tumor-derived or virus-trasformed cells. Enhancement of human natural killer cell activitu by interferon and antagonistic inhibition of suceptibility of target cells to lysis. J. Exp. Med., 147, 1314.
6. Welsh R. M., and Hallenbeck L.A., 1980, Effect of virus infections on target cell susceptibility to natural killer cell-mediated lysis. J. Immunol. 124 (5), 2491.
7. Moore M., White W.J., and Potter M.R., 1980, Modulation of target cell susceptibility to human natural killer cells by interferon. Int. J. Cancer, 25, 565.
8. Trinchieri G. Granato D., and Perussia B., 1981, Interferon-induced resistance of librblasts to cytolysis mediated by NK cells:

specificity and mechanism. J. Immunol., 126, (1), 219.

9. Welsh R.M., Karre K., Hansson M., Kunkel L.A., and Kiessling R.W., 1981, Interferon-mediated protection of normal and tumor target cells against lysis by mouse natural killer cells. J. Immunol. 126 (1), 219.

10. Sonnenfeld G., Meruelo D., Mc Devitt M.O., and Merigan T.C., 1981, Effect of type I and type II interferons on murine thymocytes surface antigen expression: induction or selection? Cell. Immunol., 57, 427.

11. Heron I., Hokland M., and Berg K., 1978, Enhanced expression of β_2-microglobulin and HLA antigens on human lymphoid cells by interferon. Proc. Natl. Acad. Sci. USA, 75, 6215.

12. Dolei A., Ameglio F., Capobianchi M.R., and Tosi R., 1981, Human β-Type interferon enhances the expression and shedding of Ia-like antigens Comparison to HLA-A, B, C and β_2-microglobulin Antiviral. Res. 1; 367.

13. Dolei A., Capobianchi M.R., and Ameglio F., 1983, Human interferon- enhances the expression of class I and class II major histocompatibility complex products in neoplastic cells more effectively then interferon- and interferon-B. Infect. Immun. 40, 172.

14. Ameglio F., Capobianchi M.R., Dolei A., and Tosi R., 1983, Differential effects of interferon-γ on expression of HLA class II molecules controlled by the DR and DC Loci. Infect. Immun., 42, 122.

15. Cikes M., Friberg S. Jr., and Klein G., 1973, Progressive loss of H-2 antigens with concomitant increase of cell- surface antigen(s) determined by Moloney leukemia virus in cultured murine lymphomas. J. Natl. Cancer Inst. 50, 347.

16. Gresser I., Tovey M.G., Bandu M.T., Maury C., and Brouty-boye D., 1976, Role of interferon in the pathogenesis of virus diseases in mice as demonstrated by the use of anti-interferon serum. I. Rapid evolution of encephalomyocarditis virus infection. J. Exp. Med. 144, 1305.

17. Julius M.H., Simpson E., and Herzenberg L.A., 1973, A rapid method for the isolation of functional thymus-derived murine lymphocytes. Europ. J. Immunol. 3, 645.

18. Stulting R.D., and Berke G., 1973, Nature of lymphocyte-tumor interaction. A general method for cellular immunoabsorption. J. Exp. Med. 137, 932.

19. Kumar V., Luevano E., and Bennett M., 1979, Hybrid resistance to EL-4 lymphoma cells. I. Characterization of natural killer cells that lyse EL-4 cells and their distinction from marrow-dependent natural killer cells. J. Exp. Med. 150, 531.

20. Herbermann R.B., Aoki T., Nunn M., Lavrin D.H., Soares N., Gadzar A., Holden H., and Chang K.S.S., 1974, Specificity of ^{51}Cr-release cytotoxicity of lymphocytes immune to murine sarcoma virus. J. Natl. Cancer Inst. 53, 1103.

Specificity of ^{51}Cr-release cytotoxicity of lymphocytes immune to murine sarcoma virus. J. Nat. Cancer Inst. 53, 1103.

21. Cerottini J.C., and Brunner K.T., 1974, Cell-mediated cytotoxicity allograft, rejection and tumor immunity. Advanc. Immunol. 18, 67.

22. Thorn R.M., and Henney C.S., 1976, Kinetic analysis of target cell destruction by effector T cells. I. Delineation of parameters related to the frequency and lytic efficiency of killer cells. J. Immunol. 117, 2213.

MEMBRANE CHANGES INDUCED BY INTERFERONS IN HUMAN NEO-PLASTIC CELLS

A. Dolei'", F.Ameglio", M.R. Capobianchi', and R. Tosi"

'Istituto di Virologia, Viale di Porta Ti-burtina 28, Roma; "Laboratorio di Biologia Cellulare del CNR, Via Romagnosi 18, Roma "Cattedra di Patologia Generale per Scienze Via Camerini, Camerino

A variety of important functions in the host have been attributed to the interferons (IFN). Among these, antiviral, cell-modulating and immunoregulatory activities are the most documented[1]. At least three antigenically distinct types of IFN have been identified so far: alpha, produced by B, natural killer cells and monocytes; beta, produced by fibroblast, epithelial cells and macrophages; and gamma, produced by sensitized or mitogen activated T lymphocytes. The antiviral effects as well as the effects on other cell functions may be activated by the three IFNs through different mechanisms of action[2]. Moreover, IFN gamma is a more potent mediator of antitumor and anticellular activities than IFN alpha and IFN beta[3-5], especially with respect to functions related to the immune system[5]. It is conceivable that at least some of these activities may be connected to modulation of major histocompatibility complex-(MHC)-controlled components.

It was previously shown that IFN alpha and beta enhance the expression as well as the shedding of Class I and Class II products[6-8,12], the magnitude of the effect depending on IFN type, dosage and timing of treatment, and on the cell type. The amount of each antigen in the cell lysates and in the supernates was tested in radioimmunoassay (RIA) as published[6-12].

211

On table I are reported some representative data obtained in human Ml4 melanoma cells treated with IFNs. In order to compare the efficacies of the three IFNs in enhancement of MHC product expression, we calculated the IFN concentration, in terms of antiviral units, which caused an enhancement corresponding to 50% of the maximal effect obtainable (P/2 value). With Ml4 cells IFN alpha and beta have similar potencies in enhancing HLA-A, B, C and beta$_2$-microglobulin (beta$_2$-m) (for HLA-A, B, C P/2 was 650 and 500, respectively with alpha and beta IFNs, while was 830 in the case of beta$_2$-m for both IFNs).

IFN gamma was more effective, as a 5-fold difference in P/2 value was observed, with respect to IFN alpha and beta.

As for Ia expression, IFN alpha had no effect on these cells. IFN gamma appeared to be 32 times more potent than IFN beta in this respect, and 14 to 16 times more effective than IFN beta and alpha in enhancing expression of HLA-A, B, C. Furthermore, we extended the studies to Namalva lymphoblastoid cells. Data were consistent with those obtained in Ml4 cells, but the differences were even more pronounced. In all three instances, the P/2 values of IFN gamma were 100 to 200 times lower than those of IFN alpha and beta. It is noteworthy that in Namalva cells, Ia expression was also stimulated by treatment with IFN alpha [7].

It is well known that Class I and Class II HLA antigens play an important role in triggering and controlling immune responses[13-14]. Ia components are involved in antigen presentation, activation of mixed lymphocytes reaction, and generation of specific cytolytic T cells, whereas HLA-A, B, C are involved in T-lymphocytes killing of virus-infected cells. IFNs are among the mediators produced during immune responses, and have immunoregulatory properties, particularly the gamma type. IFN gamma is also the most effective in enhancing MHC expression.

These findings suggest a major role of IFN gamma in the modulation of various components of the immune system. Moreover we suggest that at least some of the immunoregulatory effects of IFNs are mediated by the regulation of Ia and HLA-A, B, C expression.

Table I. MHC expression in Ml4 cells treated
          IFN alpha, beta and gamma.

Treatment (IFN U/ml)		Ia	HLA-A, B, C	beta$_2$-m
none		38	13	102
alpha	200	39	21	116
	5000	37	36	204
beta	200	37	22	117
	5000	85	37	233
gamma	200	81	42	191
	1000	79	47	270

Cells were trated for 48 h with IFN, then assayed by RIA. Data are expressed as 50% inhibition units (IU$_{50}$/10^6 cells).

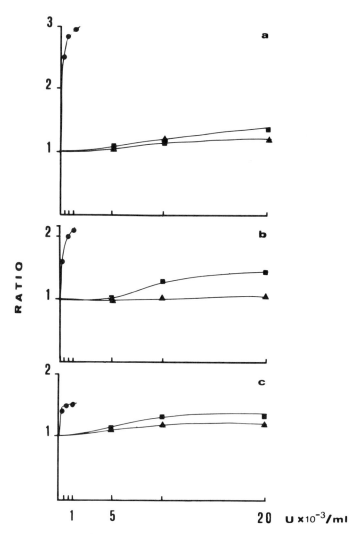

FIG 1. Expression of DC4 (a), DR4 (b) and Ia (c) in
        Namalva cells treated for 48 h with graded
        amounts of IFN alpha (▲), beta (■) and gam-
        ma (●). Data are expressed as increase over
        control values taken as 1.

AKNOWLEDGEMENTS

Work supported in part by grants from Consiglio Nazionale delle Ricerche,progetto Finalizzato Controllo della Crescita Neoplastica, Contratto 83.00304.96 and Controllo delle Malattie da Infezione, Contratto 83.00645.
52.

REFERENCES

1. S. Baron, F. Dianzani and G.J. Stanton, "The
    interferon System: a Review to 1982",Texas
    Reps. Biol. Med.. vol. 41 (1981-1982).
2. F. Dianzani, M. Zucca, A. Scupham and J.A.
    Georgiades, Immune and virus-induced inter-
    ferons may activate cells by different de-
    repressional mechanisms. Nature 283: 400-
    403 (1980).
3. W.R. Fleischmann, Potentiation of the direct
    anticellular activity of mouse interferons:
    mutual synergism and interferon concentrat-
    ion dependence. Cancer Res. 42: 869-875
    (1982).
4. B.Y. Rubin and S.L. Gupta, Differential effica-
    cies of human type I and type II interferons
    as antiviral and antiproliferative agents.
    Proc. Natl. Acad. Sci. USA 77: 5928-5932
    (1980).
5. G. Sonnenfeld, D. Meruelo, H.O. McDevitt and T.
    C. Merigan, Effect of type I and type II in-
    terferons on murine thymocyte surface antigen
    expression: induction or selection? Cell. Im-
    munol. 57: 427-439 (1981).
6. M.R. Capobianchi, F. Ameglio, A. Dolei and R.
    Tosi, Expression of MHC products in human
    cell lines treated with interferons, p. 485-
    487. In: "Expression of differentiated funct-
    ions in cancer cells" R. Revoltella, G.M.
    Pontieri, C. Basilico, G. Rovera, R.M. Gallo
    and J.H. Subak-Sharpe, ed. Raven Press, New
    York (1982).
7. A. Dolei, F. Ameglio, M.R. Capobianchi and R.
    Tosi, Human beta-type interferon enhances
    the expression and shedding of Ia-like an-
    tigens. Comparison to HLA-A, B, C and
    beta$_2$-microglobulin, Antiviral Res. 1:
    367-381 (1981).

8. A. Dolei, M.R. Capobianchi and F. Ameglio, Human
    interferon gamma enhances the expression of
    Class I and Class II major histocompatibility
    complex products in neoplastic cells more
    effectively than interferon alpha and inter-
    feron beta. Infect. Immun. 40: 172-176
    (1983).
9. I. Heron, M. Hokland and K. Berg, Enhanced ex-
    pression of beta$_2$-microglobulin and HLA
    antigens on human lymphoid cells by inter-
    feron, Proc. Natl. Acad. Sci. USA 75: 6215-
    6219 (1978).
10. G. Sonnenfeld, D. Meruelo, H.O. McDevitt and
    T.C. Merigan, Effect of type I and type II
    interferons on murine thymocyte surface an-
    tigen expression: induction or selection ?
    Cell.Immunol. 57: 427-439 (1981).
11. D. Wallach, M. Fellous, and M. Revel, Preferen-
    tial effect of gamma interferon on synthesis
    of HLA antigens and their mRNAs in human
    cells, Nature 29: 833-836 (1982).
12. F. Ameglio,M.R. Capobianchi, A. Dolei and R.
    Tosi, Differential effects of interferon
    gamma on expression of HLA Class II molecu-
    les controlled by the DR and DC loci, Infect.
    Immun. (1983).
13. S.G. Emerson, D.B. Murphy and R.E. Cone, Selec-
    tive turn over and shedding of H-2K and H-2D
    antigens controlled by the major histocompat-
    ibility complex. Implications for H-2-Re-
    stricted recognition. J. Exp. Med. 152: 783-
    785 (1980).
14. R.P. Langman and M. Cohn, Why the MHC is impor-
    tant to the immune system, Transplant.
    Proc. 13/ 1797-1799 (1981).

MODULATION OF Ia ANTIGENS BY INTERFERONS IN HUMAN LYMPHOID CELLS

M.R. Capobianchi', F. Ameglio", R. Tosi" and A. Dolei'··

'Istituto di Virologia, Viale di Porta Tiburtina 28, Roma; "Laboratorio di Biologia Cellulare del CNR, Via Romagnosi 18, Roma; "Cattedra di Patologia Generale per Scienze Via Camerini, Camerino

As long as ten years ago it was shown that treatment with interferon (IFN) enhances the expression of Class I histocompatibility antigens (HLA - A, B,C) in mouse system[1]; the same was found to be true in human cells[2]. In later times, IFN was also shown to increase the expression and release of Class II (Ia) antigens[3]. Of the three types of IFN that are known so far, α, leukocytic, β, fibroblastic, and γ, immune IFN, the latter is the most effective in both instances[4], in keeping with data from the literature, indicating that IFN γ is the most effective of the three as mediator of antitumor and anticellular activities[5-7].

In this report we present some data on the expression of products of the Ia loci in human lymphoid cells treated with IFNs. Three established cell lines were chosen: Namalva cells of B origin, MOLT4, and 1301 T cell lines. The levels of Ia antigens were measured by radioimmunoassay (RIA) as published[3,4,8]. The Namalva cell line is sensitive to IFN with respect to both the establishment of the antiviral state and the enhancing effect on the expression of Ia antigens[3,4]. The T cell lines do not express Ia antigens and treatment with IFN does not cause any induction of Ia expression (Table 1), even

217

though the cells are sensitive to the antiviral
effect of IFN (not shown).

A more detailed analysis of IFN effect was carried
out on Namalva cells, taking into account the
recognized genetic heterogeneity of Class II molecules.
Recent evidence has been provided for the existence
in humans of the two classes of Ia molecules which
have been well characterized in the mouse: I-A and
I-E. The corresponding human homologues, DR and DC,
were shown to differ from each other for both α and
β subunits[9].

In Fig. 1 are reported data obtained in Namalva
cells. Both the expression of overall Ia and that
of separate gene products are affected by IFN γ.
Moreover, this occurs to a greater extent than in
cells treated with the other two IFNs. In fact, we
found that in this respect, IFN γ is up to 200-
fold more effective than IFN α and β[4].

In table 1 are shown the levels of Ia products
in the cell lines tested after a 48 hr-treatment
with IFN γ. In addition, we report also some
preliminary data on the expression of Ia antigens
in normal circulating lymphocytes. Data from these
cells are in keeping with those from the established
cell lines.

The conclusions drawn from our results can be
summarized as follows: a) all three IFNs can
enhance the expression of Ia molecular subsets;
b) IFN γ is the most potent IFN in this respect;
c) Ia-negative cell lines are not inducible by IFN
to express Ia antigens; d) among the Ia subsets,
the DR molecules, which represent the majority of
Ia products, are expressed at levels 2 times
higher than controls; the DC antigens, which are a
minor component, are more sensitive to the action
of IFN γ, in keeping with our published data on
melanoma cells (2-3 times more DR as opposed to
7-8 times more DC antigens)[8]; e) the effect is
found also on peripheral blood lymphocytes
derived from healthy people.

The differences between these molecular species
controlled by Ia region should correspond to
differentiated functions. It has been suggested
that DC molecules are involved in the generation
of effector T cells mediating specific cytolitic

activity[10]. DR molecules, instead, play a role in the
activation of mixed lymphocyte reaction and in
antigen presentation[14]. In addition, they are
strongly related to a variety of diseases. In this
respect a relationship has been found between
some autoimmune disorders and DR. More recently
the same was suggested also for DC[12].

It seems reasonable to infer that agents such as
IFN which modify the expression of these antigens can
in some way influence the function(s) of these
molecules and the clinical conditions of patients
affected by Ia-associated diseases.

Table 1   Expression of Ia, DR and DC in human
           lymphoid cells treated with 300 U/ml
           of IFN γ for 48 hr.

cells	Ia		DR		DC	
	−	+IFN	−	+IFN	−	+IFN
Namalva	13	20	44[a]	97[a]	66[b]	195[b]
1301	−	−	ND[c]	ND	ND	ND
MOLT4	−	−	ND	ND	ND	ND
Normal lymphocytes[d]	26	41	36[e]	74[e]	4[b]	11[b]

Data are expressed as 50% inhibition units/10^6 cells.
(a) DR4; (b) DC4; (c) not done; (d) normal
lymphocytes were obtained from blood samples after
Fycoll-Hypaque gradient sedimentation[8], and deprived
of adherent cells; (e) DR7.

ACKNOWLEDGEMENTS

Work supported in part by grants from: Consiglio
Nazionale delle Ricerche, Progetto Finalizzato
Controllo della Crescita Neoplastica, Contratto
n. 83.00304.96 and Controllo delle Malattie da
Infezione, Contratto n. 83.00645.52 and from
Istituto Pasteur-Fondazione Cenci Bolognetti.

REFERENCES

1. P. Lindhal, P. Leary and I. Gresser, Enhancement
   by interferon of the expression of surface
   antigens on murine leukemia L_{1210} cells, Proc.
   Natl. Acad. Sci. USA 70: 2785-2788 (1973).
2. I. Heron, M. Hokland and K. Berg, Enhanced
   expression of β_2-microglobulin and HLA antigens
   on human limphoid cells by interferon. Proc.
   Natl. Acad. Sci. USA 75: 6215-6219 (1978).
3. A. Dolei, F. Ameglio, M.R. Capobianchi and R.
   Tosi, Human β type interferon enhances the
   expression and shedding of Ia-like antigens.
   Comparison to HLA-A,B,C and β2-microglobulin,
   Antiviral Res. 1: 367-381 (1981).
4. A. Dolei, M.R. Capobianchi and F. Ameglio, Human
   interferon-α enhances the expression of Class I
   and Class II major histocompatibility complex
   products in neoplastic cells more effectively
   than interferon-α and interferon β, Infect.
   Immun. 40: 172-176 (1983).
5. M. Fellous, M. Kamoun, I. Gresser and R. Bono,
   Enhanced expression of HLA antigens and β_2-
   microglobulin on interferon-treated human
   lymphoid cells. Immunology 9: 446-449 (1979).
6. B.Y. Rubin and S.L. Gupta, Differential
   efficacies of human type I and type II
   interferons as antiviral and antiproliferative
   agents, Proc. Natl. Acad. Sci. USA 77: 5928-
   5932 (1980).
7. G. Sonnenfeld, Modulation of immunity by interferon
   in: "Lymphokine reportes", vol. 1, E. Pick. ed.,
   Academic Press Inc. New York p. 113-131 (1980).
8. F. Ameglio, M.R. Capobianchi, A. Dolei and
   R. Tosi, Differential effects on interferon-α
   on expression of HLA class II molecules
   controlled by the DR and DC loci, Infect.
   Immun. 42 (1983).
9. N. Tanigaki, R. Tosi, R.J. Dunquesnoy and G.B.
   Ferrara, Three Ia species with different

structures and alloantigenic determinants in an HLA homozygous cell line, J. Exp. Med. 157: 231-247 (1983).

10. G. Corte, A. Moretta, E. Cosulich, D. Ramarli and A. Bargellesi, A monoclonal antibody selectively inhibits the generation of effector T cells mediating specific cytolytic activity. J. Exp. Med. 156: 1539-1544 (1982).

11. D.H. Katz and B. Benacerraf, The role of products of histocompatibility gene complex in immune responses, Academic Press Inc. New York (1979).

12. R. Tosi, D. Vismara, N. Tanigaki, G.B. Ferrara, F. Ciccimarra, W. Buffolano, D. Follo and S. Auricchio, Evidence that coeliac disease is primarily associated with a DC locus allelic specificity. Clin. Immunol. Immunopathol. 28: 395-404 (1982).

ROLE OF PGE$_2$ PRODUCED BY NEOPLASTIC CELLS AS

MODULATORS OF MACROPHAGE CHEMOTAXIS

G.M. Pontieri, L. Lenti, M. Lipari, D. Lombardi,
A. Zicari, F. Ippoliti, and A. Conforti

Institute of General Pathology
University of Rome "La Sapienza"
Viale Regina Elena 324, Rome, Italy

INTRODUCTION

The relationships between tumor cells and macrophages during tumor growth have been the subject of many investigations.
The aims were essentially the following: a) a better understanding of the mechanism(s) leading to the accumulation of macrophages within a growing tumor and b) the understanding of the
mechanism(s) responsible for the macrophages' acquisition of peculiar properties (strictly resembling those which occur during
the process of activation) in tumor-bearing subjects.

Analysis of tumor macrophage accumulation and,specifically,
the ratio of macrophages to tumor cells,furnished evidence that
macrophage infiltration does not seem to be proportional to tumor cells growth,particularly during the last half period of the
neoplastic disease (Normann and Cornelius,1978). These observations strongly support the findings of Moore and Moore (1977),
demonstrating that the percentage of macrophages to total tumor
cells clearly shows a decreased macrophage infiltration during
late tumor growth. Inhibition of macrophage infiltration within
a given tumor requires,therefore,a threshold number of tumor
cells (Eccles and Alexander,1974;Normann and Schardt,1978).
The analysis carried out by Normann and Cornelius showed that

223

the tumor cells' threshold strongly varies,not only between species for different tumors,but also for the same tumor at different
sites. The reasons for such variability have not been clarified.
Of course,cell movement plays a crucial role in the macrophages
response to neoplasms. The migration of macrophages towards neoplastic cells,or sites close to them,has been clearly demonstrated (Normann,1978;Evans,1972;Hanna et al.,1972). It has been recently postulated that the eventual survival or regression of a
tumor may be partially due to the cancer cell's ability to produce factors that either inhibit or enhance the migration of the
host's macrophages within the tumor (Normann and Sorkin,1977;
Snyderman and Pike,1976;Meltzer et al.,1975). On the other hand,
there is evidence that macrophages,besides playing a defensive
role through the acquisition of tumoricidal activity,may contribute together with the tumor cells,to suppressing the host's immune system. It has been demonstrated that prostaglandins of the
E series are the mediators of this immunosuppressive activity
(Pelus and Bockman,1979). Furthermore,it has been shown that macrophages from tumor-bearing mice amplify the degree of immunosuppres-
sion started by PGE_2 release on the part of the tumor cells
(Plescia et al.,1976). Indeed,the "in vitro" addition of tumor
cells to normal macrophages induces not only a release of PGE_2,but
also,the appearance of an immunosuppressive activity. This has
been analyzed in a "Mishell and Dutton" in vitro system (Ippoliti
et al.,1983). Cyclo-oxygenase inhibitors (Aspirin,flufenamic acid
and indomethacin) partially block the immunosuppressive capacity
displayed by both tumor cells and macrophages. It is evident that
the direct contact between tumor cells and macrophages might be
regarded as responsible for this phenomenon.

   The aims of the present investigation are threefold:
a) to observe "in vitro" the ultrastructural connections between
   Lewis Lung Carcinoma cells and normal macrophages;
b) to observe whether or not PGE_2 are responsible for these cell-
   to-cell contacts
c) to study whether or not the PGE_2,produced by the neoplastic
   cells,are modulators of macrophage chemotaxis.

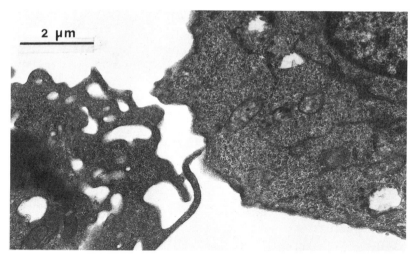

Fig. 1. A macrophage in contact with a tumor cell
via a thin cellular extension (see text).

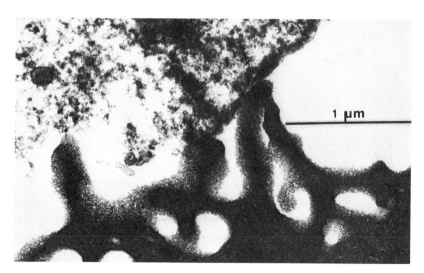

Fig. 2. A high magnification of the cell-to-cell
contact (see text).

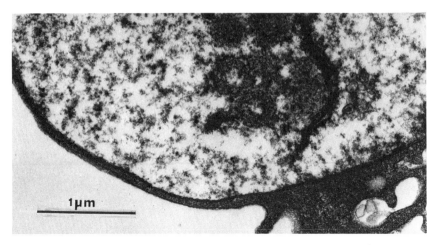

Fig. 3. A high magnification of the phagocytic
process (see text).

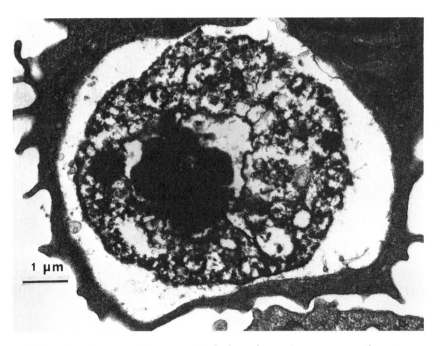

Fig. 4. A macrophage containing in a large vacuole an
entire necrotic tumor cell (see text).

Cell-to-cell contacts between Lewis Lung Carcinoma (3LL) cells and C57B1/6 mice peritoneal macrophages

The 3LL cells were added to 24-hour-old cultures of peritoneal cells,in a ratio of 1 to 1. The incubation was performed in fetal calf serum free RPMI 1640 in a 5% CO_2 humified atmosphere at 37°C. One hour later the cells were fixed in situ with a glutaraldehyde solution (2.5% w/v) in phosphate buffer 0.1M,pH 7.3 at room temperature. After 3 hrs,the cells were gently scraped from the bottom of the plates,postfixed in osmium tetraoxide,dehydrated in alcohol baths,and embedded in Epon 812 resin. Ultrasections,obtained with a Reichert Ultracut microtome,were stained with lead hydroxide and uranyl acetate and examined under a Philips EM300 microscope.

Fig.1 shows an electron photomicrograph of a peritoneal macrophage in close contact with a tumor cell. The contact is established via a thin cellular extension as described by Hibbs (1972). The same contact is shown at a higher magnification in Fig.2. The plasma membrane of the tumor cell appears disrupted. The phagocytic process of macrophage against a 3LL tumor cell,the initial phases of which are shown in Fig.1-2,continues: a thin extension of the macrophage's cytoplasm appears to engulf a necrotized tumor cell (Fig.3). It reaches its highest expression in the complete phagocytosis of a tumor cell,as shown in Fig.4. The macrophage contains now an entire necrotic tumor cell,in which nuclear material is still distinguishable as a picnotic mass.

A threshold number of tumor cells is necessary to demonstrate their macrophage chemotactic activity

In order to identify the threshold number of tumor cells exhibiting remarkable chemotactic activity towards macrophages,experiments were carried out in vitro by employing the blind-well chemotaxis chambers,as described by Snyderman and Pike (1976). The upper compartment contained 0.2 ml of peritoneal cells suspension in RPMI 1640 (1.5×10^6 macrophages/ml). The lower compartment was filled with 0.2 ml of the supernatants obtained after 1 hour of incubation of 3LL cells at concentrations varying from 4×10^5 to 8×10^6/ml,prepared as described elsewhere (Lipari et al., 1983). The two compartments were separated by a 5.0 μ polycar-

Table I. Macrophage chemotactic activity displayed by a
threshold number of tumor cells

Nr tumor cells/ml	Nr migrated macrophages/field
4×10^5	8
8×10^5	10
1.5×10^6	100
4×10^6	5
8×10^6	5

bornate (Nuclepore) filter. Chemotactic activity is expressed as
the mean value of the number of macrophages that had completely
migrated through the filter in twenty random microscopic fields at
100x magnification after 4 hours' incubation at 37°C.

Table I clearly shows that when the ratio tumor cells/macro-
phages is about 1 to 1,maximal macrophage migration occurs. With
either lower or higher number of tumor cells,no significant macrophage chemotaxis is detectable.

Effect of acetylsalicylic acid (ASA) on the tumor cells chemotactic
activity

The immunosuppressive activity of 3LL cells has been linked to
their high PGE_2 production and,furthermore,several products of arachidonic acid metabolism have either chemotactic or chemokinetic
activity (Becker et al.,1982;Higgs,1982). We decided,therefore,to
test whether or not drug interfering with cyclo-oxygenase pathway
would modify the chemotactic activity displayed by tumor cells.
The neoplastic cells were preincubated with 5.5 μM ASA. At low
concentrations,ASA acetylates PGH synthase rapidly (within minutes),
acting as a site-specific,irreversible enzyme inhibitor (Roth,1982).

As table II shows,the chemotactic activity is strongly modified when a threshold number of tumor cells (1.5×10^6) is preincubated with ASA:there is a 90% inhibition. On the other hand,
when a higher number of neoplastic cells is preincubated with
ASA,a 25% increase in chemotaxis is detectable.

Table II. Effect of ASA on the macrophage chemotactic
activity displayed by tumor cells

Nr tumor cells/ml	Nr migrated macrophages/field
1.5 x 10^6	100
1.5 x 10^6 + ASA	10
4 x 10^6	5
4 x 10^6 + ASA	32

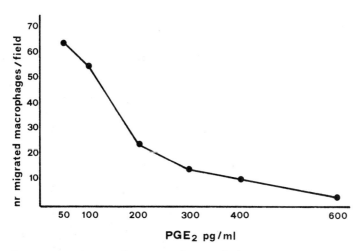

Fig. 5.   Macrophage chemotactic activity displayed by PGE$_2$
at various concentrations.

<u>PGE$_2$</u> <u>exibiting a dose-dependent chemotactic activity towards</u>
<u>macrophages</u>

In order to ascertain whether or not PGE$_2$ alone can play a
chemotactic role towards macrophages,different amounts of PGE$_2$
(Sigma) were tested. As Fig.5 shows,the highest activity is displayed at low concentrations of PGE$_2$ (100-50 pg/ml). With higher
concentrations there is a progressive decrease of chemotaxis.

DISCUSSION

The ultrastructural demonstration that the contacts between
the plasma membranes of macrophages and 3LL cells occur during the
incubation of both cell populations in a fetal calf serum free medium,strongly suggests that the contacts follow a chemoattraction
by one cell type towards the other. On the other hand, our previous
experience has shown that after such incubation,macrophages acquire immunosuppressive activity,linked to their increased biosynthesis and release of PGE$_2$ (Pontieri,1982).

There is evidence that cyclo-oxygenase products influence leukocyte function. PMNs and macrophages,when activated,produce prostaglandins. Thus,they most probably contribute to prostaglandin
synthesis in injured tissue. PGE$_1$ is chemotactic for rabbit PMNs,
and PGF$_{2\alpha}$ enhance the chemotactic responses of leukocytes to
other stimuli. Thromboxane B$_2$ is chemotactic for mouse PMNs,but not
for human leukocytes. These reports have led us to speculate that
cyclo-oxygenase products are involved in modulating cell migration
in inflammation. Generally,however,the activities reported are species specific (Higgs,1982). Cyclic-AMP concentrations influence
leukocyte function and the increase of neutrophil cyclic AMP results
in inhibiting the movement of these cells. There have been a number
of reports which claim that prostaglandins of the E series suppress
leukocyte activities,such as phagocytosis and movement,by increasing cyclic AMP (Rivkin et al.,1974;Smith et al.,1971).

On the other hand,there is also evidence that the platelet
aggregation can be inhibited by agents increasing the level of cyclic AMP. PGI$_2$,PGD$_2$ and PGE$_1$ have been demonstrated to be the most
potent endogenous inhibitors of platelet aggregation and appear to

act via stimulation of platelet adenylate cyclase. PGI$_2$ is of particular interest,since its production can be stimulated by prostaglandins endoperoxides that cause platelet aggregation. PGD$_2$ can be produced by the platelets themselves during platelet aggregation. These two prostaglandins,therefore,may act as feedback regulators (Siegl, 1982). Furthermore,it has also been shown that PGE$_1$ and PGE$_2$ can inhibit PGI$_2$-induced adenylate cyclase activation in a dose-dependent manner,suggesting that PGI$_2$ interacts with the E-type receptor (Schafer et al.,1979).

Since ASA is a potent inhibitor of prostaglandin synthesis by acetylating the PGH synthase,more arachidonic acid becomes available for the lipoxygenase pathway,resulting in the production of more chemotactic leukotrienes. However,it has been reported,that some leukotrienes have other effects,such as the stimulation of prostaglandin synthesis in macrophages (Hammarström,1983).

Our results show that the PGE$_2$,at low concentrations, are chemotactic towards macrophages. On the other hand,the macrophage chemotaxis is progressively inhibited as PGE$_2$ concentration increases. The latter observation confirms the hypothesis that systemic impairment of macrophage accumulation requires not only a threshold number of tumor cells,but also a "threshold" amount of PGE$_2$. We may therefore conclude that the PGE$_2$ might act not only as regulators of prostaglandins synthesis by tumor cells,but also might play a role as modulators of the macrophage arachidonic acid metabolism.

SUMMARY

Both the immune system and macrophage chemotaxis may be suppressed by high levels of prostaglandins of the E series. This research,however,shows that the PGE$_2$ at low concentrations are chemotactic towards macrophages. These findings confirm the hypothesis that macrophage chemotaxis also requires a "threshold" amount of PGE$_2$.

ACKNOWLEDGEMENT

This research was supported by M.P.I. (60% - 1983).

REFERENCES

Becker,E.L.,Showel,H.J.,Naccache,P.H.,Freer,R.J.,Walenga,R.W.,
     Sha'afi,R.I.,1982,Chemotactic Factors:locomotory hormones, in:
     "Phagocytosis:Past and Future", M.L.Karnovsky,L.Bolis,ed.,
     p.87, Academic Press,New York-London.
Eccles,S.A.and Alexander,P.,1974,Macrophage content of tumours in re-
     lation to metastatic spread and host immune reaction,Nature,
     250:667.
Evans,R.,1972,Macrophages in syngeneic animal tumours,Transplantation,
     14:468.
Hammarström,S.,1983,Leukotrienes,Ann.Rev.Biochem.,52:355.
Hanna,M.G.,Zbar,B.,Rapp,H.J.,1972,Histopathology of tumor regression
     after intralesional injection of Mycobacterium bovis,J.Natl.
     Cancer Inst.,48:1441.
Hibbs,J.B.,Lambert,H.L.,Remington,J.S.,1972,Macrophage mediated non-
     specific cytotoxicity possible role in tumor resistance,
     Nat.New.Biol.,235:48.
Higgs,G.A.,1982,Arachidonic acid.Metabolism in leukocytes, in:
     "Phagocytosis:Past and Future",M.L.Karnovsky,L.Bolis,ed.,p.105,
     Academic Press,New York-London.
Ippoliti,F.,Bellelli,L.,Lombardi,D.,Lenti,L.,Di Giovambattista,A.M.,
     Zicari,A.,Pontieri,G.M.,1983,In vitro PGE release from macro-
     phages during 3LL development in C57B1/6 mice.,Cong.ETCS-EURES.
Lipari,M.,Lenti,L.,Di Renzo,L.,Bellelli,L.,Catanzano,A.,Sezzi,M.,
     Pontieri,G.M.,1983,Activation of the alternative complement
     pathway by Lewis Lung Carcinoma cells,Folia Immun.Allergol.Clin
     30:252.
Meltzer,M.S.,Tucker,R.W.,Brener,A.C.,1975,Interaction of BCG-activated
     macrophages with neoplastic and non neoplastic cell lines in
     vitro:Cinemicrographic analysis,Cell.Immunol.,17:30.
Moore,M.and Moore,K.,1977,Kinetics of macrophage infiltration of ex-
     perimental rat neoplasms, in: "The Macrophage and Cancer",
     J.B.McBride and A.Stuart,ed.p.330,Econoprint,Edinburgh.
Normann,S.J.and Sorkin,E.,1977,Inhibition of macrophage chemotaxis by
     neoplastic and other rapidly proliferating cells in vitro,
     Cancer Res.,37:705.
Normann,S.J.and Cornelius,J.,1978,Concurrent depression of tumor
     macrophage infiltration and systemic inflammation by progres-
     sive cancer growth,Cancer Res.,38:3453.

Normann,S.J.,1978,Tumor cell threshold required for suppression of
     macrophage inflammation,J.Natl.Cancer Inst.,60:1091.
Normann,S.J.and Schardt,M.A.,1978,A cancer related macrophages
     dysfunction in inflamed tissues.,J.Ret.Soc.,24:147.
Pelus,L.M.and Bockman,R.,1979,Increased prostaglandin synthesis
     by macrophages from tumor-bearing mice,J.Immunology,
     123:2118.
Plescia,O.J.,Grinwich,K.,Plescia,A.M.,1976,Subversive activity of
     syngeneic tumor cells as an escape mechanism from immune
     surveillance and the role of prostaglandins.Ann.N.Y.Acad.
     Sci.,276:455.
Pontieri,G.M.,Ippoliti,F.,Lipari,M.,Fragomele,F.,Lenti,L.,Lucchesi,
     M.,1982,Subversion of the immune system and tumorigenesis,
     Bull.Eur.Inst.Ecol.Cancer,10:113.
Rivkin,I.,Rosenblatt,J.,Becker,E.L.,1974,The role of cyclic AMP in
     the chemotactic responsiveness and spontaneous motility of
     rabbit peritoneal neutrophils,J.Immunol.,115:1126.
Roth,G.J.,1982,Preparation of (acetyl-^{3}H)Aspirin and use in quan-
     titating PGH synthase, in "Methods in Enzymology",W.E.M.,
     Lands and W.L.,Smith,ed.,Academic Press,New York-London,
     86:392.
Schafer,A.I.,Cooper,B.,O'Hara,D.,Handin,R.I.,1979,Identification of
     platelet receptors for prostaglandin I$_2$ and D$_2$, J.Biol.Chem.
     254:2914.
Siegl,A.M.,1982,Receptors for PGI$_2$ and PGD$_2$ on human platelets, in:
     "Methods in Enzymology",W.E.M.Lands and W.L.Smith,ed.,
     Academic Press,New York-London,86:179.
Smith,J.W.,Steiner,A.L.,Parker,C.W.,1971,Human lymphocyte metabolism.
     Effects of cyclic and non cyclic nucleotides on stimulation
     by phytohemagglutinin,J.Clin.Invest.,50:442.
Snyderman,R.,Pike,M.,1976,An inhibitor of macrophage chemotaxis
     produced by neoplasms.,Science,192:370.
Snyderman,R.,Pike,M.,1976,Chemotaxis of mononuclear cells. in:
     "In vitro methods in cell-mediated and tumor immunity",
     B.R.,Bloom,J.R.,David,ed.,p.651,Academic Press,New York-
     London.

THE RELATIONSHIPS BETWEEN THE HIGH PRODUCTION OF PROSTAGLANDINS BY TUMORS AND THEIR ACTION ON LYMPHOCYTES AS SUPPRESSIVE AGENTS

V. Tomasi*, R. Mastacchi**, G. Bartolini*,S. Fadda°,
O. Barnabei*
R. Gatto, F. Barboni***
A. Trevisani[+] A. Capuzzo, M.E. Ferretti, M.C. Pareschi****
G. Martelli, R. Danieli, S. Rossini*****

*   Lab. of General Physiology, University of Bologna
**   Present address: Alfa Farmaceutici, Bologna
°   Present address: Neurological Clinic, University of Bologna
***   Central Laboratory of the Hospital Malpighi,Bologna
**** Institute of General Physiology, University of Ferrara, Italy
***** Istituto dei composti del Carbonio contenenti eteroatomi e loro applicazioni - C.N.R., Ozzano Emilia, Bologna
+ Deceased, June 1983

INTRODUCTION

The immune surveillance theory states that cancer cells having foreign antigens on their surfaces, are recognized and destroyed by cells of the immune system before they can grow into a life-threatening tumor. The foreign antigens would be recognized by the immune system triggering the production of cytotoxic T lymphocytes specifically directed against the antigens[1].

One major problem of this theory is that nude mice (genetic mutants that lack thymus gland) or mice whose thymuses were removed at birth, have a normal incidence of cancers despite the absence of mature T lymphocytes[2]. However, the discovery of natural killer cells (NK) breathed new life into the somewhat murimund theory of

235

immune surveillance. NK cells as a matter of fact, are a novel type
of cells distinct from conventional B cells, T cells or macrophages,
having the spontaneous ability to destroy tumor cells and cells
infected with viruses[3,4].

It has been shown that nude mice have normal or perhaps even
elevated numbers of NK cells[2,3], which is a strong argument in
favour of the possibility that these cells, rather than mature T
lymphocytes, may be performing immune surveillance.

Actually proving that NK cells carry out immune surveillance
in humans will be difficult. However, animal studies suggest that
these cells both retard the development of primary tumors and
prevent metastatic spread of the cancer, the most dangerous aspect
of the disease.

Probably the most important regulatory signal for NK activity
has been detected. It is a glycoprotein called type II or immune
interferon which appears to be formed by mitogen or antigen-stimulated T cells[2].

Interferon augments NK activity for appropriate target cells
in two ways: 1) it might activate existing NK cells, like the activation of macrophages by limphokines or 2) it could trigger the
differentiation of a precursor to the NK cell into an effector
cell[2].

But what happens when a tumor develops probably by subverting
the immune surveillance system?

In 1975 Plescia and collaborators[5] proposed that many tumors
may use prostaglandins to subvert the immune system. Two arguments
are in favour of this hypothesis: a) following the observations of
Karim and co-workers[6] many investigators have shown that tumors or
transformed cells produce higher amounts of prostaglandins (mainly
of E type) with respect to appropriate controls (Table 1);
b) lymphocytes are very sensitive to PGE which, by increasing
cyclic AMP levels, inhibits mitogen-induced cell proliferation[7].

So far most of the experiments were carried out using total
lymphocytes or T and B cells respectively. As far as we know, only
few experiments have been carried out using NK cells[8,9].

Table I

R E F E R E N C E S	PG PRODUCTION BY TUMORS	PG$_s$ INHIBIT TUMOR DEVELOPMENT	PG$_s$ INHIBITORS DEPRESS TUMOR DEVELOPMENT	CORRELATION BETWEEN PG PRODUCTION BY TUMORS AND PG EFFECTS ON LYMPHOCYTES
1) THOMAS D.R. et al.: Exp. Cell. Res. (1974) 84: 40	+	+		
2) JAFFE B.M.: PG$_s$ (1974) 6: 453-461	+	+		
3) SANTORO M.G. et al.: Nature (1976) 263: 777		+		
4) HIAL V. et al.: J. Pharmacol. Expt. Ther. (1977) 202: 446			+	
5) HAMMARSTRÖM S.: Eur. J. Biochem. (1977) 74: 7-12	+			
6) CUMMINGS K.R. et al.: J. Urol. (1977) 118: 710	+			
7) PLESCIA O.J. et al.: Prog. Biochem. Pharm. (1978) 14: 123				+
8) LYNCH N.R., SALOMON J.C.: J. Natl. Cancer. Inst. (1979) 62: 117			+	
9) BENNETT A. et al.: PG$_s$ (1979) 17: 179			+	
10) DROLLER M.J. et al.: Cell. Immunol. (1979) 47: 261	+			+
11) FITZPATRICK F.A. et al.: P.N.A.S. (1979) 76: 1765	+	+		
12) SANTORO M.G. et al.: Br. J. Cancer (1979) 39: 408		+		
13) FAVALLI C. et al.: PG$_s$ (1980) 19: 587		+		+
14) ROLLAND P.H. et al.: J. Natl. Cancer. (1980) 64: 1061	+		+	
15) BENNETT A. et al.: Br. J. Cancer (1980) 41: 204	+			
16) GOODWIN J.S. et al.: Cencer Immunol. Immunopath. (1980) 8: 3	+	+	+	+
17) FULTON A.M., LEVY J.G.: Int. J. Cancer (1980) 26: 669			+	
18) GOODWIN J.S.: J. Immunopharmacol. (1980) 2: 397			+	+
19) BRUNDA M.J. et al.: J. Immunol. (1980) 124: 2682				+
20) GOODWIN J.S.: Clinical Immun. Immunopath. (1980) 15. 106				+
21) OWEN K. et al.: Cancer Res. (1980) 40: 3167	+			+
22) TUTTON P.J.M., BARKLA D.H.: Br. J. Cancer (1980) 41: 47		+	-	
23) DROLLER M.J.: J. Urol. (1981) 125: 757			+	+
24) POLLARD M., LUCKERT P.M.: Science (1981) 214: 558			+	
25) HOKAMANA Y. et al.: Res. Comm. Chem. Path. Pharm. (1981) 31: 379	+			

HIGH PRODUCTION OF PROSTAGLANDINS BY TUMORS AND VIRUS TRANSFORMED
CELLS

Some years ago we entered the field of prostaglandins and tumors because we were interested in the biological role of prostaglandins. We had carried out studies on liver cells populations
indicating that PGE_2 produced mainly in parenchymal cells acted on
synusoidal cells increasing cyclic AMP which in turn seemed to
regulate PGI_2 synthesis[10]. Thus PGE_2 appeared to behave as an inter-
cellular messenger[11,12].

The hypothesis proposed by Plescia appeared to offer us the
possibility to examine the role of prostaglandins in a different
system, in which the communicating partners are tumor cells and
lymphocytes (Fig. 1).

Our results obtained using a transplantable rat hepatoma can
be summarized as follows[13]:
a) tumor cells produced PGE_2 as the main prostaglandin in an
amount 3 or 4 fold higher with respect to isolated hepatocytes in
suspension or cultured either in the absence or presence of
arachidonate;
b) cyclic AMP levels in these conditions were not modified
and addition of PGE_2 to cancer cells failed to augment its level;
c) indomethacin or ASA inhibited PGE_2 synthesis and at the
same time reduced cancer cell proliferation in vivo and augmented
the survival time of tumor-bearing rats.

Thus, the high production of PGE_2 by tumor cells appears to be
best explained by assuming that it is used to subvert the immune
system.

The results more recently obtained[14] using mouse hepatoma (HTC)
and virus transformed kidney cells (RKBK) are more difficult to
interpret, but they are in line with Plescia's hypothesis.

The mouse hepatoma HTC produced so high levels of PGE_2 (in the
nanogram range) that a comparison with controls (impossible to
perform) seemed to be superfluous. Again PGE_2 biosynthesis was
severely depressed in the presence of 10 μM indomethacin (see Fig.2).

The results obtained with RKBK cells are less impressive but
they clearly indicate a time- and substrate-dependent capacity for

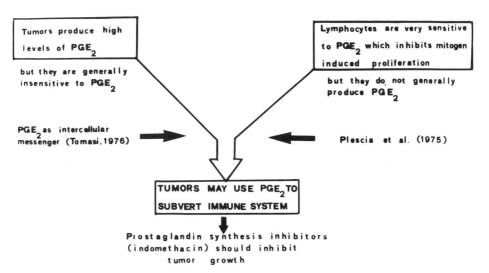

Fig. 1. Proposed role of prostaglandins as suppressive
factors in the immunological response against tumors.

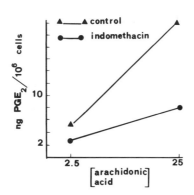

Fig. 2. The effect of indomethacin (10 μM) on PGE2 biosynthesis in
HTC cells at different substrate concentrations (μg/ml).
(From ref. 14).

PGE$_2$ biosynthesis which was strongly inhibited by indomethacin (see
Fig. 3).

THE EFFECT OF PROSTAGLANDINS ON CYCLIC AMP LEVELS OF HUMAN PERIPHERAL LYMPHOCYTES AND RAT THYMOCYTES

In 1971 Smith et al.[15] reported that PGE$_1$ and PGE$_2$ were capable
of inhibiting the incorporation of labeled thymidine into PHA-stimu-
lated lymphocytes, by an action mediated by cyclic AMP.

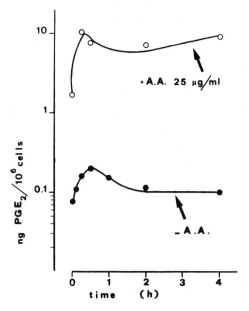

Fig. 3. Time-course of PGE_2 biosynthesis in RKBK cells, reported on semi-log scale. (Redrawn from ref. 14).

These findings have been confirmed in several laboratories and have led to the concept that cyclic AMP levels are inversely proportional to lymphocytes proliferative rates[16-19].

Our studies were aimed at:

a) investigating the details of the action of prostaglandins on human peripheral blood lymphocytes (HPBL) cyclic AMP levels

b) correlating the levels of the cyclic nucleotide with the effect of mitogens on cultured lymphocytes.

We have used in addition to the classical prostaglandins, PGE_1 and PGE_2, a novel compound, 6-keto-PGE_1 which may represent a circulating prostaglandin[20,21] (Fig. 4).

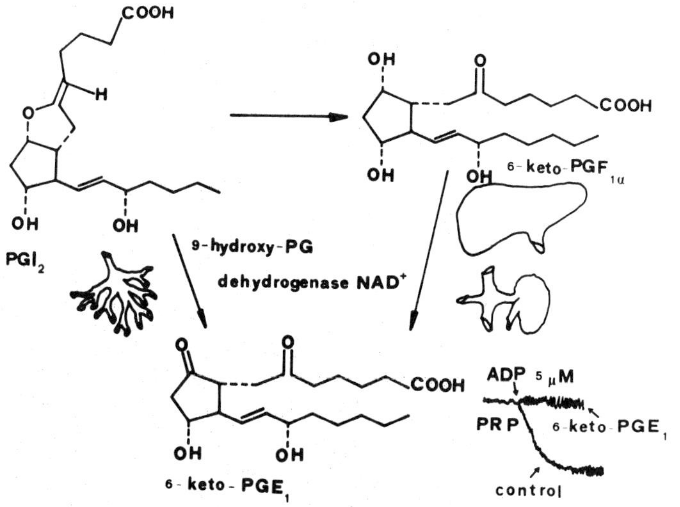

Fig. 4. Biosynthesis of 6-keto-PGE$_1$ in various tissues and its effect on platelet aggregation. (Redrawn from Quilley C.P. et
al. (1980) Hypertension).

As far as the point a) is concerned, we were mainly interested
in testing the effect of 6-keto-PGE$_1$ on lymphocyte cyclic AMP levels
and to ascertain whether or not it acts on the same receptor by
which PGE$_1$ is expressing its effects.

The results of these experiments[22,23] indicate that:
1) 6-keto-PGE$_1$ is capable of increasing lymphocyte cyclic AMP
levels being however less effective than PGE$_1$. Interestingly PGI$_2$
was practically ineffective also after short incubation times when
cyclic nucleotide levels were clearly increased by 6-keto-PGE$_1$.
2) Studies carried out using PGE$_1$ and 6-keto-PGE$_1$ alone or in
combinations indicate a lack of additivity which suggests an action
of the two prostaglandins on the same receptor (Table 2).

Table 2. Effect of combinations of PGE_1 and $6KPGE_1$ on HPBL cAMP levels

		pmoles cAMP/ /5·10^5 cells		pmoles cAMP/ /5·10^5 cells
Control		3.31±0.91		
			250 ng PGE_1 + 250 ng $6KPGE_1$	16.59±2.02
	250 ng	15.42±2.61		
PGE_1	500 ng	17.21±3.52		
			500 ng PGE_1 + 500 ng $6KPGE_1$	22.95±4.17
	750 ng	19.53±3.61		
	250 ng	8.75±3.12		
			750 ng PGE_1 + 750 ng $6KPGE_1$	16.63±2.59
$6KPGE_1$	500 ng	13.26±2.35		
	750 ng	16.53±3.81		

The results are means ± S.E. of four different experiments. Incubation and assay of cyclic AMP were carried out as described in Ref.22.

Table 3. The effect of $6KPGE_1$ and PGE_1 on cAMP levels of human T and B lymphocytes

		unseparated lymphocytes	s/b	T lymphocytes	s/b	B lymphocytes	s/b
Control		4.02±0.70		2.38±0.59		4.06±1.18	
PGE_1	250 ng	N.D.		13.60±3.37	5.7	N.D.	
	500 ng	28.80±4.38	7.16	14.46±3.27	6.1	19.61±5.94	4.8
$6KPGE_1$	250 ng	17.73±3.21	4.4	11.72±4.62	4.9	N.D.	
	500 ng	18.16±3.04	4.5	12.12±4.33	5.1	17.35±1.77	4.3

* 10 min of incubation
N.D. - not done   s/b - stimulated/basal
each value represents the mean of 4-5 experiments. Results are means ± S.E.M.

3) The last result is in accordance with the fact that PGE$_1$ and 6-keto-PGE$_1$ are equally effective on separated T and B lymphocytes (Table 3).

On the other hand we were interested in comparing the effect of prostaglandins on lymphocytes with that on lymphoblastoid cell lines which having rapid proliferative rates, should be expected to escape signals inhibiting proliferation. We found that lymphoblasts are much less sensitive than lymphocytes to the action of PGE$_1$ or PGE$_2$, but they are equally sensitive to 6-keto-PGE$_1$. This fact does not agree with the hypothesis that PGE$_1$ and 6-keto-PGE$_1$ have the same receptor on lymphoblasts. Experiments performed using thymocytes from normal and from tumor-bearing rats are in line with the findings described above (Table 4, Table 5, Fig. 5).

Table 4. The effects of some derivatives of arachidonic acid on cyclic AMP levels in thymocytes from normal and Yoshida tumor-bearing rats.

Experimental conditions	Cyclic AMP (% of control values)*			
	Normal rats		Yoshida tumor-bearing rats	
Control	6	100	5	100
PGE$_2$	6	1603 ± 279	4	863 ± 139
PGI$_2$	4	449 ± 116	3	293 ± 7
6-K-PGF$_{1\alpha}$	5	177 ± 23	4	114 ± 5
6-K-PGE$_1$	4	967 ± 184	3	657 ± 135
PGA$_1$	3	257 ± 58	2	190
PGF$_{1\alpha}$	2	168	1	100
Arachidonic acid	2	133	1	98

* Normal rats: 0.60 ± 0.08 pmol/10^6 cells; Yoshida tumor-bearing rats: 0.72 ± 0.02 pmol/10^6 cells.
PGs and Arachidonic acid were $1 \cdot 10^{-5}$ M.

Table 5. Kinetic parameters of ^{3}H -PGE$_{2}$ binding to crude
plasma membrane fraction of thymocytes from normal
and Yoshida tumor-bearing rats.

	Normal rats		Yoshida tumor-bearing rats	
High affinity binding sites	K_d	16 nM	K_d	5 nM
	R_{max}	30 fmol/mg protein	R_{max}	29 fmol/mg protein
Low affinity binding sites	K_d	0.3 µM	K_d	0.2 µM
	R_{max}	239 fmol/mg protein	R_{max}	176 fmol/mg protein

In each sample there were ^{3}H -PGE$_{2}$ (specific activity 160
Ci/mmole) 1.52×10^{-9}M and 300-400 µg of proteins.
In the samples for the non specific binding the amount of
PGE$_{2}$ was 10^{-5} M.
Incubation were carried out at 25°C for 30 minutes.

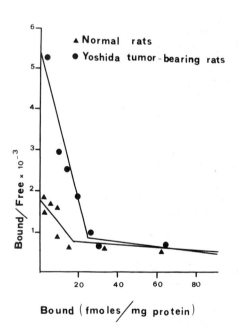

Fig. 5. Scatchard plot of the binding of ^{3}H-PGE$_{2}$ to thymocyte crude plasma membrane fraction from normal and Yoshida tumor-bearing rats. For experimental conditions see Table 5.

SOME CONSIDERATIONS ABOUT A NOVEL PROSTAGLANDIN: 6-KETO-PGE$_1$

The discovery of a novel metabolic pathway leading to the formation of 6-keto-PGE$_1$[20,21] has aroused much interest.

This compound has properties similar to PGI$_2$ but is character-ized by a higher stability <u>in vivo</u>. On the other hand PGE$_1$ which in several systems (except platelets) is equipotent with PGI$_2$ or PGE$_2$ does not appear to be produce <u>in vivo</u> to any significant extent since the concentration of its precursor is generally low[24,25]. Therefore there is the possibility that PGE$_1$ behaves as an agonist on a 6-keto-PGE$_1$ receptor. The results reported in Table 2 and 3 support this possibility. We measured the increase of cyclic AMP in the presence of either PGE$_1$ or 6-keto-PGE$_1$ alone and when com-bined. We have observed that the effect of combinations of the two prostaglandins at different concentrations was never additive, which constitutes a strong argument in favor of an action of the two compounds on the same receptor coupled to adenylate cyclase.

Experiments carried out using separated T and B lymphocytes are in partial agreement with this possibility. We found that the effect on cyclic AMP levels of T lymphocytes was similar to that exerted on unseparated cells. On the other hand, B lymphocytes had a response to PGE$_1$ similar to that exhibited by 6-keto-PGE$_1$.

Previous studies[22] do not support the hypothesis postulating a single receptor: it has been found comparing lymphoblasts with lymphocytes that the formers were much less sensitive to PGE$_1$ than the latters while they were equally sensitive to 6-keto-PGE$_1$.

CONTROL BY PROSTAGLANDINS OF MITOGEN-INDUCED LYMPHOCYTE PROLIFERATION

Regarding the correlation between the action of prostaglandins on cyclic AMP levels in cultured lymphocytes and the inhibition of mitogen-induced proliferation, there are reports which either con-firm or oppose it. However, it is now reasonably clear that E type prostaglandins are capable, at least as far as T lymphocytes are concerned, to inhibit mitogen-induced proliferation[7,26].

Also the involvement of cyclic AMP in the process has been doubted[7,26]. Recently, however, Goodwin and co-workers[18] established that cyclic AMP increase precedes and it is well correlated with the inhibitory effect of prostaglandins. Thus, the process appears

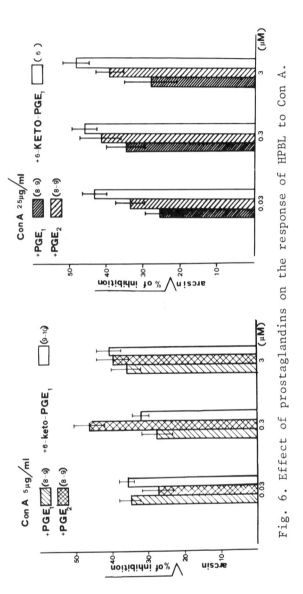

Fig. 6. Effect of prostaglandins on the response of HPBL to Con A.

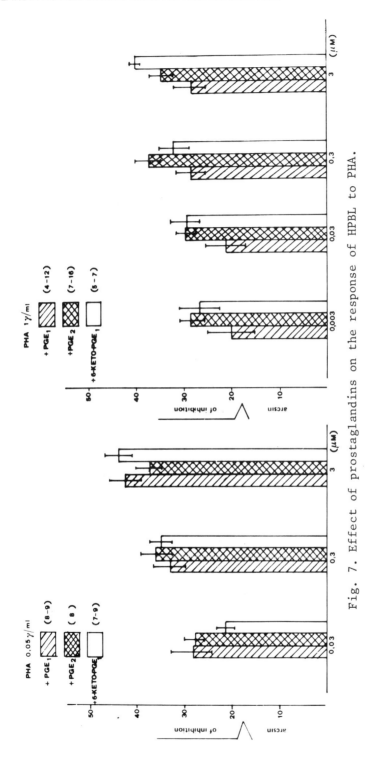

Fig. 7. Effect of prostaglandins on the response of HPBL to PHA.

to meet all the criteria needed to establish cyclic AMP as the second messenger of PGE effects on lymphocytes.

We have compared the effects of PGE_1, PGE_2 and 6-keto-PGE_1 on
the responsiveness to mitogens of human lymphocytes.

When prostaglandins were added to cultured lymphocytes stimulated by Con A (Fig. 6) or PHA (Fig. 7) a dose-related inhibition
of labeled thymidine incorporation was observed. 6-keto-PGE_1 had a
potency very similar to that of PGE_1 or PGE_2 in reducing the proliferation. Moreover prostaglandins were effective at doses which
are in good agreement with those needed to affect cyclic AMP
levels[7,26].

Having previously observed that cultured lymphoblasts had a
reduced response to PGE while maintaining a normal response to 6-
keto-PGE_1[22], we considered of interest to extend these findings to
leukemic lymphocytes. Using a B cell-leukemia lymphocytes we have
observed (Table 6) that not only the sensitivity to prostaglandins
but also that to isoproterenol and histamine were severely reduced
with respect to normal lymphocytes. Although these data are in
agreement with the findings of Polgar et al.[27], we plan to repeat
the experiments by using fresh lymphocytes instead than cells stored
at low temperatures. It is well known, as a matter of fact, that
many adenylate cyclase systems became de-sensitized when cells are
stored even at low temperatures[28].

We were unable to correlate these findings with a possible
lack of effect of prostaglandins on the control of cell proliferation, because the mitogens we have used (including LPS) had little
effect on proliferative rates of leukemic lymphocytes as shown in
Table 7. We plan to try the use of spontaneous proliferation in
culture or to employ the pokeweed mitogen, which has been reported
to be effective mainly on B lymphocytes[29].

STUDIES WITH INHIBITORS OF PGE ACTION:
STRUCTURE-ACTIVITY RELATIONSHIPS

In several areas of endocrinological research the progress has
been often facilitated by the availability of synthetic compounds
having the capacity to block hormone receptors (for example alfa
and beta receptor blocking agents). In the field of prostaglandins
several attempts have been pursued to synthesize receptor blockers

Table 6. Production of cAMP by leukemic lymphocytes

		pmoles cAMP/ $5 \cdot 10^5$ cells	Stimulation index Leukemic lymphocytes	Stimulation index Normal lymphocytes
Control		6.52±1.27 (9)		
PGE$_1$	250 ng/ml	7.74±1.92 (8)	1.45±0.12	
	500 ng/ml	8.84±1.98 (9)	1.30±0.11	10.1
	750 ng/ml	9.86±1.37 (7)	1.68±0.40	
6-K-PGE$_1$	250 ng/ml	8.76±1.71 (5)	1.70±0.37	3.03
	500 ng/ml	8.91±1.70 (7)	1.60±0.28	4.34
	750 ng/ml	9.52±1.77 (5)	1.30±0.17	-
Isoproterenol 10^{-5}M		11.45±1.93 (7)	1.51±0.08	3.8
Histamine 10^{-4}M		8.43±2.20 (7)	1.27±0.09	4.99

The results are means ± S.E.; in the brackets is the number of the experiments.
Stimulation index is the ratio of cAMP produced in stimulated samples to control samples.
For the other experimental conditions, see Ref. 22.

Table 7. Effect of mitogens on ^{3}H-thymidine incorporation by normal and leukemic lymphocytes.

	Lymphocytes	
	Normal	Leukemic
Control	856 ± 71 (8)	174 ± 18 (5)
+ PHA 1γ/ml	54147 ± 4392	209 ± 64
Control	928 ± 173 (9)	179 ± 18 (5)
+ ConA10γ/ml	13714 ± 2549	219 ± 70
Control	1365 ± 259 (8)	595 (2)
+ LPS100γ/ml	1667 ± 312	836

Mitogens are used at the concentrations reported. The results are given as means ± S.E. and the number of the experiments is reported in the brackets.

by modifying the prostaglandin structure[30]. However, the results so
far obtained were unsatisfactory mainly because of the low potencies
and lack of specificity of the analogues available (see for example
the analogues derived from 7 oxa-prostynoic acids[31,32]).

It is well known that the biological activity of prostaglandins
is linked to a flexible hairpin configuration[33,34]; therefore, it
is reasonable to trace the activity of prostaglandin analogues to
their own spatial conformation rather than to mere structural anal-
ogies.

In these last years it resulted that modifications of the
structure of a compound which often results in the synthesis of
analogues capable of modifying an enzyme activity, is an approach
which has not much success as far as hormone receptors are concerned.
Thus, alfa and beta receptors blocking agents are structurally different from catecholamines; endorphins and enkephalins are very
different from morphine ecc.

We have recently prepared, starting from biliary acids, a number
of steroidal derivatives having in vivo some properties which could
be explained by assuming that they inhibit prostaglandin biosynthesis
or their effects. On the basis of structural examinations of these
compounds, a similarity with prostaglandins is observable, since
they can be considered prostaglandin derivatives blocked in a tight
conformation[35,36]. Thus, it was considered of interest to test their
effects as possible prostaglandin E receptor antagonists.

The results reported here indicate that some of the compounds
tested behaved as inhibitors of prostaglandin E effects on cyclic
AMP levels of peripheral human lymphocytes. Fig. 8 shows the inhibition of the PGE_1 effect on cyclic AMP levels when three different
antagonists were added to the incubation system. The dose-dependent
inhibition was evaluated using concentrations ranging from 1 to
100 μg per ml and the ID 50 was calculated. In the fig. 9 the
structures of compounds tested as well as their relative ID 50 are
reported. The activity seems to be linked to the presence of a
keto group in the pentatomic ring in position A (MG_9 having an
hydroxy group is not active) and to the presence of conjugated
double bonds (MG_1, MG_3 and MG_5 lacking double bonds are not active).
The most active compounds MG_2, MG_8 and MG_{10} had ID 50 ranging from
15 to 42 μg per ml. The presence of additional OH groups in the

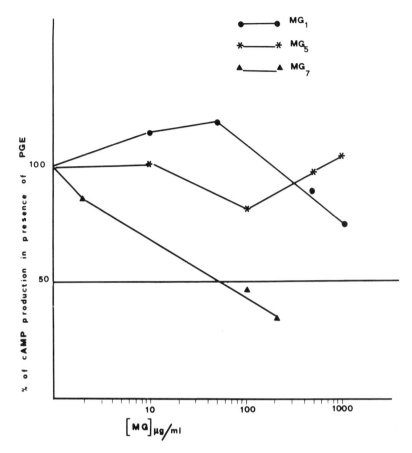

Fig. 8. The effects of MG_1, MG_5 and MG_7 on the response to PGE_1 of human peripheral blood lymphocytes (HPBL). The potencies of antagonists were evaluated by calculating the amounts required to inhibit 50% of the response to prostaglandin E (ID 50).

molecule does not seem to be critically involved.

These compounds had no antiaggregating effects nor influenced prastacyclin action when evaluated according to the platelet aggregation test, some of them were weak agonists (results not shown).

We have no formal evidence that the compounds tested inhibit PGE-induced increase of cyclic AMP levels by an action exherted only at the receptor level. As a matter of fact such an action could be explained also on the basis of an intracellular effect

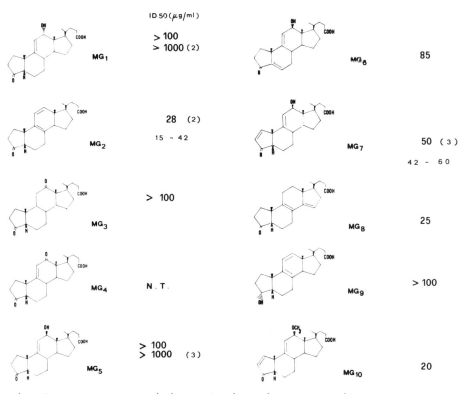

Fig. 9. Structure-activity relationships of 10 different prostaglandi
        E receptor antagonists.
        ID 50 was calculated as described in Fig. 1. In the brackets
        is the number of experiments performed; N.T., not tested.

(i.e. activation of cyclic AMP phosphodiesterase) or by an effect on
membrane fluidity. The former possibility is not very likely since
we blocked phosphodiesterase by using classical inhibitors as
aminophylline and more potent inhibitors such as IBMX. The latter
possibility is, in our opinion, too not very likely since any
modification of membrane fluidity does not seem to be so critically
dependent on the structure of a lipophilic molecule.

    In other words it would be difficult to explain why MG_1 and MG_5
have little effects at concentrations of 1000µg per ml under conditions in which 15 µg per ml of MG_2, 25 µg per ml of MG_8 or 20 µg
per ml of MG_{10} inhibit 50% of the response to PGE_1 (see Fig. 9).

    Thus, the most likely explanation is that these steroid-like
molecules act as PGE receptor blocking agents. However, this can

be proved only by performing binding studies using membrane preparations, an approach which we will try to carry out.

It is interesting that recently Milne and Johnson on the basis of a structural homology between PGE and levonantradol, a cannabinoid, suggested that it may be acting at the PGE receptor level[37]. Fitzpatrick et al.[38] have found that an epoxyimino derivative of prostanoic acid behaves as a thromboxane A_2 antagonist with an ID 50 lower than 200 ng per ml. This antagonist is thus much more potent than ours, however we feel that further structural modifications could lead to an improvement of the potency of our antagonists.

FINAL REMARKS

It seems appropriate now to emphasize the points which, in our opinion, have to be clarified before establishing that two apparently unrelated facts, high production of prostaglandins by tumors and suppression of immune system, are actually interconnected.

If the Plescia's hypothesis is true one would expect that prostaglandins are produced by tumors but not by lymphocytes. Conflicting reports have been published. Thus, while according to Ferraris and De Rubertis[39] mitogens release prostaglandins from cultured lymphocytes, Okasaki et al.[40] more recently were unable to confirm this finding. This discrepancy could be, at least in part, overcome considering that Goodwin et al.[41] have found that in peripheral lymphocytes a minor part of the cell population, isolated by its adherence to glass wool, was responsible for the major production of PGE_2. In Hodgkin's disease these glass adherent suppressor cells, producing 4 fold more PGE_2 than normal lymphocytes do, appear to be the cause of the hyporesponsiveness to mitogens observed in Hodgkin's lymphocytes[42].

A second important point is where prostaglandins receptors are localized in HPBL[43]. Prostaglandins could in principle inhibit directly the cell activated by mitogens or act via an intermediate cell. For example prostaglandins could activate a suppressor cell population which in turn would inhibit the responding cell through a pathway not related to prostaglandins. According to Webb and co-workers[19] adherent mouse splenocytes produce PGE which acting on non adherent splenocytes produces a release of suppressor factors which in turn inhibit T cell proliferation. Goodwin and collaborators[44] have shown that a small percentage of human periferal T cells possesses receptors for PGE.

On the other hand, we have found that both T and B cells have a similar sensitivity to the action of PGE_1 and 6-keto-PGE_1, at least as far as cyclic AMP levels are concerned. It is difficult to explain these data on the basis of a response restricted to a subpopulation of T cells.

The dramatic effects of anti-inflammatory drugs in the control of tumor growth can be best explained considering also the effects of prostaglandins on macrophages. It has been clearly shown that PGE_1 and PGE_2 (but not $PGF_{2\alpha}$) are capable of inhibiting tumoricidal activity of activated macrophages. Prostaglandins can be produced not only by tumors but also by the macrophages themselves which, when stimulated, can release high amounts of PGE_2[45]. Thus, indomethacin could act also by inhibiting PGE_2 production by activated macrophages, which favours their tumoricidal action[46-50]. However at the moment some discrepancy exists at this regard[51].

In conclusion, the hypothesis proposed by Plescia and collaborators[5,52] has stimulated a tremendous amount of work. Most of the experimental data do in fact support this hypothesis. The most recent observations regarding the role of natural killer activity which has been shown to be under negative control by PGE_2[8,9,53] and the role of other prostaglandins as TXB_2[54,55] and 6-keto-PGE_1 contribute to make more convincing the approach towards the use of cycloxygenase inhibitors[56] or of prostaglandin receptor-antagonists, as immunoadjuvants, in the treatment of some malignancies.

A third approach, more difficult to carry out in vivo, could consists in the immunization against PGE_2[57,58].

REFERENCES

1. H. Friedman, S. Specter, I. Kamo, and J. Kateley, Tumor-associated immunosuppressive factors, Ann. N.Y. Acad. Sci. 276: 417 (1976)
2. B.R. Bloom, Interferons and the immune system, Nature 284: 593 (1980).
3. R. Kiessling, E. Klein and H. Wigzell, Natural Killer cells in the mouse. Cytotoxic cells with specificity for mouse maloney leukemia cells: specificity and distribution according to genotype, Europ. J. Immunol. 5: 112 (1975).

4. R. B. Herberman and H. T. Holden, Natural Killer cells as anti-tumor effector cells, J. Natl. Cancer Inst. 62: 441 (1979).

5. O. J. Plescia, A. H. Smith and K. D. Grinwich, Subversion of immune system by tumor cells and the role of prostaglandins, Proc. nat. Acad. Sci. USA 72: 1848 (1975).

6. S. M. M. Karim and B. Rao, Prostaglandins and tumors, Adv. Prostaglandin Res. 3: 303 (1976).

7. J. S. Goodwin and D. R. Webb, Regulation of the immune response by prostaglandins, Clin. Immunol. Immunopath. 15: 106 (1980).

8. J. C. Roder and M. Klein, Target effector interaction in the natural killer cell system, J. Immunol. 123: 2785 (1979).

9. M. J. Brunda, R. B. Herberman and H. T. Holden, Inhibition of murine natural killer cell activity by prostaglandins, J. Immunol. 124: 2682 (1980).

10. V. Tomasi, G. Bartolini, M. Orlandi, C. Meringolo and O. Barnabei, Mechanism of action and biological significance of pro-staglandin E_2 and prostacyclin in the liver, in: "Lipoprotein metabolism and Endocrine regulation", L. W. Hessel and H. M. J. Krans, eds., Elsevier-North Holland, Amsterdam, 279 (1979).

11. G. Bartolini, C. Meringolo, M. Orlandi and V. Tomasi, Biosynthesis of prostaglandins in parenchymal and non-parenchymal rat liver cells, Biochim. Biophys. Acta 530: 325 (1978).

12. V. Tomasi, C. Meringolo, G. Bartolini and M. Orlandi, Biosynthesis of prostacyclin in rat liver endothelial cells and its control by prostaglandin E_2, Nature 273: 670 (1978).

13. A. Trevisani, A. Ferretti, A. Capuzzo and V. Tomasi, Elevated levels of prostaglandin E_2 in Yoshida hepatoma and the inhi-bition of tumor growth by non steroidal anti-inflammatory drugs, Br. J. Cancer 41: 341 (1980).

14. A. Capuzzo, A. Corallini, E. Fabbri, M. E. Ferretti, M. Pareschi, V. Tomasi and A. Trevisani, Osservazioni preliminari sulla biosintesi in vitro di prostaglandine di tipo E in cellule tumorali e trasformate da virus, Boll. Soc. It. Biol. Sper. 57: 2104 (1981).

15. J. W. Smith, A. L. Steiner and C. W. Parker, Human lymphocytic metabolism. Effects of cyclic and non cyclic nucleotides on stimulation by phytohaemagglutinin, J. Clin. Invest. 50: 442 (1971).

16. J. D. Stobo, M. S. Kennedy and M. E. Goldyne, Prostaglandin E modulation of the mitogenic response of human T cells, J. Clin. Invest. 64: 1188 (1979).

17. A. Novogrodsky, A. L. Rubin and K. H. Stenzel, Selective sup-
    pression by adherent cells, prostaglandin and cyclic AMP
    analogues of blastogenesis induced by different mitogens,
    J. Immunol. 122: 1 (1979).
18. J. S. Goodwin, S. Bromberg and R. P. Messner, Studies on the
    cyclic AMP response to prostaglandin in human lymphocytes,
    Cell. Immunol. 60: 298 (1981).
19. D. R. Webb, T. J. Rogers and I. Nowowiesky, Endogenous prosta-
    glandin synthesis and the control of lymphocyte function,
    Proc. N.Y. Acad. Sci. 332; 262 (1980).
20. P. Y. K. Wong, J. C. McGiff, F. F. Sun and W. H. Lee, 6-keto-
    prostaglandin E_1 inhibits the aggregation of human platelets,
    Eur. J. Pharmacol. 60: 245 (1979).
21. P. Y. K. Wong, K. U. Malik, D. M. Desiderio, J. C. McGiff and
    F. F. Sun, Hepatic metabolism of prostacyclin (PGI_2) in the
    rabbit: formation of a potent novel inhibitor of platelet
    aggregation, Biochem. Biophys. Res. Commun. 93: 486 (1980).
22. S. Fadda, R. Mastacchi, G. Romeo, V. Tomasi and O. Barnabei,
    Regulation of cyclic AMP levels in human lymphocytes and
    lymphoblasts by prostaglandins, Prost. and Med. 5: 477 (1980).
23. R. Mastacchi, S. Fadda, V. Tomasi and O. Barnabei, The effect
    of 6-keto-PGE_1 on human lymphocyte cyclic AMP levels, Prost.
    and Med. 5: 487 (1980).
24. W. E. Lands and B. Samuelsson, Phospholipids precursors of
    prostaglandins, Biochim. Biophys. Acta 164: 426 (1968).
25. M. Hamburg, B. Samuelsson, On the metabolism of PGE_1 and PGE_2
    in man, J. Biol. Chem. 246: 6713 (1971).
26. K. V. Honn, R. S. Bockman and L. J. Marnett, Prostaglandins and
    cancer. A review of tumor initiation through tumor metastasis,
    Prostaglandins 31: 833 (1981).
27. P. Polgar, J. Carlos Vera and A. M. Rutenburg, An altered
    response to cyclic AMP stimulating hormones in intact human
    leukemic lymphocytes, Proc. Soc. Exp. Biol. Med. 154: 493
    (1977).
28. C. R. Kahn, Membrane receptors for hormone and neurotransmitters,
    J. Cell Biol. 70: 261 (1976).
29. C. W. Parker, Control of lymphocyte function, New Engl. J. of
    Medic. 295 (21): 1180 (1976).
30. J. H. Sanner and K. E. Eakins, Prostaglandin antagonists in:
    "Prostaglandins: Chemical and biochemical aspects", S. M. M.
    Karim, ed., MTP, Lancaster, 139-187 (1976).

31. D. E. Mac Intyre and J. L. Gordon, Discrimination between platelet prostaglandin receptors with a specific antagonist of bisenoic prostaglandins, Thrombosis Res. 11: 705 (1977).
32. G. C. Le Breton, D. L. Venton, E. S. Enke and P. V. Halushka, 13 Azoprostanoic acid: a specific antagonist of the human blood platelet thromboxane/endoperoxide receptor, Proc. Natl. Acad. Sci. USA 76: 4097 (1979).
33. D. A. Langs, M. Erman and G. T. De Titta, Conformations of PGF$_{2\alpha}$ and recognition of prostaglandins by their receptors. Science 197: 1003 (1977).
34. N. H. Andersen, S. Inamoto, N. Subramanian, D. H. Picker et al., Molecular basis forp prostaglandin potency. III. Tests of the significance of the "Hairpin conformation" in biorecognition phenomena, Prostaglandins 22 (5): 841 (1981).
35. D. Brewster, M. Myers, J. Ormerod, A. C. B. Smith, M. E. Spinner and S. Turber, Prostaglandin synthesis design and execution, J. Chem. Soc. Perkin 1: 2796 (1973).
36. M. Baumgarth and K. Irmscher, Secoandrostansäuren als enantiomere prostaglandin-analoga-I, Tetrahedron 31: 3109 (1975).
37. G. M. Milne and M. R. Johnson, Levonantradol: a role for central prostanoid mechanisms, J. Clin. Pharmacol. 21(S): 367S (1981).
38. F. A. Fitzpatrick, G. L. Bundy, R. R. Gorman and T. Honohan, 9,11 Epoxy-Iminoprosta-5,13-Dienoic acid is a thromboxane A$_2$ antagonist in human platelets, Nature 275: 764 (1978).
39. V. A. Ferraris and F. R. De Rubertis, Release of prostaglandin by mitogen- and antigen-stimulated leukocytes in culture, J. Clin. Invest. 54: 378 (1974).
40. T. Okasaki,S. Masatoshi, C. E. Arbesman and E. Jr. Middleton, Prostaglandin E and mitogenic stimulation of human lymphocytes in serum-free medium, Prostaglandins 15 (3): 423 (1978).
41. J. S. Goodwin, A. D. Bankhurst, R. P. Messner, Suppression of human T cell mitogenesis by prostaglandin E. Existence of a prostaglandin producing suppressor cell, J. Exp. Med. 146: 1719 (1977).
42. J. S. Goodwin, R. P. Messner, A. D. Bankhurst, G. T. Peake, J. H. Saiki and R. C. Williams Jr, Prostaglandin producing suppressor cells in Hodgkin's disease, New Eng. J. Med. 297: 263 (1977).
43. J. S. Goodwin, A. Wiik, M. Lewis, A.D. Bankhurst and C. R. Williams Jr, High affinity binding sites for prostaglandin E on human lymphocytes, Cell Immunol. 43: 150 (1979).

44. J. S. Goodwin, P. A. Kaszubowski and C. R. Williams Jr, Cyclic
    adenosine monophosphate response to prostaglandin E_2 on sub-
    population of human lymphocytes, J. Exp. Med. 150: 1260
    (1979).
45. K. H. Leung, D. G. Fischer and H. S. Koren, Erythromyeloid tumor
    cells (K 562) induce PGE synthesis in human peripheral blood
    monocytes, J. Immunol. 131 (1): 445 (1983).
46. R. M. Schultz, N. A. Pavlidis, W. A. Stylos and M. A. Chirigos,
    Regulation of macrophage tumoricidal function: a role for
    prostaglandins of the E series, Science 202: 320 (1978).
47. W. F. Stenson and C. W. Parker, PG_s, Macrophages and Immunity,
    J. Immunol. 125: 1 (1980).
48. M. E. Goldyne and J. D. Stobo, PGE_2 as a modulator of macrophage-T
    lymphocyte interactions, J. Invest. Dermatol. 74: 297 (1980).
49. D. S. Snyder, D. I. Beller and E. R. Unanne, Prostaglandins
    modulate macrophage I_a expression, Nature 299: 163 (1982).
50. M. E. Snider, R. H. Fertel, and B. S. Zwilling, Prostaglandin
    regulation of macrophage function: effect of endogenous and
    exogenous prostaglandins, Cell Immunol. 74: 234 (1982).
51. S. M. Taffet and S. W. Russell, Macrophage-mediated tumor cell
    killing: regulation of expression of cytolytic activity by
    PGE, J. Immunol. 126: 424 (1981).
52. O. J. Plescia, K. Grinwich, J. Sheridan and A. M. Plesia, Sub-
    version of the immune system by tumors as a mechanism of
    their escape from immune rejection, Prog. Biochem. Pharmacol.
    14: 123 (1978).
53. T. Goto, R. B. Herberman, A. Maluish and D. M. Strong, Cyclic
    AMP as a mediator of Prostaglandin E-induced suppression of
    human natural killer cell activity, J. Immunol. 130 (3):
    1350 (1983).
54. I. Mahnud, N. Fukui and Y. Miura, Arachidonic acid metabolism
    in normal and regenerating liver and hepatoma, Adv. Enzyme
    Regul. 18: 27 (1980).
55. Y. Kanzeki, I. Mahnud, M. Asanagi, N. Fukui and Y. Miura,
    Thromboxane B_2 as possible trigger of liver regeneration,
    Cell Mol. Biol. 25: 147 (1979).
56. J. S. Goodwin, Prostaglandin synthetase inhibitors as immuno-
    adjuvants in the treatment of cancer, J. Immunopharmacol.
    2: 397 (1980).
57. M. R. Young and S. Henderson, Enhancement in immunity of tumor
    bearing mice by immunization against PGE_2, Immunol. Commun.
    11: 345 (1982).

58. A. Fischer, A. Durandy and C. Griscelli, Role of prostaglandin
    E$_2$ in the induction of non specific T lymphocyte suppressor
    activity, J. Immunol. 126: 1452 (1981).

ACKNOWLEDGEMENTS

    This work was supported partly by grants from the C.N.R. (Rome)
project "Control of neoplastic growth" n. 81.01474.96 to V.T. and
partly by grants from C.N.R. (Rome) project "Chimica fine e secon-
daria" Cb 1.
    The authors are grateful to prof. G. Cainelli, Institute of
Chemistry, Bologna, for continuous advice and encouragement.

ONCOGENES AND THE NEOPLASTIC PROCESS

Stuart A. Aaronson, Yasuhito Yuasa, Keith C. Robbins,
Alessandra Eva, Rosita Gol, and Steven R. Tronick

Laboratory of Cellular and Molecular Biology
National Cancer Institute
Bethesda, Maryland 20205

RETROVIRUSES AS MODELS FOR STUDYING HUMAN CANCER

The quest to understand the mechanisms by which normal human
cells become malignant has been aided immeasurably by research
on oncogenic retroviruses (oncoviruses). Two major groups of
oncoviruses have been recognized based on their biological
properties[1]. One group, termed chronic transforming retroviruses,
causes mostly leukemias when inoculated into susceptible animals
but only after a latent period of several months. These viruses
replicate in known assay cells in tissue culture without causing
apparent transforming effects. The other group, known as acute
transforming viruses, induces a variety of tumors within a very
short time of days to a few weeks. The types of malignancies they
cause include sarcomas, hematopoietic tumors, and even carcinomas.
Cells infected with acute viruses undergo morphologic transformation, acquire the ability to grow in soft agar, and cause tumors
when inoculated into susceptible hosts.

STRUCTURE OF RETROVIRAL GENOMES

The relationships between chronic and acute viruses have been
uncovered by the use of molecular hybridization, molecular cloning,
and nucleotide sequence analysis. The general structure of a
retrovirus consists of three genes which code for the internal
virion structural proteins (gag), the reverse transcriptase (pol),
and the envelope glycoproteins (env), respectively[2]. These genes
are flanked by long terminal direct repeats, termed LTRs, which

contain signals for the initiation, enhancement, and termination
of transcription. Thus, retroviruses closely resemble transposable
elements that have been isolated from procaryotic and eucaryotic
species[3].

Whereas the chronic viruses have always been found to possess
this structure, the acute viruses usually lack portions of one or
all of the three chronic viral genes and characteristically contain
a discrete unique sequence. This latter piece of genetic information has been shown to possess homology with the chromosomal DNA
of the species from which the acute virus was isolated. When
incorporated into a retroviral genome, this sequence is designated
v-onc and its cellular counterpart c-onc. The structures of some
acute transforming viruses isolated from mice are shown in Fig. 1.
Our own studies, as well as those of other laboratories, have led
to the understanding that recombination between chronic retoviruses
and cellular genes has resulted in the genesis of acute transforming retroviruses (for reviews see refs. 2, 4, 5).

TRANSFORMING GENES OF ACUTE RETROVIRUSES

Although the mechanisms of transformation by chronic viruses
are not well understood, genetic and molecular approaches have
demonstrated that v-onc genes are required for transforming
functions of acute viruses. Thus, classic genetic experiments
demonstrated that transformation-defective mutants of Rous sarcoma
virus have specifically deleted their v-onc gene (src). Furthermore, cells infected with viruses possessing temperature sensitive
onc sequences lose the transformed phenotype at the non-permissive
temperature (for reviews see refs. 2, 4).

The availability of molecularly cloned retroviral genomes has
made it possible to construct mutants with precisely defined
deletions[6,7]. To illustrate, an analysis of a series of such
mutants of simian sarcoma virus (SSV), a primate-derived acute
transforming virus, is shown in Fig. 2. The deletions that
destroyed the ability of SSV DNA to transform NIH/3T3 mouse cells
in DNA transfection assays were localized to its v-onc sequences,
designated sis. Analogous studies with the DNAs of other acute
retroviruses have firmly established that their onc genes are
required for induction and maintenance of the virus transformed
state[2,7].

The transforming functions of v-onc genes appear to be
mediated by proteins encoded by v-onc sequences. Onc-specific
proteins have been identified by the use of sera obtained from
animals bearing virally induced tumors. By use of such sera, the

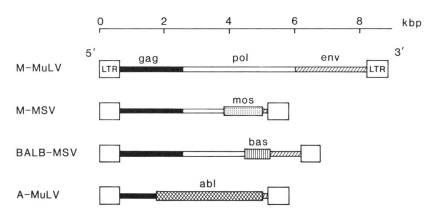

Fig. 1.   Relationship of three murine transforming retroviral genomes
to the chronic transforming virus genome. The onc gene of
each retrovirus is indicated by a differently shaded box to
denote the different cellular origin of each.

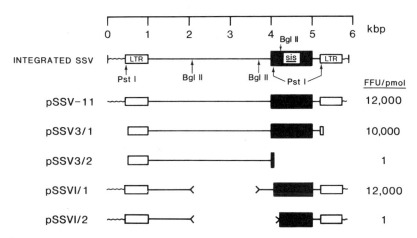

Fig. 2.   Biological analysis of SSV deletion mutants. Mutants were
constructed from the integrated form of SSV. NIH/3T3 cells
were transfected with plasmid DNAs containing each of the
genomes illustrated. Wavy lines represent host cellular
flanking sequences, and the SSV onc gene, sis, is designated
by the black box.

translational product of v-src was shown to be a protein kinase
with the unique substrate specificity for tyrosine residues[8,9].
Since this discovery, the transforming proteins of several other
viruses have been shown to possess a similar activity[5].

Another approach that our laboratory has used to identify the
onc gene product of SSV has been to prepare antisera to peptides
synthesized on the basis of the nucleotide sequences of sis[6,10].
Such antisera specifically precipitated a 28,000 MW protein from
SSV-transformed cells (Fig. 3). This molecule corresponds in size
to the predicted length of the sis gene product.

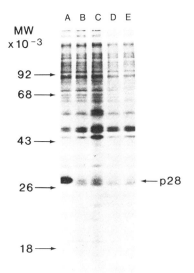

Fig. 3. In vivo detection of a v-sis translational product by
         immunoprecipitation analysis. Cells nonproductively
         transformed by SSV clone 11 were metabolically labeled
         with ^{35}S-methionine. Cell extracts were treated with an
         anti-sis peptide serum and the immunoprecipitates were
         analyzed by polyacrylamide gel electrophoresis. Extracts
         were pre-incubated with 0, 0.1, 0.3, 1.0 or 10 μg (lanes
         A-E, respectively) of the sis peptide.

BIOLOGICAL SPECIFICITY OF RETROVIRAL ONC GENES

Although all mammalian acute viruses transform cultured mouse fibroblasts, they can also be extraordinarily specific in their actions on other cells. BALB and Harvey murine sarcoma viruses (MSV), whose oncogenes (v-H-ras) are closely related and encode a 21,000 MW transforming protein (p21), induce sarcomas and erythroleukemias in mice or rats (for review see 11). Using an in vitro bone marrow colony assay[12], it was possible both in culture and in vivo to demonstrate that these acute viruses transform a novel hematopoietic cell with the properties of an early lymphoid progenitor.

Snyder-Theilen feline sarcoma virus (ST-FeSV) codes for a tyrosine-specific protein kinase. In the same bone marrow colony assay as that used to analyze the action of BALB and Harvey MSVs, ST-FeSV transforms hematopoietic blast cells that appear to be at an early stage in B-cell differentiation[13]. Interestingly, Abelson murine leukemia virus (A-MuLV), whose oncogene product has functional similarities to that of FeSV, transforms pre-B lymphoblasts that are indistinguishable from those transformed by FeSV[14]. These findings indicate that the in vitro functional similarities in onc gene products may reflect common pathways by which they exert their oncogenic potential.

CELLULAR ORIGIN OF RETROVIRAL ONC GENES

Studies performed by several laboratories using v-onc specific cDNAs indicated that certain avian and murine v-onc sequences are well-conserved in the genomes of evolutionarily diverse species[2,4,5]. Subsequently, the availability of molecularly cloned v-onc probes made it possible to take advantage of the great sensitivity of filter hybridization techniques. By use of such techniques, it has been shown that v-onc probes derived from mammalian acute viruses hybridize to specific restriction fragments of highly diverged species such as Drosophila[15]. The high degree of conservation of onc sequences strongly suggests that c-onc genes serve important normal physiological functions.

Of the more than two dozen acute transforming viruses studied to date, viruses isolated not only from the same, but also from widely diverged species, have been shown to contain highly related onc genes[2,4,5]. Thus, acute transforming viruses have incorporated only a very few cellular genes from a potential battery of many thousands. These findings argue that the number of cellular genes that can be altered to become transforming genes when incorporated into the retroviral genome is not unlimited.

CHROMOSOMAL LOCALIZATION OF ONC RELATED GENES IN HUMAN CELLS

Since genes related to retroviral onc genes are well conserved in human DNA, it became possible to assess the role of onc genes in the etiology of human cancers. One approach we have used in this regard is chromosomal mapping of human c-onc genes. We utilized panels of human-rodent somatic cell hybrids possessing varying numbers of human chromosomes. It was possible to distinguish rodent and human onc sequences by digestion of cellular DNAs with appropriate restriction enzymes. To enhance the signal intensity of human sequences, we utilized cloned DNAs from human onc loci as the molecular probes.

The results of these studies are summarized in Table I. It is apparent that onc genes are widely distributed throughout the human genome. Thus, sis has been assigned to chromosome 22[16], mos and myc to chromosome 8,[17],[18] and myb to chromosome 6[19]. Members of the ras oncogene family are found on chromosomes 1 (N-ras), 6 (K-ras), 11 (H-ras-1), and 12 (K-ras-2)[19],[20]. Other groups have made similar observations and have mapped additional onc genes to chromosomes 15 (fes), 22 (abl), and X (H-ras-2)[21-30].

Table 1. Chromosomal Assignments of the Human Homologues (Proto-oncogenes) of Retroviral onc Genes.

Chromosome Number	Onc Gene	Chromosomal Aberration	Tumor[1]
1	N-ras	del 1p	Neuroblastoma
6	K-ras-1; myb	6q⁻; t(6:14)	ALL, Ovarian CA
8	mos; myc	t(8;14); t(8;22); t(2;8)	Burkitt's Lymphoma
		t(8;21)	AML
9	abl	t(9;22)	CML
11	H-ras-1	11p⁻	Wilms' Tumor
12	K-ras-2	12+	CLL
15	fes	t(9;22)	CML
20	src	-	-
22	sis	t(9,22)	CML

[1]Cancers with chromosomal aberrations affecting chromosome to which onc gene homologues have been localized.

ONCOGENE ACTIVATION BY CHROMOSOMAL TRANSLOCATIONS

Klein[31] speculated that onc genes might be activated by chromosomal translocations, since specific chromosomal rearrangements
were known to occur in the cells of certain human tumors. As shown
in Table 1, chromosomes harboring onc related genes are involved
in several such diseases. It has been possible to show that, in
the case of Burkitt's lymphoma, the c-myc locus is translocated
from chromosome 8 to chromosome 14[18,21] into the immunoglobulin
(μ chain) α switch region[18]. Evidence has been obtained indicating
that these tumor cells express increased levels of the myc gene[32].
Other examples of onc gene translocations have been observed in
cells of patients with chronic myelogenous leukemia[33,34] (abl and
sis) and acute promyelocytic leukemia (fes)[35]. However, the
relevance of these rearrangements to the etiology of such hematopoietic neoplasms is not as yet known.

ISOLATION OF TRANSFORMING GENES FROM HUMAN TUMOR CELLS

An independent approach for the detection of transforming
genes has been provided by the development of DNA-mediated gene
transfer techniques (transfection) (for review see ref. 5). Thus,
certain cell lines could be stably transformed by DNAs from a
variety of tumors, including some of human orgin, whereas normal
DNAs showed no such effect. Investigations in several laboratories
led to the identification and molecular cloning of a human oncogene
from the T24 human bladder carcinoma cell line[36-38]. It was of
interest to determine whether any viral oncogenes were related to
the human bladder oncogene. The T24 human bladder tumor oncogene
hybridized strongly and reciprocally with a v-H-ras onc gene
probe[39-41]. Moreover, restriction endonuclease mapping of the T24
gene in the region required for its transforming activity demonstrated that it was indistinguishable from that of the normal H-ras
human homolog. These results implied that the cellular sequences
transduced by retroviruses could be activated by subtle genetic
alteration, within naturally occurring human cancers independent
of retroviral involvement.

FREQUENT ACTIVATION OF RAS ONCOGENES IN HUMAN TUMOR CELLS

The linkage between retroviral and human cellular oncogenes
precipitated an intensive search for more examples of such relationships. A high fraction of the transforming genes of solid
tumors were found to be related to the oncogene (v-K-ras) of
Kirsten MSV (KiMSV)[42]. The transforming gene of Ki-MSV is
distantly related to those of BALB and Harvey MSVs at the nucleo-

tide level; however, the amino acid sequences of the p21 protein
encoded for by these oncogenes are highly homologous[43,44]. Oncogenes related to the retroviral ras sequences have also been found
to be present frequently in human hematopoietic tumors[45]. Of
these, we found a high percentage to be a new member of the ras
gene family, initially isolated from a human neuroblastoma cell
line[46]. Not all oncogenes detected by transfection have been shown
to be ras related. In fact, Cooper and co-workers have identified
and, in one case molecularly cloned, oncogenes that are not related
to known retroviral oncogenes[47].

ACTIVATION OF RAS ONCOGENES BY SINGLE POINT MUTATIONS

   The virtual identity between the T24 oncogene and its normal
cellular counterpart suggested that the high transforming activity
of this bladder oncogene could be due to very subtle alterations
in its structure[39]. By construction of appropriate recombinants,
the transforming activity of the T24 oncogene was localized to a
small region. Nucleotide sequence analysis of the gene yielded
the startling result that a single base change in the 12th codon
of the p21 coding sequence resulted in the substitution of valine
for glycine in the T24 gene and was therefore responsible for the
acquisition of its transforming properties[48-51].

   Further evidence for the importance of single point mutations
in activating ras genes has been derived from sequence analysis of
the corresponding domains of Ha-, BALB- and Ki-MSVs. The first
37-residue amino acid sequence encoded by each of these onc genes
is almost identical to the first exon of the human cellular H-ras
allele despite the fact that BALB and Harvey MSVs are of mouse and
rat origin, respectively, and v-K-ras originated from a different
proto-oncogene of rat origin. Yet, at position 12 each v-onc has
substituted a different amino acid: that is, lysine (E. Reddy et
al., unpublished), arginine[44] and serine[45], respectively.

   An H-ras-related oncogene (designated Hs242) was isolated from
cells of a human lung tumor explant[52]. By the approach utilized
for the analysis of the T24 gene, a 450-bp segment of the Hs242
gene was shown to be responsible for its transforming activity. In
contrast to the T24 oncogene, nucleotide sequence analysis revealed
that a single point mutation resulted in the incorporation of a
leucine instead of a glutamine in the 61st amino acid residue of
the N-ras p21 coding sequence. Thus, the Hs242 oncogene was
activated to become a transforming gene by a mechanism totally
different from that found for the T24 oncogene. A transforming
N-ras-related gene was molecularly cloned from NIH/3T3 cells transfected by the DNA of a human lung carcinoma (SW1271)[53]. A series

of recombinants between the SW1271 and N-ras genes were constructed
and tested for their transforming activity in the NIH/3T3 assay.
The transforming sequences in SW1271 could be localized to a region
encompassing the first and second exons of the gene. By nucleotide
sequence analysis, it was shown that the only change in these exons
between the normal and transforming alleles was a point mutation
that led to the replacement of glutamine by an arginine residue
in the 61st codon[53].

Recent studies by several groups[54-56] have also localized the
lesions that activate ras genes to become transforming genes to
these same specific codons. Thus, codons 12 and 61 appear to be
hot spots for activating members of the ras family of oncogenes.
Presumably, these mutations alter the site at which p21 interacts
with its normal substrates. The p21 proteins coded for by the
Hs242, T24, and SW1271 genes exhibit altered electrophoretic
mobilities when analyzed on polyacrylamide gels[39,48,52,57]. This
suggests that the mutations in either positions 12 or 61 cause a
conformational change in the protein. All of these findings argue
that qualitative rather than quantitative alterations are probably
the most common cause of these genes acquiring malignant properties
under natural conditions.

Of critical importance to the understanding of how human
cancers arise is the determination of the functions of transforming
proteins. Although much is known about how ras oncogenes become
activated as transforming genes of human tumors, virtually nothing
is known about their in vivo function(s). In vitro studies have
shown that certain p21 species bind GDP and GTP and do not possess
tyrosine-specific protein kinase activity as do many other onc
gene products[5].

IDENTIFICATION OF THE FUNCTION OF AN ONCOGENE ENCODED PROTEIN

Because proto-oncogenes are so well conserved in evolution,
it is likely that they serve important functions in normal cell
growth and development. However, identification of the function
of proto-oncogenes from which oncogenes have arisen has until
recently eluded efforts of scientists. For a number of years,
our laboratory has been investigating the properties of SSV. As
indicated earlier, the determination of its complete nucleotide
sequence allowed us to identify its transforming gene (sis) and
to study the physical and biochemical properties of the sis gene
product. Independently, other investigators were studying the
structure of human platelet-derived growth factor (PDGF), a potent
mitogen for connective tissue culture[58-60]. This protein is of
biological importance because it is thought to be involved in

wound healing. PDGF is a heat-stable, cationic protein which is
normally stored in the α granules of platelets. Its biologically
active forms are disulfide-bonded and range in size from 28,000-
35,000 daltons. Upon reduction, the molecule loses biologic
activity, yielding two distinct polypeptides, 1 and 2, each around
18,000 daltons in size[61].

Antoniades and Hunkapiller[62] recently reported the N-terminal
amino acid sequences of PDGF polypeptides 1 and 2. Upon entering
these newly published sequences into his computer bank of genetic
sequences, Doolittle made the striking observation that the amino
acid sequence of PDGF peptide 2 matched very closely, without
the introduction of gaps, with a stretch of the putative v-sis
protein[63] (Fig. 4). Studies by another group working on PDGF
structure[64] led to similar conclusions concerning the relationship
of the two proteins. The fact that v-sis is of New World primate
origin[65], while the sequence was derived from the PDGF human
protein, likely explained the very close but not perfect sequence
match. This strongly suggests that sis and PDGF have arisen from
the same cellular genes.

A tentative model emerges from the findings. In the normal
wound healing process, platelets disrupt and release PDGF at the
site of a wound. This leads to the transient stimulation of proliferation of connective tissue cells involved in wound healing.
However, if the sis/PDGF gene were abnormally derepressed, or
derepressed and/or qualitatively altered as well, in a cell
responsive to its growth stimulating actions, it might set in
motion a cycle of continuous cell growth. Thus, activation of sis
might be a step in the progression of events that leads certain
cell types along the pathway toward malignancy. This is a testable
model. It should be possible to clone the human c-sis gene transcribed in connective tissue tumors and determine whether it is
activated as a transforming gene in such tumors.

IMPLICATIONS

The normal cell possesses thousands of genes. The interactions between these genes and their products define cellular
developmental pathways as well as the regulation of normal cellular
growth. The malignant process appears to irreversibly alter
certain growth controls. Until recently, there have been very few
clues as to the mechanisms involved in malignant conversion. However, the research approaches summarized here have implicated what
appears to be a rather limited set of cellular genes as targets

```
p28sis    1   M T L T W Q G D P I P E E L Y K M L S G H S I R S F D D L Q R L L Q G D S G K E D G A E L D L N M T   50

p28sis   51   A S H S G G E L E S L A R G K R S L G S L S V I A E P A M I A E C K T R T E V F E I S R R L I D R I T N   100
PDGF-2    1                             S L G S L I T I I A E P A M I A E C K T R I E V F C I I C R R L ? D R I ? ?   34
PDGF-1    1                             S T E E A V P A I V C K T R T V T Y E I I S R R I E L I D I ? ? ?   28

p28sis  101   A N F L V W I P P C V E V Q R I C S I G C C N N I R N V Q I C I R I P I T I Q V Q L R I P I V I Q V I R I K I E I T V R I K I K   P I F   150
PDGF-2   35   ? ? ? ? P P C V E V K A I C I T I G C C N N I A N V I K I C I A I P I S I Q Y Q L I A I P I ? I Q V I A I K I E I I V I A I K I L   80
PDGF-1   29   A N F L I L   32

p28sis  151   K K A T V T L E D H L A C K C E I V A A A A R A V T R S P G T S Q E Q R A K T T Q S R V T I R T V R V   200

p28sis  201   R R P P K G K H A K C K H T H D K T A L K E T L G A   226
```

A, alanine; C, cysteine; D, aspartic acid; E, glutamic acid; F, phenylalanine; G, glycine; H, histidine; I, isoleucine; K, lysine; L, leucine; M, methionine; N, asparagine; P, proline; Q, glutamine; R, arginine; S, serine; T, threonine; V, valine; W, tryptophan; Y, tyrosine.

Fig. 4. Comparison of the amino acid sequences of PDGF peptides with the predicted amino acid sequence of the v-sis transforming protein (p28). Regions of identity are indicated by shaded boxes.

for genetic alterations that can lead normal cells to become
malignant. These genes were initially detected as transforming
genes captured by transforming retroviruses. Independent of retrovirus involvement, they appear to be activated by a variety of
mechanisms including chromosomal rearrangements and even extraordinarily subtle genetic alterations affecting their structure.

It is likely that new oncogenes will be discovered. Nonethe-
less, it is believed from evidence obtained so far that the problem
of deciphering the neoplastic process is becoming less complex and,
thus, more approachable. If so, it is likely that by studying the
small set of proto-oncogenes initially discovered as components of
a small group of RNA tumor viruses, insight will be gained into
strategies that may eventually be useful in the diagnosis, treatment and even prevention of human cancer.

REFERENCES

1. L. Gross, "Oncogenic Viruses", 2nd edit, Pergamon Press, Oxford (1970).
2. R. A. Weiss, N. Teich, H. Varmus, and R. J. Coffin, eds., "Molecular Biology of Tumor Viruses, RNA Tumor Viruses," 2nd edit., Cold Spring Harbor Laboratory, New York, N. Y. (1982).
3. H. Temin, Function of the retrovirus long terminal repeat, Cell 28:3 (1982).
4. P. H. Duesberg, Retroviral transforming genes in normal cells?, Nature 304:219 (1983).
5. J. M. Bishop, in: "Ann. Rev. Biochemistry," E. E. Snell, P. D. Boyer, A. Meister, and C. C. Richardson, eds., Academic Press, Palo Alto, CA. (1983).
6. K. C. Robbins, S. G. Devare, E. P. Reddy, and S. A. Aaronson, In vivo identification of the transforming gene product of simian sarcoma virus, Science 218:1131 (1982).
7. A. Srinivasan, C. Y. Dunn, Y. Yuasa, S. G. Devare, E. P. Reddy, and S. A. Aaronson, Abelson murine leukemia virus: structural requirements for transforming gene function, Proc. Natl. Acad. Sci. USA 79:5508 (1982).
8. M. S. Collet and R. L. Erickson, Protein kinase activity associated with the avian sarcoma virus src gene product, Proc. Natl. Acad. Sci. USA 75:2021 (1978).
9. A. D. Levinson, H. Opperman, L. Levintow, H. E. Varmus, and J. M. Bishop, Evidence that the transforming gene of avian sarcoma virus encodes a protein kinase associated with a phosphoprotein, Cell 15:561 (1978).
10. S. G. Devare, E. P. Reddy, J. D. Law, K. C. Robbins, and S. A. Aaronson, Nucleotide sequence of the simian sarcoma virus genome: demonstration that its acquired cellular sequences encode the putative transforming gene product p28sis, Proc. Natl. Acad. Sci. USA 80:731 (1983).
11. S. A. Aaronson, E. P. Reddy, K. Robbins, S. G. Devare, D. C. Swan, J. H. Pierce, and S. R. Tronick, in: "Human Carcinogenesis," C. C. Harris and H. N. Autrup, eds. Academic Press, N. Y., in press.
12. J. H. Pierce and S. A. Aaronson, BALB- and Harvey-MSV transformation of a novel lymphoid progenitor cell, J. Exp. Med. 156:873 (1982).
13. J. H. Pierce and S. A. Aaronson, In vitro transformation of murine pre-B lymphoid cells by Snyder-Theilen sarcoma virus, J. Virol. 46:993 (1983).
14. N. Rosenberg and D. Baltimore, A quantitative assay for transformation of bone marrow cells by Abelson murine leukemia virus, J. Exp. Med. 143:1453 (1976).

274   S. A. AARONSON ET AL.

15. B-Z. Shilo and R. A. Weinberg, DNA sequences homologous to vertebrate oncogenes are conserved in Drosophila melanogaste, Proc Natl. Acad. Sci. USA 78:6789 (1981).
16. D. C. Swan, O. W. McBride, K. C. Robbins, D. A. Keithley, E. P. Reddy, and S. A. Aaronson, Chromosomal mapping of the simian sarcoma virus onc gene analogue in human cells, Proc. Natl. Acad. Sci. USA 79:4691 (1982).
17. K. Prakash, O. W. McBride, D. C. Swan, S. G. Devare, S. R. Tronick, and S. A. Aaronson, Molecular cloning and chromosomal mapping of a human locus related to the transforming gene of Moloney murine sarcoma virus, Proc. Natl. Acad. Sci. USA 79:5210 (1982).
18. R. Taub, I. Kirsch, C. Morton, G. Lenoir, D. C. Swan, S. Tronick, S. A. Aaronson, and P. Leder, Translocation of the c-myc gene into the immunoglobulin heavy chain locus in human Burkitt's lymphoma and murine plasmacytoma cells, Proc. Natl. Acad. Sci. USA 79:7837 (1982).
19. O. W. McBride, D. S. Swan, K. C. Robbins, K. Prakash, and S. A. Aaronson, Chromosomal mapping of tumor virus transforming gene analogues in human cells, in: "Gene Transfer and Cancer 1982," M. L. Pearson and N. L. Sternberg, eds., Raven Press, New York, in press.
20. O. W. McBride, D. C. Swan, E. Santos, M. Barbacid, S. R. Tronick, and S. A. Aaronson, Localization of the normal allele of T24 human bladder carcinoma oncogene to chromosome 11, Nature 300:773 (1982).
21. R. Dalla Favera, R. C. Gallo, A. Giallongo, and C. M. Croce, Chromosomal localization of the human homolog (c-sis) of the simian sarcoma virus onc gene, Science 218:686 (1982).
22. R. Dalla-Favera, M. Bregni, J. Erikson, D. Patterson, R. C. Gallo, and C. M. Croce, Human c-myc onc gene is located on the region of chromosome 8 that is translocated in Burkitt lymphoma cells, Proc. Natl. Acad. Sci. USA 79:7824 (1982).
23. B. G. Neel, S. C. Jhanwar, R. S. K. Chaganti, and W. S. Hayward, Two human c-onc genes are located on the long arm of chromosome 8, Proc. Natl. Acad. Sci. USA 79:7842 (1982).
24. B. De Martinville, J. Giacalone, C. Shih, R. A. Weinberg, and U. Francke, Oncogene from human EJ bladder carcinoma is located on the short arm of chromosome 11, Science 219:498 (1983).
25. A. Y. Sakaguchi, S. L. Naylor, T. B. Shows, J. J. Toole, M. McCoy, and R. A. Weinberg, Human c-Ki-ras-2 proto-oncogene on chromosome 12, Science 219:1081 (1983).
26. A. Hall, C. J. Marshall, N. I. Spurr, and R. A. Weiss, Identification of transforming gene in two human sarcoma cell lines as a new member of the ras gene family located on chromosome 1, Nature 303:396 (1983).

27. M. E. Harper, G. Franchini, J. Love, M. I. Simon, R. C. Gallo, and F. Wong-Staal, Chromosomal sublocalization of human c-myb and c-fes cellular onc genes, Nature 304:169 (1983).
28. B. De Martinville, J. M. Cunningham, M. J. Murray, and U. Francke, The N-ras oncogene assigned to the short arm of human chromosome 1, Nucleic Acids Res. 11:5267 (1983).
29. J. Ryan, P. E. Barker, K. Shimizu, M. Wigler, and F. Ruddle, Chromosomal assignment of a family of human oncogenes, Proc. Natl. Acad. Sci. USA 80:4460 (1983).
30. S. J. O'Brien, W. G. Nash, J. L. Goodwin, D. R. Lowy, and E. H. Chang, Dispersion of the ras family of transforming genes to four different chromosomes in man, Nature 302:839 (1983).
31. G. Klein, The role of gene dosage and genetic transpositions in carcinogenesis, Nature 294:313 (1981).
32. A. Ar-Rushdi, K. Nishikura, J. Erikson, R. Watt, G. Rovera, and C. M. Croce, Differential expression of the translocated and the untranslocated c-myc oncogene in Burkitt lymphoma, Science 222:390 (1983).
33. A. de Klein, A. G. Van Kessel, G. Grosveld, C. R. Bartram, A. Hagemeijer, D. Bootsma, N. K. Spurr, N. Heisterkamp, J. Groffen, and J. R. Stephenson, A cellular oncogene is trans-located to the Philadelphia chromosome in chronic myelocytic leukaemia, Nature 300:765 (1982).
34. J. Groffen, N. Heisterkamp, J. R. Stephenson, A. G. Van Kessel, A. de Klein, G. Grosveld, and D. Bootsma, C-sis is trans-located from chromosome 22 to chromosome 9 in chronic myelocytic leukemia, J. Exp. Med. 158:9 (1983).
35. D. Sheer, L. R. Hiorns, K. F. Stanley, P. N. Goodfellow, D. M. Swallow, S. Povey, N. Heisterkamp, J. Groffen, J. R. Stephenson, and E. Solomon, Genetic analysis of the 15;17 chromosome translocation associated with acute promyelocytic leukemia, Proc. Natl. Acad. Sci. USA 80:5007 (1983).
36. C. Shih, and R. A. Weinberg, Isolation of a transforming sequence from a human bladder carcinoma cell line, Cell 29:161 (1982).
37. S. Pulciani, E. Santos, A. V. Lauver, L. K. Long, K. C. Robbins, and M. Barbacid, Oncogenes in human tumor cell lines: molecular cloning of a transforming gene from human bladder carcinoma cells, Proc. Natl. Acad. Sci. USA 79:2845 (1982).
38. M. Goldfard, K. Shimizu, M. Perucho, and M. Wigler, Isolation and preliminary characterization of a human transforming gene from T24 bladder carcinoma cells, Nature (London) 296:404 (1982).
39. E. Santos, S. R. Tronick, S. A. Aaronson, S. Pulciani, and M. Barbacid, The T24 human bladder carcinoma oncogene is an activated form of the normal human homologue of BALB- and Harvey-MSV transforming genes, Nature 298:343 (1982).

40. L. F. Parada, C. J. Tabin, C. Shif, and R. A. Weinberg, Human
    EJ bladder carcinoma oncogene is homologue of Harvey
    sarcoma virus ras gene, Nature 297:474 (1982).
41. C. J. Der, T. G. Krontiris, and G. M. Cooper, Transforming
    genes of human bladder and lung carcinoma cell lines are
    homologous to the ras genes of Harvey and Kirsten sarcoma
    viruses, Proc. Nat. Acad. Sci. USA 79:3637 (1982).
42. S. Pulciani, E. Santos, A. V. Lauver, L. K. Long, S. A.
    Aaronson, and M. Barbacid, Oncogenes in solid human tumors,
    Nature 300:539-542 (1982).
43. R. Dhar, R. W. Ellis, T. Y. Shih, S. Oroszlan, B. Shapiro, J.
    Maizel, D. Lowy, and E. Scolnick, Nucleotide sequence of the
    p21 transforming protein of Harvey murine sarcoma virus,
    Science 217:934 (1982).
44. N. Tsuchida, R. Ryder, and E. Ohtsubo, Nucleotide sequence of
    the oncogene encoding the p21 transforming protein of
    Kirsten murine sarcoma virus, Science 217:937 (1982).
45. S. Eva, S. R. Tronick, R. A. Gol, J. H. Pierce, and S. A.
    Aaronson, Transforming genes of human hematopoietic
    tumors: frequent detection of ras-related oncogenes whose
    activation appears to be independent of tumor phenotype,
    Proc. Natl. Acad. Sci. USA 80:4926 (1983).
46. K. Shimizu, M. Goldfarb, M. Perucho, and M. Wigler, Isolation
    and preliminary characterization of the transforming gene
    of a human neuroblastoma cell line, Proc. Natl. Acad. Sci.
    USA 80:383 (1983).
47. G. Goubin, D. S. Goldman, J. Luce, P. E. Neiman, and G. M.
    Cooper, Molecular cloning and nucleotide sequence of a
    transforming gene detected by transfection of chicken
    B-cell lymphoma DNA, Nature 302:114 (1983).
48. C. J. Tabin, S. M. Bradley, C. I. Baugmann, R. A. Weinberg,
    A. G. Papageorge, E. M. Scolnick, R. Dhar, D. R. Lowy, and
    E. H. Chang, Mechanism of activation of a human oncogene,
    Nature 300: 143 (1982).
49. E. P. Reddy, R. K. Reynolds, E. Santos, and M. Barbacid, A
    point mutation is responsible for the acquisition of
    transforming properties by the T24 human bladder carcinoma
    oncogene, Nature 300:149 (1982).
50. E. Taparowsky, Y. Suard, O. Fasano, K. Shimizu, M. Goldfard,
    and M. Wigler, Activation of the T24 bladder carcinoma
    transforming gene is linked to a single amino acid change,
    Nature 300:762 (1982).
51. D. J. Capon, E. Y. Chen, A. D. Levinson, P. H. Seeburg, and
    D. V. Goeddel, Complete nucleotide sequences of the T24
    human bladder carcinoma oncogene and its normal homologue,
    Nature 302:33 (1983).

52. Y. Yuasa, S. K. Srivastava, C. Y. Dunn, J. S. Rhim, E. P. Reddy, and S. A. Aaronson, Acquisition of transforming properties by alternative point mutations within c-bas/has human protooncogene, Nature 303:775 (1983).
53. Y. Yuasa, et. al., Manuscript in preparation, (1983).
54. K. Shimizu, D. Birnbaum, M. A. Ruley, O. Fasano, Y. Suard, L. Edlund, E. Taparowsky, M. Goldfard, and M. Wigler, Structure of the Ki-ras gene of the human lung carcinoma cell line Calu-1, Nature 304:497 (1983).
55. D. J. Capon, P. H. Seeburg, J. P. McGrath, J. S. Hayflick, U. Edman, A. D. Levinson, and D. V. Goeddel, Activation of Ki-ras-2 gene in human colon and lung carcinomas by two different point mutations, Nature 304:507-513 (1983).
56. E. Taparowsky, K. Shimizu, M. Goldfarb, and M. Wigler, Structure and activation of the human N-ras gene, Cell 34:581 (1983).
57. C. J. Der and G. M. Cooper, Altered gene products are associated with activation of cellular ras genes in human lung and colon carcinomas, Cell 32:201 (1983).
58. R. Ross, J. Glomset, B. Kariya, and L. Harker, A platelet-dependent serum factor that stimulates the proliferation of arterial smooth muscle cells in vitro, Proc. Natl. Acad. Sci. USA 71:1207 (1974).
59. C. D. Scher, R. C. Shepard, H. N. Antoniades, and C. D. Stiles, Platelet-derived growth factor and the regulation of the mammalian fibroblast cell cycle, Biochim. Biophys. Acta 560:217 (1979).
60. C. H. Heldin, B. Westermark, and A. Wasteson, Platelet-derived growth factor: Purification and partial characterization, Proc. Natl. Acad. Sci. USA 76:3722 (1979).
61. H. N. Antoniades and L. T. Lewis, Human platelet-derived growth factor: structure and function, Fed. Proc. 42:2630 (1983).
62. H. N. Antoniades and M. W. Hunkapiller, Human platelet-derived growth factor (PDGF): amino-terminal amino acid sequence, Science 220:963 (1983).
63. R. F. Doolittle, M. W. Hunkapiller, L. E. Hood, S. G. Devare, K. C. Robbins, S. A. Aaronson, and H. N. Antoniades, Simian sarcoma virus onc gene, v-sis, is derived from the gene (or genes) encoding a platelet-derived growth factor, Science 221:275 (1983).
64. M. D. Waterfield, G. T. Scrace, N. Whittle, P. Stroobant, A. Johnsson, A. Wasteson, B. Westermark, C. H. Heldin, J. S. Huang, and T. F. Deuel, Platelet-derived growth factor is structurally related to the putative transforming protein p28^{sis} of simian sarcoma virus, Nature 304:36 (1983).
65. K. C. Robbins, R. L. Hill, and S. A. Aaronson, Primate origin of the cell-derived sequences of simian sarcoma virus, J. Virol. 41:721 (1982).

MODULATION OF THYROID EPITHELIAL DIFFERENTIATION BY TWO VIRAL

ONCOGENES

P.P. Di Fiore, A. Fusco, G. Colletta, A. Pinto,
M. Ferrentino, V. De Franciscis, and G. Vecchio

Centro di Endocrinologia ed Oncologia Sperimentale del
C.N.R., c/o Dipartimento di Biologia e Patologia
Cellulare e Molecolare, II Facoltà di Medicina e
Chirurgia dell' Università di Napoli, Via S. Pansini
5, 80131, Napoli, Italy

The loss of the expression of a differentiated phenotype is one of the most interesting features of many tumors, either spontaneously occurring in humans, or experimentally induced into laboratory animals.

The molecular analysis of the relationships between cellular transformation and the expression of the differentiated functions is complicated by the lack of in vitro systems of cell lines continuously growing in culture, but stably expressing a differentiated phenotype. In particular, although in the last few years many systems have been developed of mesenchimal origin, which allowed to study the effect of transformation on cellular differentiation such as chondroblasts (1,2), fibroblasts (3,4) and hemopoietic precursors (5,6,7), very few epithelial systems have been so far available for such studies (8,9).

Recently in our laboratory a system has been developed of rat epithelial thyroid cells, established as a continuously growing cell line (10). This cell line, called FRT-L, displays in vitro several of the highly specific differentiated functions of the gland from which it has been obtained, i.e. the thyroid gland. FRT-L cells, in fact, are able to concentrate iodide from the culture medium, to synthesize and secrete thyroglobulin (the major thyroid protein); moreover, they possess a specific membrane receptor for the thyroid physiological regulatory hormone (the thyrotropin, TSH) and are dependent on a mix of six growth factors (including TSH) for optimal growth.

279

This cell system represents, then, an excellent model to study the relationships between the epithelial cell transformation and the expression of the differentiated phenotype. The use of such a model could be also interesting on the ground of the hypothesis which considers cancer as a "differentiation disease" rather than a "proliferation disease" (5).

These cells have been successfully infected and transformed with the Kirsten murine sarcoma virus (11-13) as well as with several isolates of other murine sarcoma viruses. A detailed outline of the latter work is presented elsewhere in this volume (14). Since one of the most impressive effect of transformation by these viruses is the loss of the differentiated functions we decided to focus our attention on this problem. We, therefore, infected and transformed FRT-L cells with two different isolates of murine sarcoma viruses, both temperature sensitive (ts) for transformation.

Murine sarcoma viruses ts for transformation possess a transforming protein which is thermosensitive, in that it is functional at a given temperature (33 °C, permissive temperature), whereas it is inactivated at a higher temperature (39 °C, nonpermissive temperature). Consequently, a cell infected by such a virus is expected to behave as malignant at the permissive temperature and as normal at the nonpermissive one. The use of such mutants allowed us to study whether the loss of differentiation of FRT-L cells was a phenomenon linked to cell transformation or somehow only triggered by this latter event, but essentially independent from the continuous presence and functionality of the viral transforming protein.

In a first series of experiments we infected FRT-L cells with a ts mutant of the Kirsten murine sarcoma virus (KiMSV). A detailed analysis of such a work has been already published elsewhere (13); only summary data will be presented here togheter with some new experimental data.

The KiMSV possesses an oncogene called Ki-ras, which encodes for the transforming protein p21 (15,16). This viral oncogene is particularly interesting in the light of its strict structural homology with several transforming genes isolated from human tumors. In Table 1 are shown the effects of infection of FRT-L cells with KiMSVts. FRT-L cells grown at permissive temperature after the infection, became rapidly morphologically transformed and behaved as truly malignant in that they showed anchorage independent growth (as tested by soft agar assay, see also Fig. 2). The cells were able to grow as solid tumors when injected subcutaneously into syngeneic rats (Table 1).All of the tumors induced showed the histological features of carcinomas with a

Table 1: Transformation of epithelial differentiated rat thyroid cells by a wild type and a temperature sensitive strain of the Kirsten sarcoma virus.

CELL LINE	VIRUS PRODUCTION		TRANSFORMATION MARKERS		DIFFERENTIATION MARKERS		
	RT[a]	FFU[b]	Growth in soft agar	Tumor induction	TG production[c]	TG mRNA	Iodide uptake
FRT-L	−	−	−	−	+	+	+
FRT-L KiMSV wt	+	+	+	+	−	−	−
FRT-L KiMSV ts 33 °C	+	+	+	+	−	−	−
FRT-L KiMSV ts 39 °C	+	+	+	NT[d]	−	−	−

[a] RT: reverse transcriptase assay

[b] FFU: focus forming unit; the assay was performed on RAT-2 cells at 37 °C

[c] Thyroglobulin production was measured either by immunoprecipitation/gel electrophoresis or a radio-immunoassay

[d] NT: Not tested

moderate degree of differentiation, as evidenced by the formation
of glandular-like structures (Fig. 1).

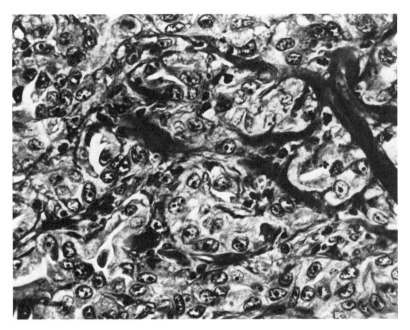

Fig. 1: Histological appearance of a tumor induced by injecting
        subcutaneously FRT-L cells transformed by KiMSVts into
        a syngeneic newborn Fischer rat (courtesy of Dr G.
        Tajana).

The epithelial origin of the induced tumors was also confirmed by
an electron microscopy study, which showed typical epithelial
tight junction (desmosomes) between cells (17).

      As far as the expression of the differentiation markers is
concerned we observed, after transformation with KiMSVts at the
permissive temperature, a complete loss in the expression of the
differentiated functions by FRT-L cells. Cells were unable to trap
iodide and to synthesize and secrete thyroglobulin; in particular
the results of the analysis of thyroglobulin production were
constantly negative either when the search was performed by
immunoprecipitation by anti-TG antibodies and subsequent gel
electophoresis, or when a more sensitive radio-immunoassay for rat
thyroglobulin (courtesy of Dr. A. Schneider, Chicago, USA) was
employed (Table 1).

When the KiMSVts-transformed cells were shifted to the nonpermissive temperature (39 °C), a complete reversion of the transformed phenotype was observed: cells reacquired a morphology closely resembling that of normal epithelial cells growing in vitro, and were unable to grow in soft agar.

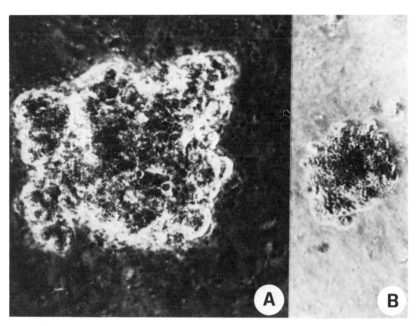

Fig. 2: Anchorage-independent growth of FRT-L cells transformed with KiMSVts, in soft agar either at permissive (A) or nonpermissive temperature (B).

In Fig. 2 is shown the appearance of the soft agar assay performed on FRT-L KiMSVts cells grown either at permissive (Fig. 2A) or nonpermissive temperature (Fig. 2B). It is interesting to notice that the cells grown at 33 °C displayed a very high cloning efficiency (> 80%), and formed very large colonies; in contrast, cells grown at the nonpermissive temperature displayed a very low cloning efficiency (< 2-3%), and the few colonies which they formed were very small.

The residual ability of FRT-L KiMSVts cells, grown at 39 °C, (non- permissive temperature) to form colonies in agar might be attributed to their provenience from the permissive temperature, prior to seeding in agar at 39 °C. When the assay was performed on cells grown at 39 °C for many generations, no colony formation was observed in agar plates incubated at the same temperature (data not shown).

Interestingly, the reversion of the transformation markers was not paralleled by the reversion of differentiation. FRT-L KiMSVts cells, in fact, did not reacquire either the ability to synthesize thyroglobulin or that of concentrating iodide from the supernatant fluid (Table 1).

Therefore we conclude that the loss of the differentiated phenotype, which took place upon infection and transformation of FRT-L cells by KiMSVts is irreversible, in that it is independent from the continuous expression of the ras oncogene and from the presence of the specific transforming product of this oncogene, i.e. the p21 protein.

A molecular analysis was then initiated to identify the molecular site in which the damage has occurred which led to the block in the expression of the differentiated phenotype.We focused our attention on the expression of the TG gene, taking advantage from cDNA clones, specific for the thyroglobulin messenger RNA, recently obtained in our laboratory (18) (courtesy of Dr. R. Di Lauro, Naples, Italy).

Cytoplasmic RNA (Table 1) and nuclear RNA (data not shown), extracted from normal FRT-L and KiMSVts transformed cells (either grown at 33 °C or 39 °C), were spotted onto nitrocellulose filters and then hybridized with a nick-translated cDNA clone, which recognizes the 3' end of the thyroglobulin mRNA; no TG-specific mRNA was detected, by this technique, in transformed cells at both temperatures, whereas positive results were observed with RNA extracted from normal FRT-L cells (Table 1).The absence of TG mRNA at cytoplasmic and nuclear level allowed us to conclude that the loss of the expression of the specific thyroid protein is attributable to a block in the transcription of the TG gene.

A study is now in progress in our laboratory to ascertain whether any change is detectable in the TG gene of transformed cells (vs. the TG gene present in normal cells) which can account for the block in the transcriptional process. This study includes:

1. Analysis of the presence and conformational status of TG gene (by means of restriction endonucleases digestion, Southern blotting and hybridization to specific probes) in normal and transformed cells;
2. analysis of the methylation pattern in and around the TG gene in both types of cells;
3. Chromatin structure analysis by means of DNase I and micrococcal nuclease probes.

Preliminary results revealed that the TG gene is present in the same conformational status either in normal or transformed cells, thus the block in its expression cannot be attributed to gross rearrangements in the gene structure. An example of these results is given in Fig. 3, where a restriction analysis of a region located toward the 3' end of the TG gene is shown; from the comparison of the Southern blot analysis performed on DNA extracted from normal and transformed cells and digested with the indicated endonucleases, is evident that no gross alterations in the gene structure was caused by the transformation event.

N   T

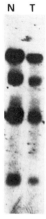

Pvu II

Fig. 3: Conformational status of the Tg gene in normal and KiMSVts transformed cells.
High molecular weight DNA was extracted from normal (N) or transformed cells (T) and digested with Pvu II restriction endonuclease. Southern blot hybridization was performed with a cDNA cloned probe (p36) of 1.8 Kb wich recognizes a region located 1.2 Kb far from the 3' end on the TG mRNA.

The data here reported show that the TG gene, normally expressed in rat thyroid cells, is repressed by the transformation event caused by the KiMSV. Studies are now in progress, in our laboratory, to analyze in detail other sequences that are regulated by the presence of an active transforming protein p21, which is the product of the Ki-ras oncogene. To this purpose, a cDNA bank obtained from normal rat thyroid glands (courtesy of Drs. R. Di Lauro and V. Ursini) has been hybridized with RNA prepared from KiMSVts-infected cells, grown at both temperatures, in order to isolate clones representative of sequences that are modulated (activated or repressed) by the transformation event.The isolated clones can be assigned to one of the following four different categories which represent different sequences:

a. those negatively regulated by the transformation event, which disappear after transformation, both at 33° and 39° C (TG like sequences);

b. those also negatively regulated, but which disappear at 33°C and reappear at 39°C;

c. those positively regulated by the transformation event, which are expressed at high level at 33°C and remain expressed at 39°C;

d. those also regulated positively by the transformation event, but which are expressed at high levels at 33°C and disappear almost completely at 39°C.

Table 2. Transformation of epithelial differentiated rat thyroid cells by various strains of the myeloproliferative sarcoma virus

CELL LINE	GROWTH IN SOFT AGAR	TUMOR INDUCTION	TG[a] mRNA	IODIDE UPTAKE
FRT-L	−	−	+	+
FRT-L MPSVwt	+	+	−	−
FRT-L MPSVts 33 °C	+	NT[b]	−	−
FRT-L MPSVts 39 °C	−	NT	−	−

[a] TG: Thyroglobulin
[b] NT: Not Tested.

Further studies are in progress aimed to the full characterization of such clones (V. De Franciscis, V.E. Avvedimento, G. Colletta, V. Zimarino, V. Ursini, unpublished experiments).

A similar study has been undertaken with another retrovirus, the myeloproliferative sarcoma virus (MPSV), of which a ts mutant for transformation is available (19), in order to generalize the effect of retroviral transformation on the differentiation of thyroid epithelial cells. One can in fact postulate that the irreversible block in the expression of the mature phenotype is a general consequence of the transformation of FRT-L cells or, alternatively, that it might be attributable to a peculiar interaction of the ras oncogene with the epithelial thyroid cell. The use of MPSVts can help us to distinguish between these hypotheses: MPSV, in fact, possesses an oncogene belonging to the mos family (20), a group of oncogenes which is distinct from the ras family. Thus far the MPSV specific transforming protein is different from the p21-ras protein and it can be supposed to act through different mechanisms and/or interactions with different cellular substrates.

FRT-L cells infected with MPSVts (FRT-L MPSVts) rapidly became tranfromed, when grown at the permissive temperature, undergoing morphological changes and acquiring the typical transformation properties (growth in soft agar and tumorigenicity into syngeneic animals) (Table 2). Also in this case, transformation was followed by a complete disappearance of the differentiation markers (TG production and iodide uptake) (Table 2).

Upon shifting from the permissive to the nonpermissive temperature, FRT-L MPSVts cells exibited the typical dissociation between transformed and differentiated phenotypes. In fact, while we observed the complete regression of the transformation markers (Table 2), the differentiated functions remained suppressed. Also in the case of MPSV transformation, then, the loss of the expression of the differentiated phenotype is irreversible in our system of differentiated epithelial thyroid cells.

The results reported here, togheter with those previously obtained, demonstrate that:

1. Murine sarcoma viruses, such as KiMSV and MPSV, have an oncogenic potential not only towards cells of mesenchimal origin, but also towards epithelial cells, such as thyroid cells. Results obtained with other murine sarcoma viruses, presented elsewhere in this volume (14) further strenghten this point.
2. Thyroid epithelial differentiation is modulated in a negative fashion by murine sarcoma viruses, i.e. thyroid differentiation markers are expressed by normal untransformed thyroid cells, but their expression is blocked after transformation.
3. In contrast to transformation which can be reverted by infecting the thyroid cells with temperature sensitive strains of either KiMSV or MPSV at the permissive temperature (33°C) and then shifting the cultures at the non permissive temperature (39°C), the block in differentiation cannot be reverted by such a temperature shift. Other biochemical events must have occurred, therefore, after transformation, which are responsible for the lack of reversion of the differentiated phenotype and which do not necessarily require the expression of the p21 product of the ras oncogene.

ACKNOWLEDGEMENTS

This work was supported by the Progetto Finalizzato Controllo della Crescita Neoplastica of the Consiglio Nazionale delle Ricerche (C.N.R.)

REFERENCES

1. M. Pacifici, D. Boettiger, K. Roby and H. Holtzer, Transformation of chondroblasts by Rous sarcoma virus and synthesis of the sulphated proteoglycan matrix, Cell 11:891 (1977).
2. E. Gionti, O. Capasso and R. Cancedda, The culture of chick embryo chondrocytes and the control of their differentiated functions, J. Biol. Chem. 258:7190 (1983).
3. S.L. Adams, M.E. Sodel, B.H. Howard, K. Olden, K.M. Yamada, B. de-Crombrugghe and I. Pastan, Levels of translatable mRNAs for cell surface protein, collagen precursors, and two membrane proteins are altered in Rous sarcoma virus-transformed chick embryo fibroblasts, Proc. Natl. Acad. Sci. USA 74:3399 (1977).
4. M.I. Parker, K. Judge and W. Gevers, Loss of type I procollagen gene expression in SV40-transformed human fibroblasts is accompanied by hypermethylation of these genes, Nucl. Acids Res. 10:5879 (1982).
5. T. Graf, N. Ade and H. Beug, Temperature sensitive mutant of avian erythroblastosis virus suggests a block of differentiation as mechanism of leukemogenesis, Nature 275:496 (1978).
6. J. Pierce and S.A. Aaronson, Balb and Harvey murine sarcoma virus transformation of a novel lymphoid progenitor cell, J. Exp. Med. 156:876 (1982).
7. J. Pierce and S.A. Aaronson, In vitro transformation of murine pre-B lymphoid cells by Snyder-Theilen feline sarcoma virus, J. Virol. 46:993 (1983).
8. B.E. Weissman and S.A. Aaronson, Balb and Kirsten murine sarcoma viruses alter growth and differentiation of EGF-dependent Balb/c mouse epidermal cheratinocyte lines, Cell 32:599 (1983).
9. N. Auersperg, J.B. Hudson, E.G. Goddard and V. Klement, Transformation of cultured rat adrenocortical cells by Kirsten murine sarcoma virus (Ki MSV), Int. J. Cancer 19:81 (1977).
10. F.S. Ambesi-Impiombato, L.A.M. Parks and H.G. Coon, Culture of hormone-dependent epithelial cells from rat thyroids, Proc. Natl. Acad. Sci. USA 77:3455 (1980).
11. A. Fusco, A. Pinto, F.S. Ambesi-Impiombato, G. Vecchio and N. Tsuchida, Transformation of rat thyroid epithelial cells by Kirsten murine sarcoma virus, Int. J. Cancer 28:655 (1981).
12. A. Fusco, A. Pinto, D. Tramontano, G. Tajana, G. Vecchio and N. Tsuchida, Block in the expression of differentiation markers of rat thyroid epithelial cells by transformation with Kirsten murine sarcoma virus, Cancer Res. 42:618 (1982).
13. G. Colletta, A. Pinto, P.P. Di Fiore, A. Fusco, M. Ferrentino, V.E. Avvedimento, N. Tsuchida and G. Vecchio, Dissociation between transformed and differentiated phenotype in rat thyroid epithelial cells after transformation with a temperature-sensitive mutant of the Kirsten murine sarcoma virus, Mol. Cell. Biol. 3:2099 (1983).

14. A. Fusco, P.P. Di Fiore, M.T. Berlingieri, G. Colletta, A.M. Cirafici, G. Portella and M. Santoro, Thyroid neoplastic transformation in vivo and in vitro, this volume.

15. T.Y. Shih, M.O. Weeks, H.A. Young and E.M. Scolnick, Identification of a sarcoma virus-coded phosphoprotein in nonproducer cells transformed by Kirsten or Harvey murine sarcoma viruses, Virology 96:164 (1979).

16. T.Y. Shih, M.O. Weeks, H.A. Young and E.M. Scolnick, P21 of Kirsten murine sarcoma virus is thermolabile in a viral mutant temperature sensitive for the maintenance of transformation, J. Virol. 31:546 (1979).

17. G. Vecchio, L. Nitsch, G. Tajana, A. Pinto and A. Fusco, Experimental thyroid carcinogenesis by RNA tumor viruses, in "Advances in thyroid neoplasia 1981", M. Andreoli et al. eds., Field Educational Italia, Roma, 1981.

18. R. Di Lauro, S. Obici, A.M. Acquaviva and C. G. Alvino, Construction of recombinant plasmids containing rat thyroglobulin mRNA sequences, Gene 19:117 (1982).

19. W. Ostertag, I.B. Pragnell, A. Fusco, D. Hughes, M. Freshney, B. Klein, C. Jasmin, J. Bilello, G. Warnecke and K. Vehemeyer, Studies on the biology and genetics of murine erythroleukemia viruses, in "Expression of differentiated functions in cancer cells", R. F. Revoltella et al. eds., Raven Press, New York (1982).

20. I.B. Pragnell, A. Fusco, C. Arbuthnott, F. Smadja-Joffe, B. Klein, C. Jasmine and W. Ostertag, Analysis of Myeloproliferative sarcoma virus genome: limited changes in the prototype lead to altered target specifity, J. Virol. 38:952 (1981).

THYROID NEOPLASTIC TRANSFORMATION IN VITRO AND IN VIVO

A. Fusco, P.P. Di Fiore, M.T. Berlingieri, G. Colletta,
A.M. Cirafici, G. Portella, and M. Santoro

Centro di Endocrinologia ed Oncologia Sperimentale del
C.N.R., c/o Dipartimento di Biologia e Patologia
Cellulare e Molecolare, II Facoltà di Medicina e
Chirurgia dell' Università di Napoli, via S. Pansini 5
80131, Napoli, Italy

Oncogenic RNA viruses (retroviruses) can be classified, according to their biological and molecular features, into two broad groups: acute transforming retroviruses and chronically transforming retroviruses (1,2). Viruses from the latter group are able to induce tumors (above all lymphoid leukemias) with a long latency period and with low efficiency; they are not capable of transforming cells in culture and do not possess the specific genetic information coding for a transforming protein. The acute transforming retroviruses, on the other hand, induce tumors (above all sarcomas and non lymphoid leukemias) with a high efficiency and a short latency period; they are able to transform cells in culture and possess genomic sequences encoding for the transforming proteins (oncogenes) (1).

Retroviruses from this latter class originate from recombination events, occurred in the host cell, between the genome of a non transforming retrovirus and the cellular genome; the sequences thus transduced are responsible for the transforming property of the acute retroviruses (1).The cellular sequences are called "cellular oncogenes" and "viral oncogenes" the homologous ones present in the viral genome.

It is generally assumed that the specific targets for transformation either in vivo or in vitro of acute retroviruses are fibroblasts as well as other cells of mesenchimal derivation, including haemopoietic cell lineages (3). Some investigators reported the transformation of epithelial cells with acute retroviruses. It has been reported that rat adrenocortical epithelial cells can be transformed by the Kirsten murine sarcoma virus (Ki MSV) (4); rat liver epithelial cells by the Harvey murine sarcoma virus (Ha MSV) and Ki MSV (5,6); mouse cheratinocytes by the Balb/c murine sarcoma virus (Balb MSV) (7). Nevertheless, no systematic studies have been performed to determine whether the ability of transforming epithelial cytotypes is a general feature of these viruses or it is restricted to some of them.

This study is of high importance in the light of the fact that the epithelial malignancies (carcinomas) account for the great majority of human tumors whereas sarcomas and leukemias are a minor fraction of the malignant growth in man. Moreover, it has been possible to isolate from human carcinomas, by the transfection assay, genes capable to induce morphological changes and tumorigenicity in the NIH 3T3 cells(1,8-10). These genes are, in most cases, homologous to the viral oncogenes of two murine sarcoma viruses, the Ha MSV and the Ki MSV. These genes are called ras Ha and ras Ki, respectively.

In a previous work we demonstrated that the Ki MSV is able to transform epithelial thyroid cells from Fischer rats(11-13). These cells, called FRT-L, are a suitable model system to study the interaction of oncogenic viruses with an epithelial cytotype. FRT-L cells, in fact, are normal cells established in culture, they are definitely of epithelial origin and show in vitro a dependance from a mix of six growth factors (including the thyrotropic hormone, which is the thyroid physyological stimulator) for an optimal growth (14). Moreover, they display in culture the differentiated properties of the thyroid gland; this system is however described in detail elsewhere in this volume (15).

In the present study we report the infection and tranformation of FRT-L cells with a panel of murine sarcoma viruses. The viruses used are: the Ki MSV, the Ha MSV, the Balb/c MSV, the AF1 murine sarcoma virus (AF1 MSV), the Moloney murine sarcoma virus (Mo MSV), the myeloproliferative sarcoma virus (MPSV), the FBJ murine sarcoma virus (FBJ MSV) and the Abelson murine leukemia virus (Ab MLV). All the above mentioned viruses are able to transform fibroblasts with high efficiency.The results obtained are shown in Table 1.

Epithelial cell transformation was tested by morphological criteria and anchorage-independent growth. The results reported in Table 1 indicate that not all of the viruses are able to transform FRT-L cells: in detail the Ki MSV, Ha MSV, Balb/c MSV, AF1 MSV and the MPSV are able to initiate and maintain transformation, while Mo MSV, FBJ MSV and Ab MLV are not.

Thus the transforming ability seems to be restricted to those viruses which possess an oncogene from the ras family, with the only exception of MPSV which possesses a mos-family oncogene. These results are particularly interesting in the light of the

Table 1. Transformation markers in FRT-L cells infected by murine sarcoma retroviruses.

VIRUS	ONCOGENE FAMILY	VIRUS PRODUCTION		GROWTH IN SOFT AGAR	MORPHOLOGICAL CHANGE
		RT(a)	FFU(b)		
Ki MSV	ras	+	+	+++	+
Ha MSV	ras	+	+	+	+
Balb/c MSV	ras	+	+	+	+
AF1 MSV	ras	+	+	+	+
MPSV	mos	+	+	+++	+
Mo MSV	mos	NT^c	NT	−	−
FBJ MSV	fos	NT	NT	−	−
Ab MLV	abl	NT	NT	−	−
None		−	−	−	−

a Reverse transcriptase.
b Focus formig units as assayed on RAT-2 fibroblasts.
c NT: Not tested.

fact that the oncogenes isolated from human epithelial tumors (carcinomas), by means of the transfection assay, are all from the ras family (1). It is also interesting to point out that MPSV, which possesses a mos oncogene is able to transform FRT-L cells, whereas Mo MSV, which possesses a very similar oncogene, cannot transform these cells. This could be due to some molecular differences between the mos oncogenes of MPSV and Mo MSV; in particular one codon of the mos oncogene of Mo MSV is deleted in the MPSV oncogene (W. Ostertag, personal communication), this deletion also leads to significant biological in vivo differences between these viruses. Here we report, for the first time, that these in vivo differences are paralleled by in vitro ones.

It is interesting to notice that similar results have been obtained by using another epithelial system consisting of Fischer rat epatocytes in culture. Also in this system we have demonstrated that the transforming ability on epithelial cells is restricted to viruses possessing a ras oncogene.

Thus it appears that the ras oncogenes share the general property to be able to initiate and maintain the transformation of epithelial cells growing in vitro. On the other hand, fos and abl oncogenes seem to lack this ability. The problem is more intriguing with regard to the mos oncogene; one can postulate that minor molecular changes in this oncogene can confere different biological activities and target specificities either in vivo or in vitro.

Since we have demonstrated a correlation between types of oncogenes and in vitro transformation of thyroid epithelial cells, we decided to widen our analysis to study whether these oncogenes (in particular the ras oncogenes) are also expressed in rat thyroid tumors developing in vivo. In our laboratory several thyroid transplantable tumors are available, induced by goitrogens (16).

These experimental tumors can represent a suitable model system for such a study; they exhibit, in fact, a certain degree of differentiation ranging from moderately differentiated tumors to very undifferentiated ones. This system could then also allow the analysis of the relationships between oncogenes expression and the loss of the differentiated phenotype.

The expression of oncogenes in this experimental tumors was assayed hybridizing, by means of a dot blot hybridization, mRNA (purified by affinity chromatography on oligo dT cellulose) extracted from the tumors with a panel of oncogene-specific DNA probes. The results of this study are summarized in Table 2. An increase in Ha-ras, Ki-ras and myc specific mRNA was evidenced.

Table 2. Oncogenes expression in experimental rat thyroid tumors

Poly A$^+$ RNA from	ONCOGENES				
	v-ras Ki	v-ras Ha	c-myc	v-abl	c-sis
Normal rat thyroid	−	−	−	−	−
Normal rat liver	−	−	−	−	−
1-5 G Tumor	+	+	+	−	−
1.8 Tumor	+	+	+	−	−
16.5 Tumor	+	+	+	−	−

Northern blot hybridizations have then been performed to determine the molecular size of the specific transcripts of the c-ras oncogenes in thyroid experimental tumors. From this analysis it is clear that c-ras-ki oncogene encodes for only one class of messenger RNA whose size is about 5.4 Kb; c-ras-Ha, on the other hand, encodes for a single mRNA of about 2.0 Kb.

These results, although not yet conclusive, may prompt further studies aimed to verify, by means of a transfection assay on NIH 3T3 cells, whether transforming sequences are present in the genome of these experimental thyroid tumors, belonging to ther ras family or to other oncogene families.

ACKNOWLEDGEMENTS

This work was supported by the Progetto Finalizzato Controllo della Crescita Neoplastica of the Consiglio Nazionale delle Ricerche (C.N.R.), contracts n° 82.00431.96 and n° 83.00974.96

REFERENCES

1. R. Weiss, N. Teich, H.E. Varmus and J. Coffin (eds.), "The molecular biology of tumor viruses", Cold Spring Harbor Laboratory, New York (1982).
2. P. Duesberg, Retroviral transforming genes in normal cells?, Nature 304:219 (1983).
3. S.A. Aaronson, Unique aspects of the interactions of retroviruses with vertebrate cells, Cancer Res. 43:1 (1983).
4. N. Auersperg, G.B. Addison, E.G. Goddard and V. Klement, Transformation of cultured rat adrenocortical cells by Kirsten murine sarcoma virus (Ki MSV), Int. J. Cancer 19:81 (1977).
5. Y. Ikawa, Transformation of cultured rat liver cells by murine sarcoma virus, in: "Comparative leukemia research 1973, Leukemogenesis, Bibl. Haemat. 40", Y. Ito and R.M. Dutcher eds., University of Tokio Press, Tokio/Karger Basel (1975).
6. J.S. Rhim, C.M. Kim, J. Okigaki and R.J. Huebner, Transformation of rat liver epithelial cells by Kirsten sarcoma virus, J. Natl. Cancer Inst. 59:1509 (1977).
7. B.E. Weissman and S.A. Aaronson, Balb and Kirsten murine sarcoma viruses alter growth and differentiation of EGF-dependent balb/c mouse epidermal keratinocyte lines, Cell 32:599 (1983).
8. C. Shih, B.Z. Shilo, M.P. Goldfarb, A.Dannemberg and R.A. Weinberg, Passage of phenotypes of chemically transformed cells via transfection of DNA and chromatin, Proc. Natl. Acad. Sci. USA 76:5714 (1979).
9. C. Shih, M. Padhy and R.A. Weinberg, Transforming genes of carcinomas and neuroblastomas introduced into mouse fibroblasts, Nature 290:261 (1981).
10. M.J. Murray, B.Z. Shilo, C. Shih, D. Cowing, H.W. Hsu and R.A. Weinberg, Three different human tumor cell lines contain different oncogenes, Cell 25:355 (1981).
11. A. Fusco, A. Pinto, F.S. Ambesi-Impiombato, G. Vecchio and N. Tsuchida, Transformation of rat thyroid epithelial cells by Kirsten murine sarcoma virus, Int. J. Cancer 28:655 (1981).
12. A. Fusco, A. Pinto, D. Tramontano, G. Tajana, G. Vecchio and N. Tsuchida, Block in the expression of differentiation

markers of rat thyroid epithelial cells by transformation with
Kirsten murine sarcoma virus, Cancer Res. 42:618 (1982).
13. G. Colletta, A. Pinto, P.P. Di Fiore, A. Fusco, M. Ferrentino,
V.E. Avvedimento, N. Tsuchida and C. Vecchio, Dissociation
between transformed and differentiated phenotype in rat
thyroid epithelial cells after transformation with a
temperature-sensitive mutant of the Kirsten murine sarcoma
virus, Mol. Cell. Biol. 3:2099 (1983).
14. F.S. Ambesi-Impiombato, L.A.M. Parks and H.G. Coon, Culture of
hormone-dependent epithelial cells from rat thyroid, Proc.
Natl. Acad. Sci. USA 77:3455 (1980).
15. P.P. Di Fiore, A. Fusco, G. Colletta, A. Pinto, M. Ferrentino
V. De Franciscis and G. Vecchio, Modulation of thyroid
epithelial differentiation by two viral oncogenes, this volume
16. S.H. Wollman, Production and properties of transplantable
tumors of the thyroid gland in the Fischer rat. Recent Prog.
Hormone Res. 19:579 (1963).

IMMUNOLOGICAL DETECTION OF CELLULAR TARGETS FOR V-ONC GENE CODED

TYROSINE KINASES

F.G. Giancotti, M.F. Di Renzo, P.C. Marchisio, G. Tarone,
G. Tarone, L. Naldini, S. Giordano, and P.M. Comoglio

Department of Histology, School of Medicine
University of Torino
Torino, Italy

INTRODUCTION

The induction of transformed phenotype by retrovirus-infec-
ted cells is triggered by the action of unique genetic sequences,
named onc genes. The protein products coded by a family of viral
onc genes - v-src, v-ros, v-fps, v-yes, v-abl, v-fes - are known
to be phosphokinases endowed with the unusual property of pho-
sphorylating tyrosine residues (1). Since phosphotyrosine (P-TYR)
constitutes less than 0.1% of the phosphoaminoacids in normal
cells and it is only 5 to 10 fold increased in virally transformed cells, identification of cellular substrates for tyrosine
kinases has been hampered by difficulties in distinguishing proteins containing P-TYR from those containing only phosphoserine
(P-SER) and phosphothreonine (P-THR)(2).

A larger body of information is available for the protein
product of Rous Sarcoma Virus src gene (pp60src), which is found
in the detergent insoluble cell fraction (3), the active form
being associated with the cytoplasmic face of plasma membrane
within adhesion plaques (4). A number of phosphotyrosyl proteins,
including three glycolytic enzymes, have been described in Rous
Sarcoma Virus (RSV) transformed avian fibroblasts, by a method
that combines two-dimensional gel electrophoresis with alkaline
hydrolysis in order to destroy the relatively base-labile P-SER
(5, 6). This method, however, failed to detect a prominent
phosphotyrosyl protein such as the pp60src itself. A completely

different approach has been used by Sefton et al (7), who immunoprecipitated vinculin from chicken cells and demonstrated that
its P-TYR content increases 5 to 10 fold upon transformation by
RSV, but even in transformed cells only 1% of the isolated
vinculin molecules contain the modified aminoacid.

Recently, we have described the use of antibodies raised
against azobenzyl-phosphonate (ABP)- a hapten known to crossreact
with P-TYR residues (8) - to identify and to localize P-TYR
containing proteins within the detergent insoluble fraction of
RSV transformed mammalian fibroblasts (9). The "in vitro" phosphorylation has proved to be a powerful system to amplify the
transfer of phosphate groups to detergent insoluble substrates,
that are then immunoprecipitated by ABP antibodies.

Here we extend the work to cells transformed by Fujinami
Sarcoma Virus (FSV) and by Feline Sarcoma Virus either of the
Snyder-Theilen (ST-FeSV) or the Gardner-Arnstein strain (GA-
FeSV). The onc genes of these viruses (v-fps and v-fes) code for
tyrosine phosphokinases, that are known to be associated with the
plasma membrane and/or the cytoskeleton. Moreover we provide
evidence that ABP antibodies, used for immunofluorescence microscopy, decorate structures located where plasma membrane and
cytoskeleton are known to interact.

METHODS AND RESULTS

Immunoprecipitation of in vitro phosphorylated detergent insoluble proteins

Mouse and rat fibroblasts, either control or transformed,
were extracted by the non-ionic detergent NP40 (1%) to fractio-
nate cell proteins according to their solubility. Under conditions allowing the kinase reaction catalized by viral transforming proteins, 32P-γ-ATP was added to the detergent insoluble
fraction, which included nuclear chromatin components, cytoskeletal proteins and large fragments of plasma membrane with associated molecules, among which vinculin (10). P-TYR containing
proteins were precipitated by ABP antibodies, according to a
previously described procedure (11). After elution from Protein
A-Sepharose, proteins were separated by SDS-PAGE.

In mouse fibroblasts transformed by the SR-D strain of RSV
(SR-BALB), three major phosphorylated components of approximately 130, 70, and 65 Kd and minor bands of 85, 60, 55,

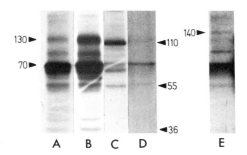

Fig. 1. Immunoprecipitation by ABP antibodies of "in vitro"
phosphorylated detergent insoluble proteins from:

(A) SR-BALB mouse fibroblasts;

(B) SR-A Rat fibroblasts;

(C) ST-FeSV transformed Fisher rat embryo cells;

(D) GA-FeSV transformed Fisher rat embryo cells;

(E) FSV transformed rat fibroblasts.

The autoradiogram of gel E was exposed four times longer
than those of gels A-D.

39 and 34 Kd were observed (Fig.1, lane A). An identical pattern
was obtained on rat fibroblasts transformed by the SR-A strain of
RSV (SRA-Rat) (Fig.1, lane B). The 60 Kd protein - partially
overlapping with the more radioactive faster component of the
70-65 Kd doublet - strictly comigrated with pp60src immunoprecipitated from 35S-Methionine labeled cells by TBR serum (not
shown). The 130 Kd protein was not identified with vinculin on
the basis of lack of crossreactivity with a vinculin antiserum
(not shown).

The pattern was different in FeSV transformed rat
fibroblasts. The major components precipitated from cells transformed by the Snyder-Theilen (ST) strain were of approximately
110, 70, 65 and 55 KD, while detergent insoluble phosphotyrosyl
proteins precipitated from cells transformed by the Gardner-
Arnstein (GA) strain displayed a molecular weight of 110, 70 and
55 Kd (Fig.1, lanes D and E).

In Fujinami sarcoma virus (FSV) transformed rat fibroblasts
the overall amount of radioactive phosphate transferred to
detergent insoluble proteins was significantly lower than that

transferred to the proteins phosphorylated in RSV transformed fibroblasts. A major component of 70 Kd and three minor bands of 140, 90, and 55 Kd were observed (Fig.1, lane C).

No radioactive band was immunoprecipitated by normal rabbit IgG in all the transformed cell lines examined, nor by ABP antibodies in all the control non transformed cell lines (not shown).

Phosphoaminoacid analysis

SDS-PAGE separated proteins were extracted and, after acid hydrolysis, their phosphoaminoacids were analyzed by electrophoresis and chromatography, as described by Frackelton et al. (12). This analysis provided direct evidence of the presence of P-TYR in all the proteins precipitated by ABP antibodies from detergent insoluble fractions of all the cell lines examined . Only the 70 Kd protein from RSV transformed rat cells and the 110 Kd protein from FeSV transformed rat cells contained additional P-SER residues (not shown).

Immunofluorescence microscopy

The intracellular distribution of molecules crossreacting with ABP antibodies was studied in control and SR-D-RSV transformed mouse fibroblasts fixed, permeabilized and examined by indirect immunofluorescence microscopy, as described by Nigg et al (13).

In normal fibroblasts, beside a faint cytoplasmic background, staining was observed within the nucleus, possibly due to the antibody crossreaction with nucleoside triphosphates (not shown). In transformed cells, a moderate diffuse fluorescence was found in the cytoplasm; moreover, intensely fluorescent streaks were observed in the cell periphery (Fig.2, A). The latter showed morphological features and distribution similar to the adhesion plaques visualized by interference reflection microscopy (Fig. 2, B). Specific decoration with ABP antibodies was also observed at the level of cell-to-cell contacts, that appeared lined by multiple intensely fluorescent dots (Fig. 2, C) and at filopodial tips, where the interference reflection microscopy demonstrates that the ventral plasma membrane is tightly close to the substratum (Fig. 2, A and B).

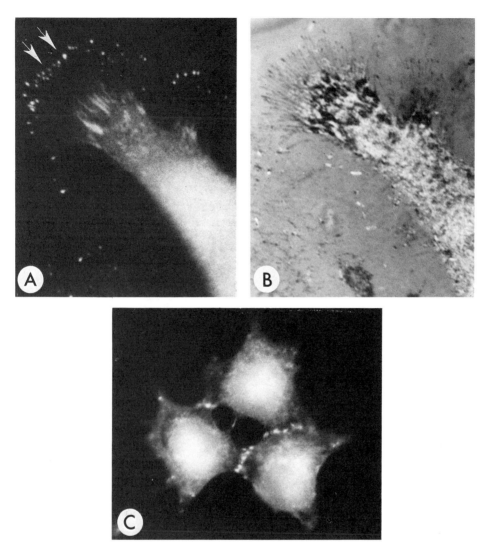

Fig. 2. Decoration of RSV transformed mouse fibroblasts by ABP
         antibodies. (A): the specific fluorescence is diffusely
         distributed within the cytoplasm and concentrated at cell
         edges (arrowed) and in restricted areas in the ventral
         plasma membrane. The latter correspond to dark areas in
         interference reflection microscopy (B). (C):intensely
         fluorescent spots line cell-to-cell contacts.

DISCUSSION

ABP antibodies precipitate from each examined transformed cell line a phosphotyrosyl protein of molecular weight identical to that of the expressed viral oncoprotein: namely pp60 in cells transformed by v-src, pp140 in cells transformed by v-fps and pp110 in cells transformed by v-fes. These data are consistent with the evidence that these kinases coded by onc genes phosphorylate themselves at tyrosine (1). Moreover ABP antibodies precipitate proteins of different molecular weight from cells transformed by different viruses. Conversely, two proteins with molecular weight 70 and 55 Kd were found to be phosphorylated at tyrosine in all the cell lines tested.

The data presented in this report provide evidence for different "in vitro" substrate specificity of the tyrosine kinases coded by v-src, v-fps and v-fes. When an "in vivo" functional role is assigned to the proteins here described, it will be possible to speculate wether these oncoproteins use different transformation strategies.

The localization of P-TYR containing proteins at adhesion plaques, filopodial tips and cell to cell contacts suggests that in RSV transformed cells the acquisition of neoplastic phenotype involves the modification of sites where interaction between cytoskeleton and plasma membrane occurs.

ACKNOWLEDGEMENTS

This work has been supported by the Italian National Research Council (C.N.R.),P.F.C.C.N. no.82.00277.

The skillful technical assistance of M.R. Amedeo and P. Rossino is gratefully acknowledged.

REFERENCES

1) J.M. Bishop, Cellular Oncogenes and Retroviruses, Ann. Rev. Biochem. 52:301-354 (1983).
2) K. Beemon, T. Ryden, and E.A. Mc Nelly, Transformation by Avian Sarcoma Viruses leads to Phosphorylation of Multiple Cellular Proteins on Tyrosine Residues, J.Virol. 42:742-747 (1982).

3) J. Burr, G. Dreyfuss, S. Penman, and J. Buchanan, Association
   of the src gene product with cytoskeletal structures of
   chicken embryo fibroblasts, Proc.Natl.Acad.USA 77:3484-3488
   (1980).
4) L.R. Rohrschneider, Adhesion plaques of Rous sarcoma virus-
   transformed cells contain the src gene product, Proc. Natl.
   Acad. USA 77:3514-3518 (1980)
5) J.A. Cooper, and T. Hunter, Four different classes of retroviruses induced phosphorylation of tyrosines present in
   similar cellular proteins, Mol.Cell.Biol. 1:394-407 (1981).
6) T. Hunter, and B.M. Sefton, Transforming gene product of Rous
   sarcoma virus phosphorylates tyrosine, Proc.Natl.Acad.USA
   77:1311-1315 (1980).
7) B.M. Sefton, T. Hunter, E.A. Ball, and S.J. Singer, Vinculin:
   a Cytoskeletal Target of the Transforming Protein of Rous
   Sarcoma Virus, Cell 24:165-174 (1981).
8) A.H. Ross, D. Baltimore, and H.N. Eisen, Phosphotyrosine-
   containing proteins isolated by affinity chromatography with
   antibodies to a synthetic hapten, Nature 294:654-656 (1981).
9) P.M. Comoglio, M.F. Di Renzo, G. Tarone, F.G. Giancotti, L.
   Naldini, and P.C. Marchisio, Detection of phosphotyrosine
   containing proteins in the detergent insoluble fraction of
   RSV transformed fibroblasts by azobenzene phosphonate
   antibodies, EMBO J. (in press).
10) G. Gacon, S. Gisselbrecht, J.P. Piau, M.Y. Fiszman, and S.
    Fischer, Phosphorylations of the Subcellular Matrix in Cells
    Transformed by Rous'Sarcoma Virus, Eur.J.Biochem. 125:453-
    456 (1982).
11) G. Tarone, P. Ceschi, M. Prat, and P.M. Comoglio,
    Transformation-sensitive Protein with Molecular Weight of
    45,000 secreted by Mouse Fibroblasts, Cancer Res. 41:3648-
    3652 (1981).
12) A.R. Frackelton, A.H. Ross, and H.N. Eisen, Characterization
    and Use of Monoclonal Antibodies for Isolation of Phospho-
    tyrosyl Proteins from Retrovirus-Transformed Cells and
    Growth Factor-Stimulated Cells, Mol.Cell.Bilo. 3:1343-1352
    (1983).
13) E.A. Nigg, J.A. Cooper, and T. Hunter, Immunofluorescent
    Localization of a 39,000-dalton Substrate of Tyrosine
    Protein Kinases to the Cytoplasmic Surface of the Plasma
    Membrane, J.Cell.Biol. 96:1601-1609 (1983).

NUCLEOTIDE SEQUENCES HOMOLOGOUS TO A CLONED REPEATED

HUMAN DNA FRAGMENT IN HUMAN LEUKEMIC DNA'S

Luca Ceccherini Nelli and Gianmarco Corneo

Cattedra di Patologia Medica II, Università di di Milano
via F. Sforza 35 , 20122 Milano

The human genome contains repetitive nucleotide sequences that are in part organized in blocks in the heterochromatin and partly interspersed among single copy genes. It is known that chromosome deletions and rearrangements occur frequently in leukemias and cancers at cytogenetic analysis. Methods of genome investigation such as analysis of DNA by restriction enzyme digestion and Southern blot hybridization could demonstrate finer genome rearrangements. Human total DNA centrifuged to equilibrium in Ag^+-Cs_2SO_4 shows four satellite DNAs and a shoulder on the light side. From this shoulder a DNA fraction, by us previously called homogeneous main band DNA[1], made up mainly by highly repeated DNA[2] other than satellite DNAs, can be separated by a subsequent CsCl centrifugation.

We have used purified homogeneous DNA as a probe to recognize homologous nucleotide sequences complementary to inserts of a human genomic library constructed through digestion of total human DNA with MboI restriction enzyme and in vitro packaging of the digested fragments in the BamHI site of the Charion 28 of λ phage competent for E. coli LE392. As expected a high percentage of phages scored positive for inserts homologous to human homogeneous main band DNA. Three steps of purification were made picking up lysis plaques definitively positive by duplicate filter

305

hybridization until all lysis plaques were single clone
originated and all uniformely positive for hybridization
to human main band DNA. At this point large amounts of
human main band DNA phage could be grown, purified by
polyethylenglycole, CsCl equilibrium banding, extracted
with phenol-chloroform and ethanol precipitated.

In fig. 1 restriction enzyme digestion products of
the phage with different restriction enzymes, migrated
by electrophoresis on agarose gels, are shown. The 1.5
kilobases BamHI, 7 kilobases EcoRI and 1.6 kilobases KpnI
fragments, that are part of the insert, were isolated from
the remaining part of the phage. Each of these fragments

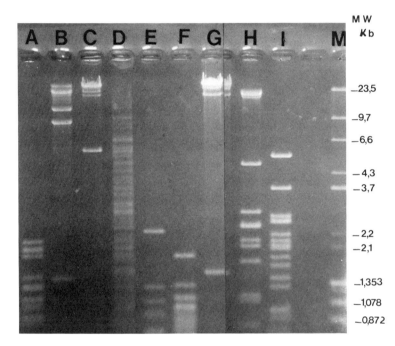

Fig. 1 Purified recombinant phage DNA, containing nucleotide sequences homologous to human main band DNA, digested with the following restriction enzymes: AluI (lane A),
BamHI (lane B), EcoRI (lane C), EcoRII (lane D), HaeIII
(lane E), HinfI (lane F), KpnI (lane G), PstI (lane H),
Ava II (lane I), run on 1% agarose gels. Molecular weights
were determined by comparison with a mixture of HindIII
digested λ phage DNA and HpaI digested and HaeIII digested φX174 phage, used as a marker (lane M).

was cut from a preparative gel, fragmented and put in
dialysis tubing. The DNA was extracted from the gel
through electrophoresis and purified. The three fragments
come from a region of the human main band phage that
partially overlaps.Total human DNA from placenta or leukemic leucocytes was digested with different restriction
enzymes, run on agarose gels through electrophoresis,
transferred to genescreen paper and hybridized to the
homogeneous human main band BamHI fragment DNA, P_{32} nick
translated at high specific activity. Dark bands on autoradiographic films show the homology of the radioactive
probe to bands specifically complementary in the examined
DNA. Fig. 2 shows the hybridization pattern of cloned
human main band DNA BamHI fragment to a human normal DNA
from placenta, digested with a battery of different
restriction enzymes. At the digestion with AluI are obtained three bands of 2 - 1.1 and 0.7 kilobases, with BamHI
four bands of 7.8 - 6.8 - 5.6 and 1.6 kilobases, with EcoRI
a band of 7.8 kilobases, with EcoRII three bands of 1.5 -

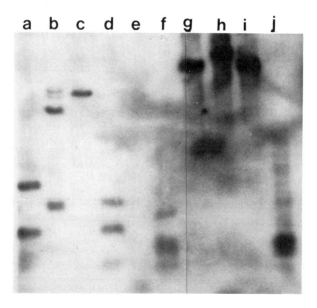

Fig. 2 Autoradiographic film of human placenta DNA
digested with: AluI (a), BamHI (b), EcoRI (c), EcoRII (d),
HaeIII (e), HinfI (f), XbaI (g), KpnI (h), PstI (i) and
AvaII (j).

0.9 and 0.55 kilobases, with HaeIII a band of 0.35 kilobases, with HinfI two bands of 1.2 and 0.55 kilobases,
with XbaI a band of 15 kilobases, with KpnI a band of 23
kilobases, with PstI a band of 16 kilobases and with AvaII
three bands of 1.3 - 1.1 and 0.7 kilobases. Fig. 3 shows
the pattern of hybridization of the 1.5 kilobases BamHI
DNA fragment to the DNA of several human leukemic bone
marrows, digested with AluI. The 0.7 kilobases band is
not visible, but the 1.1 and 2 kilobases bands are well
marked. In the DNA of a chronic myeloid leukemia in blast
crysis (lane c) the 2 kilobases band was lacking and an
additional 3 kilobases band was present. This band was
present also in the DNA from a patient affected by promyelocytic leukemia (lane i) and two patients affected
by acute lymphatic leukemia (lanes k and l).

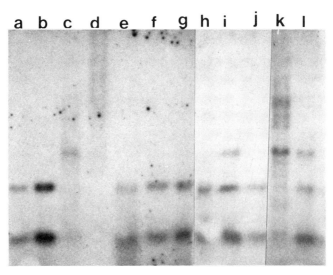

Fig. 3 Autoradiographic films of human leukemia bone
marrow DNAs digested with AluI, run on 1% agarose gel
electrophoresis, transferred to a nitrocellulose filter
and hybridized to P32 nick-translated 1.5 kilobases BamHI
human DNA fragment: acute myeloid leukemia (a and d to h),
non Hodgkin lymphoma (b), chronic myeloid leukemia in
blast crysis (c), promyelocytic leukemia (i) and acute
lymphatic leukemia (j to l).

Fig. 4 shows the hybridization pattern of the 1.5 kilobases BamHI cloned human DNA fragment to the DNA of leukemic bone marrows digested with BamHI and run on agarose gels. The DNA of three acute myeloid leukemias (lanes b,c .and h) shows remarkable differences in the size and relative amount of the upper bands (molecular weights from 5.7 to 9.6 kilobases) compared to the normal placenta DNA.

Changes in human repeated DNAs might be due to constitutional genetic polymorphism or to the leukemic process itself or to antiblastic treatment. It is premature to draw general conclusions from these preliminary data on human DNA, although it has been recently reported polymorphism of repetitive DNA both in the mouse and primates[3,4]. It will be especially interesting to detect repeated DNA polymorphism, if any, which might be associated with genetic predisposition to cancer.

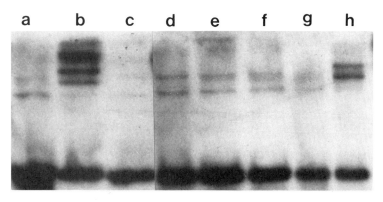

Fig. 4 As in fig. 3, except that human leukemia bone marrow DNAs were digested with BamHI: acute lymphatic leukemia (a), acute myeloid leukemia (b,c,e and h), chronic myeloid leukemia (d and f), hypereosinophilic syndrome (g).

Acknowledgments : This work was supported by grant no.
82.00281.96 from the Finalized Project 'Control of neoplastic growth' of the Consiglio Nazionale delle Ricerche
(Rome) and, in part, by funds of the M.P.I. (Rome) .

REFERENCES

1. G. Corneo, E. Ginelli and E. Polli, Renaturation
    properties and localization in heterochromatin
    of human satellite DNAs, Biochim. Biophys. Acta
    247 : 528 (1971).
2. G. Corneo, D. Meazza, M. Bregni, P. Tripputi and
    L. Ceccherini Nelli, Restriction enzyme studies
    on human highly repeated DNAs, Experientia 38 :
    454 (1982).
3. A. Maresca and M. F. Singer, Deca-satellite : a
    highly polymorphic satellite that joins α-
    satellite in the African green monkey genome,
    J. Mol. Biol. 164 : 493 (1983).
4. R. Kominami, Y. Urano, Y. Mishima, M. Muramatsu,
    K. Moriwaki and H. Yoshikura, Novel repetitive
    sequence families showing size and frequency
    polymorphism in the genomes of mice, J. Mol. Biol.
    165 : 209 (1983).

REARRANGEMENT AND ABNORMAL EXPRESSION OF HUMAN c-myc IN ACUTE LYMPHOCYTIC LEUKEMIA

C. Peschle[1], F. Mavilio[1], N.M. Sposi[1], A. Giampaolo[1], A. Carè[1],
L. Bottero[1], M. Bruno[1], G. Mastroberardino[2], R. Gastaldi[2],
M.G. Testa[2], G. Alimena[3], S. Amadori[3] and F. Mandelli[3]

1) Dept. of Hematology, Istituto Superiore di Sanità
2) Istituto Patologia Medica (VI)
3) Chair of Hematology, University of Rome, Italy

ABSTRACT

We have studied a case of acute lymphocytic leukemia (L_3 type) with 8;14 chromosome translocation. DNA obtained from peripheral blood leukemic cells was analyzed by restriction endonuclease mapping and hybridization with genomic or c-DNA human c-myc probes. The breakpoint of the translocation has been localized within the first intron of the c-myc gene, thus leaving the first untranslated exon on chromosome 8q- and rearranging the whole protein-coding region in the IgH locus on chromosome 14q+. Northern blot analysis showed high levels of two different c-myc transcripts originated from the translocated gene, which were not detected in WBC in remission phase. These studies demonstrate for the first time rearrangement and abnormal expression of a cellular onc-gene (c-myc) in primary cells from an acute leukemia patient.

INTRODUCTION

The human cellular homologue (c-myc) of the MC-29 avian myelocytomatosis virus oncogene (v-myc) is located on the distal end of the long arm of chromosome 8 (q24.13) (1, 2). Amplification of the c-myc gene and elevated levels of c-myc transcripts are detectable in human cell lines derived from acute promyelocytic (HL-60) and chronic myelogenous leukemia (K562) (3, 4). In Burkitt lymphoma, reciprocal translocations involving chromosomes 8 and 14, 22 or 2 bring the c-myc gene in close proximity to respectively Ig heavy (H), λ and κ chain loci (2, 5-10). In 8;14 translocations, c-myc is either not rearranged or rearranged "head to head" with either the Cμ or the Cγ_1 gene (5- 9). The c-myc transcripts generated by the translocated gene are expressed at high levels in these cells, if compared with EBV-transformed

311

lymphoblastoid cell lines (11-13).

Altogether, these data lead to the hypothesis that c-myc translocation into the Ig gene loci might induce its abnormal
expression, which would in turn play a key role in the oncogenic
process (see 14, 15 for a review).

We report a case of acute lymphocytic leukemia (ALL)(L_3 type)
with 8;14 chromosome translocation, whereby the c-myc is
rearranged into the IgH locus. Two different c-myc transcripts
are detectable at high levels in primary leukemic cells. Both virtually disappear in the remission phase. These data extend and
enhance the significance of the translocation-mediated c-myc activation in the genesis of B-cell neoplasias.

MATERIALS AND METHODS

Leukemic blast cells were obtained from peripheral blood and
enriched up to > 90% by standard Ficoll-Paque centrifugation.
Surface antigen characterization by commercially available monoclonal antibodies and karyotype determination were carried out by
standard techniques. DNA extraction, digestion with restriction
endonucleases, agarose gel electrophoresis, Southern transfer and
hybridization were carried out as previously described (16, 17).
Genomic and cDNA human c-myc fragments used as hybridization
probes were: i) a 449 bp Xho I - Pvu II sequence containing most
of the first untranslated exon (probe "a") (18); ii) a 3.3 Kb Pst
I fragment containing the first, most of the second exon and the
first intron (probe "b") (6); iii) a 1.5 Kb Cla I - Eco Rl fragment containing the third exon (probe "c") (6); iv) a 1029 bp cDNA
sequence (pRyc 7.4) (11) containing the third exon and the 3' end
of the second one (probe d). The Ig probes were the J, S μ and Cμ
human genomic fragments (6) and a 2.9 Kb Sma I genomic fragment of
the C α_1 locus (kindly provided by Dr. C. Croce, Wistar Institute,
Philadelphia). RNA extraction, poly-A selection by oligo-dT cellulose chromatography, agarose electrophoresis, Northern transfer
and hybridization were carried out by standard techniques (19).

RESULTS

A 13-yr-old male patient with ALL of L_3 type showed a typical
surface antigen pattern of the leukemic cells (representing > 60%
of total nucleated elements in peripheral blood) (Table 1).
Analysis of leukemic cells karyotypes showed a reciprocal 8;14
chromosome translocation (8q24 → ter; 14q32 → ter) similar to those
described in Burkitt's lymphoma (15). DNA and RNA analysis was
carried out on leukemic cells prior to initiation of therapy. The
patient underwent a partial remission (i.e., leukemic cells
disappeared from peripheral blood, but ∿ 10% of blast cells were
still present in bone marrow),which lasted less than three weeks,
and died four months after diagnosis.

In order to establish if the chromosomal translocation had
caused rearrangement of the c-myc gene, leukemic cell DNA was

TABLE I

Surface marker phenotype of malignant cells of the ALL patient at diagnosis.

IgM	90%	OKT3	–
IgG	–	OKT4	–
Igκ	90%	OKT6	–
Igλ	–	OKT9	–
IgF(ab)$_2$	98%	OKT10	90%
		OKIa	90%
		OKMI	–
		J5	10%

digested with Eco Rl, Hind III and Bam Hl (see Fig.1), and hybridized with the c-DNA probe ("d" in Fig.1). All enzymes yielded both abnormal bands (of 19.00, 15.0 and 20.6 Kb respectively) and normal c-myc fragments (Fig.2), thus indicating alterations involving their recognition sequences 5' or 3' to the structural gene. Single and double digestions with Bgl II, which cuts between the second and third exon (Fig.1), and hybridization with 5' and 3' specific probes ("b" and "c" in Fig.1) allowed to establish that the structural abnormality involved the 5' region of the myc locus (Fig.1). This may be obviously attributed to the chromosome translocation, as in some 8;14 Burkitt lymphoma lines (See 15).

In order to localize the breakpoint within the c-myc locus, DNA was digested with Pst I, Sac I and Xba I, which cut progressively 5' to 3' starting from the Hind III site (see Fig.1). Pst I digestion yielded an abnormal 3.3 band with the "b" probe, whereas both Xba I and Sac I patterns were normal (Fig.4). Hybridization with the "a" probe (not shown) of the same DNA digests allowed to establish that the breakpoint was between the first Sac I site 3' to the first exon and the Xba I site 0.4 Kb downstream. This breakage leaves the first untranslated exon of the myc gene on chromosome 8q⁻, while the second and third ones are translocated on chromosome 14q+. The restriction map of the myc locus on the 14q+ chromosome is shown in Fig.5.

Southern hybridization with different Ig probes was carried out in order to investigate if the myc gene was rearranged in proximity to any of the structural genes of the IgH locus. The restriction map of the DNA region on chromosome 14 adjacent to the translocated myc gene was not compatible with the presence therein of J, S or coding portions of the Cμ locus, as otherwise demonstrated in several Burkitt lymphoma lines (see above). Indeed, the abnormal Eco Rl and Hind III c-myc fragments did not hybridize with J, S and two different Cμ probes (data not shown). Instead, co-hybridization was observed with a Igα probe, and the restriction map is compatible with a rearrangement "head to head"

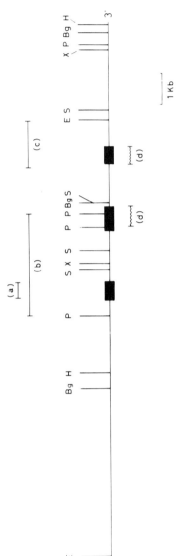

Fig. 1. Restriction endonuclease map of the human c-myc locus.
Black boxes indicate exons. Letters (a), (b) and (c) indicate ge-
nomic probes ,(d) indicates the cDNA probe (see methods). E=Eco 1,
Bg=Bgl II, H=Hind III, P=Pst I, S=Sac I, X=Xba I.

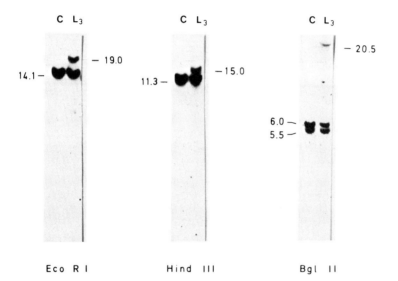

Fig. 2. Eco Rl, Hind III and Bgl II restriction pattern of DNA from the leukemic cells (L$_3$), as compared to a normal control (C) which was hybridized to the cDNA "d" probe. Sizes are in Kbp.

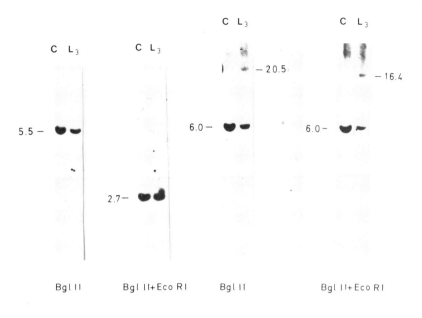

Fig.3. Bgl II and Bgl I + Eco Rl restriction pattern of DNA from the leukemic cells (L_3) as compared to a normal control (C) which was hybridized to 3' (left) and 5' (right) c-myc genomic probes (respectively "c" and "b" in Fig.1).

of the translocated myc to the α_1 locus. Further studies are now in progress in order to define the molecular details of the gene rearrangement.

Northern blot analysis of poly-A$^+$ RNA and hybridization with the c-DNA "d" probe showed high levels of c-myc transcripts in leukemic cells, which were undetectable in remission phase WBC (Fig.6). Two RNA bands of different size in a roughly 1:1 ratio were detected in leukemic cells, in contrast to what observed in HL-60, K562 and several ALL without 8;14 chromosome translocations, in which a single 2.3 kb band is observed. This band contains, in fact, two different transcripts of 2.2 and 2.4 kb (8).Both transcripts failed to hybridize with the "a" probe, indicating that they are transcribed from the myc gene translocated on chromosome 14, which lacks the first exon. No additional transcripts originating from the truncated myc on chromosome 8q- was detected by hybridization with the "a" probe.

DISCUSSION

In Burkitt lymphoma lines, translocation and rearrangement of c-myc into the Cμ or Cγ locus on chromosome 14 may underlie its

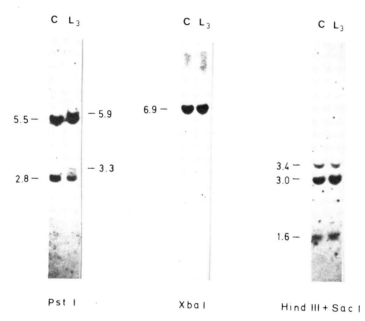

Fig. 4. Pst I, Xba I and Hind III + Sac I restriction pattern of leukemic (L₃) and control (C) DNA, hybridized to both 5' and 3' genomic c-myc probes ("b"+"c", see Fig.1).

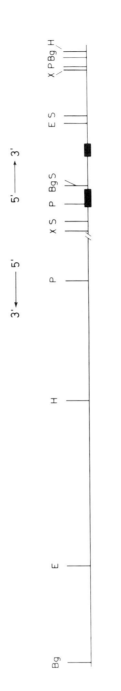

Fig. 5. Restriction endonuclease map of the c-myc translocated on chromosome 14q+ in L_3 leukemic cells. (See legend of Fig.1).

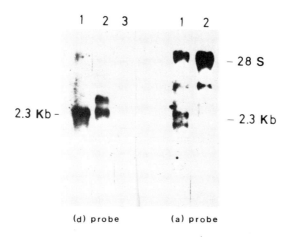

Fig.6. Northern blot analysis of poly-A$^+$ RNA extracted from L$_3$ leukemic cells and hybridized to "d" and "a" probes. RNA obtained from the HL-60 promyelocytic line is shown as a control marker (lane 1). Lane 3 is the RNA obtained from WBC in remission phase.

deregulation (20), which could in turn play a key role in neoplastic transformation of B-cells (see 14, 15, 20). However, c-myc activation cannot be attributed to a single molecular mechanism. In some Burkitt lines the myc gene is translocated virtually intact, whereas in other ones only the second and third exons move to chromosome 14. Similarly, the breakpoints of Cμ or Cγ loci are widely variable.

The present case represents the first report of c-myc translocation in primary cells from an acute leukemia. The breakpoint occurs within the first intron, leaving the first, non-coding exon on chromosome 8 and rearranging the second and third ones on chromosome 14. The breakpoint is comprised in a 0.4 Kb region, which is not involved in translocations reported so far in Burkitt lines (See 20). Furthermore, neither Cμ or Cγ Ig genes have been mapped in the rearranged DNA region on chromosome 14. Instead, preliminary evidence indicates that one of the two C loci (possibly C α$_1$) is involved. Thereby, this may be the first case of c-myc-Cα rearrangement in human neoplastic B-cells.

Two major poly-A RNA molecules are transcribed from the translocated myc. The first is slightly shorter than the normal one (i.e., 2.3 Kb) while the second is ∿ 0.7 Kb longer. Most likely, at least one and perhaps both are transcribed from cryptic promoters localized within the first intron, downstream from the translocation breakpoint (see 15).

Further studies, including cloning and sequencing of the translocated c-myc and S1 nuclease mapping of the abnormal transcripts, are now in progress in an attempt to fully elucidate the multiple molecular abnormalities of this unique case.

ACKNOWLEDGEMENTS

This work has been partially supported by CNR grants, Progetti Finalizzati "Ingegneria Genetica" (Contract No.83.01019.51) "Controllo Crescita Neoplastica" (Contract No.83.00908.96), and "Medicina Preventiva e Riabilitativa" (Contract No.83.02772.56).

REFERENCES

1)   Neel, B.G., Jhanwar, S.C., Chagauti, R.S.K. and Hayward, W.S., (1982) Proc. Natl. Acad. Sci. USA 79, 7842-7846.
2)   Dalla Favera, R., Bregni, M., Erikson, J., Patterson, D., Gallo, R.C. and Croce, C.M. (1982) Proc. Natl. Acad. Sci. USA 79, 7824-7827.
3)   Westin, E.H., Wong-Staal, F., Gelmann, E.P., Dalla Favera, R., Papas, T.S., Lauterberger, J.A., Eva, A., Reddy, E.P., Tronick, S.R., Aaronson, S.A. and Gallo, R.C. (1982) Proc. Natl. Acad. Sci. USA 79, 2490-2494
4)   Dalla Favera, R., Wong-Staal, F. and Gallo, R.C. (1982) Nature, 299, 61-63.
5)   Taub, R., Kirsch, I., Morton, C., Lenoir, G., Swan, D., Tronick S., Aaronson, S. and Leder, P. (1982) Proc. Natl. Acad. Sci. USA 79, 7837-7841.
6)   Dalla Favera, R., Martinotti, S., Gallo, R.C., Erikson, J. and Croce C.M. (1983) Science 219, 963-967.
7)   Adams, J.M., Gerondakis, S., Webb, E., Corcoran, L.M., and Cory, S. (1983) Proc. Natl. Acad. Sci. USA 80, 1982- 1986.
8)   Hamlyn, P.H. and Rabbitts, T.H. (1983) Nature 304, 135-139.
9)   Battey, J., Moulding, C., Taub, R., Murphy, W., Stewart, T.,Potter, H., Lenoir, G. and Leder, P. (1983) Cell 34, 779-787.
10) Croce, C.M., Thierfelder, W., Erikson, J., Nishikura, K., Finan, J., Lenoir, G.M. and Nowell, P.C. (1983).Proc. Natl. Acad. Sci. USA 80, 6922-6926.
11) Erikson, J., ar-Rushdi, A., Drwinga, H.L., Nowell, P.C. and Croce, C.M. (1983) Proc. Natl. Acad. Sci. USA 80, 820-824. 820-824.
12) Nishikura, K., ar-Rushdi, A., Erikson, J., Watt, R., Rovera, G., and Croce, C.M. (1983) Proc. Natl. Acad. Sci USA 80, 4822- 4826.
13) ar-Rushdi, A., Nishikura, K., Erikson, J., Watt, R., Rovera, G. and Croce, C.M. (1983) Science 222, 390-393.
14) Perry, (1983) Cell, 33, 647-649.
15) Leder, P., Battey, J., Lenoir, G., Moulding, C., Murphy,

W., Potter, H., Stewart, T. and Taub, R. (1983) Science 222, 765-771.

16) Mavilio, F., Giampaolo, A., Caré, A., Sposi, N.M. and Marinucci, M. (1983) Blood, 62, 230-233.

17) Mavilio, F., Giampaolo, A., Caré, A., Migliaccio, G., Calandrini, M., Russo, G., Pagliardi, G.L., Mastroberardino, G., Marinucci, M. and Peschle, C. (1983) Proc. Natl. Acad. Sci. USA 80, 6907-6911.

18) Watt, R., Nishikura, K., Sorrentino, J., ar-Rushdi, A., Croce,C.M. and Rovera, G. (1983) Proc. Natl. Acad. Sci. USA 80, 6307-6311.

19) Maniatis, T., Fritsch, E.F. and Sambrook, J. Molecular Cloning A Laboratory Manual. Cold Spring Harbor. (1982) New York.

20) Robertson, M. (1983) Nature, 306, 733-736.

A NEW HUMAN ERYTHROLEUKEMIC LINE: INITIAL CHARACTERIZATION AND

HEMIN-INDUCED ERYTHROID DIFFERENTIATION

G. Migliaccio[1], L. Avitabile[1], A.R. Migliaccio[1],
S. Petti[1], R. Guerriero[1], G. Mastroberardino[2], G. Saglio[5],
A. De Capua[3], A. Baldini[3], P. Markelaj[3], S. Amadori[4],
F. Mandelli[4], and C. Peschle[1]

[1]Department of Hematology, Istituto Superiore di Sanità
[2]Istituto Patalogia Medica (VI)
[3]Department of Genetics and Molecular Biology
[4]Chair of Hematology, University of Rome, Rome, Italy
[5]Istituto Medicina Interna, University of Turin
Turin, Italy

ABSTRACT

A new erythroleukemic line, designated IDA, has been established from a non-lymphoid acute leukemia of M6 type. This line is characterized by a doubling time of 35.9 ± 2.5 h and a saturation density of $\sim 3 \times 10^6$ cells/ml. Interestingly it is essentially euployd (modal No. of chromosomes, 46), although it may generate occasionally polyploid cells and elements with aberrations often involving chromosome 21. When treated with hemin $\pm$DMSO, cells are induced to massive erythroid dfferentiation (up to $\geq$ 90% benzidine positive cells). The IDA line is characterized by spontaneous and induced production of embryonic ζ- and ε-globin chains, as evaluated by analytical isoelectric-focusing of the haptoglobin-Sepharose purified globin fraction.

INTRODUCTION

Human cell lines from non-lymphoid acute leukemias have been rarely reported (for a review see 1). In particular, only two erythroleukemic lines, designated K562 and HEL, have been established (2,3). The former derives from the pleural effusion of a chronic myeloid leukemia in blastic crisis (2), the latter from peripheral blood mononuclear cells of a Hodgkin's lymphoma who developed erythroleukemia (3). K562 and HEL cells show a marked

323

tendency for polyploidy (3,4). Both lines display multiple features of erythroleukemic progenitors (1), the differentiation of which is apparently "crystallized" by the neoplastic process: they represent therefore the human counterpart of murine Friend erythroleukemic lines (5).In particular, K562 and HEL cells are induced by hemin to differentiate into normoblast-like cells. They are capable of both spontaneous and induced synthesis of globin chains (respectively, 0.3-0.5 and 3-8 pg/cell, the latter levels being detectable with benzidine staining). Interestingly, they produce embryonic (ζ ϵ) and fetal (α γ) chains, but not adult β-globin (6-10). It must be emphasized that K562 cells also express membrane antigens normally present in the granulo-macrophage (11) or megakaryocytic lineage (12), thus indicating that this line is endowed with a multi-lineage differentiation program.

We report here the establishment and the initial characterization of a new erythroleukemic line.

MATERIALS AND METHODS

Establishment of the line

Bone marrow aspirated from a 32-year-old female (I. IDA) affected by acute non-lymphoid leukemia (erythroleukemia,M6 type) was diluted in Hanks' solution (1:1). The monocellular suspension was subjected to standard Ficoll separation. Light-density cells, diluted in Iscove's modified Dulbecco medium (Gibco Bio Cult Ltd, Paisley) supplemented with streptomycin (200 ng/ml), penicillin (200 units/ml), Fungizone (0.5 ng/ml), nucleosides (1 μg/ml of each one) and heat inactived fetal calf serum (FCS, 20% of a selected batch, Gibco Bio Cult Ltd., No. 25K721-2) were incubated in a fully humidified atmosphere at 5% CO_2 and 37°C (10^6 cells/ml/ 8 ml/flask). After 15 days, non adherent cells were removed and incubated in fresh medium under the same conditions. Twice a week, cells were resuspended in fresh medium (adherent elements were never observed). After 2 months the line showed a consistent growth pattern, and was considered established 1 month thereafter. The cells are now maintained by weekly passages in fresh culture medium supplemented with 10% FCS.

Karyotype analysis

Cells were harvested on the 4th and 18th passage. Colchicine (10^{-5} M) was added in the last 3 h of culture. Standard Giemsa staining was utilized for both chromosome counting and analysis of chromosome aberrations. Chromosome identification was carried out on slides stained with quinachrine mustard (Q.M., Sigma Co., St. Louis).

Morphology and cytochemistry

A cell suspension, cytocentrifuged on FCS-precoated slides, was analyzed by May-Grünwald + Giemsa staining and routine cytochemical reactions (periodic acid-Schiff (PAS), Sudan black, α-naphtyl acetate esterase (α NAE), acid phospatase, naphtol AS-D cloracetate (NASDCA) (Sigma Co.), and Graham-Knoll peroxidase reaction (13)).

Erythroid differentiation upon hemin and/or DMSO addition
    Cultures were treated with hemin (0.05 mM) (Sigma Co.) and/or DMSO (1%, v/v) on day 0. Hb content and synthesis were evaluated on day 4, by means of respectively (a) standard benzidine staining and (b) analytical isoelectric-focusing in absence of NP40 of the haptoglobin-Sepharose purified globin fraction (14).

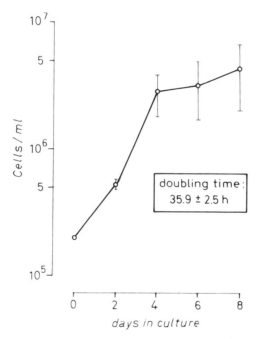

Fig.1 Growth curve of the IDA line.

RESULTS AND DISCUSSION

Initial characterization
    The IDA line has now undergone more than 60 passages over 13 months of culture. Cells in log phase growth show a doubling time of 35.9 ± 2.5 h, and reach their saturation density at approximately 3×10^6 cells/ml (Fig. 1). They grow in clusters (Fig. 2A), but never adhere to plastic surfaces.

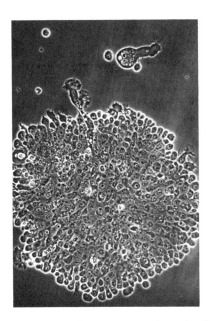

Fig. 2A   Cell cluster growing in liquid
suspension, as observed under contrast
phase microscopy (x250).

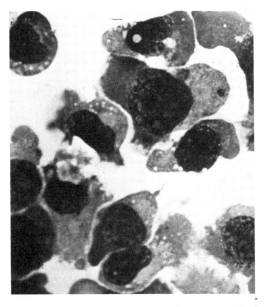

Fig. 2B   May-Grünwalg + Giemsa staining
of centrifuged IDA cells (x1500).

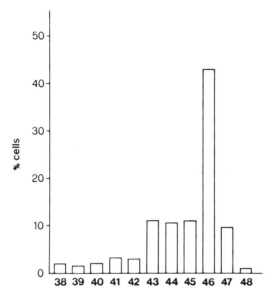

Fig. 3A   Chromosome number per cell.

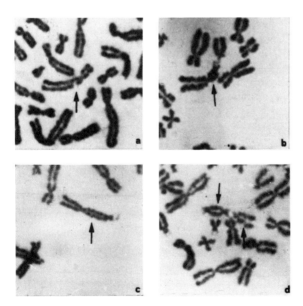

Fig. 3B   a: Chromatid break in a B-group chromosome;
          b: dicentric chromosome involving an acrocentric chromosome
             engaged in satellite association;
          c: dicentric chromosome;
          d: isodicentric chromosome and chromatid break.

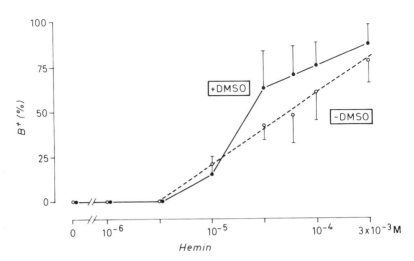

Fig. 4. Hemin ± DMSO dose/response curves (means ± SEM values).

Cells are of heterogenous size, with a mean diameter of ∿15μ (Fig. 2B), the larger ones being always polynucleated. If stained with May-Grünwald + Giemsa, they show the morphology of undiffe-rentiated blasts (i.e., a lax chromatin, 1-5 nucleoli, etc.).

Chromosome counting and analysis was performed twice, on 207 and 68 cells respectively. In both cases the modal number of chromosomes was 46, with occasional hypo- and hyper-diploid cells (Fig. 3A). However, the number of polyploid cells observed in the second sample (5.9%) was more elevated as compared to the first one (1.4%) : this may reflect chromosome instability in liquid culture. The modal karyotype obtained on Q-banded chromosomes confirms a 46, XX chromosome complement (results not shown), with no evidence for stable specific chromosome rearrangements.

Finally, 227 cells of the second sample have been investigated for chromosome aberrations. The results can be summarized as follows: 8.8% of gaps, 5.3% of chromatid and chromosome breaks, 3.5% of dicentrics (Fig. 3B). Further analysis of these aspects is now in progress.

The cytochemical analysis showed a pattern resembling that of normal monocytes (PAS, α NAE, acid phospatase positive; Sudan, peroxidase, NASDCA and benzidine negative).

Hemin induction studies

Following hemin ± DMSO addition in culture, benzidine positive cells (B^+) are already detectable after 2 h (results not

shown), and their relative number peaks after 3-4 days ($\geqq 90\%$).
Interestingly, the hemin effect can be enhanced by DMSO addition.
It is noteworthy that the doubling time is unaffected by hemin
addition, but is markedly reduced by treatment with DMSO (not
shown).

The morphology of B^+ cells is heterogeneous. Small normoblast-like cells show a diffuse benzidine staining, while larger
blasts are often characterized by intra-cytoplasmic B^+ areas,
which may be concentrated in para-golgian vescicles (results not
presented here).

Globin synthesis in IDA cells has been evaluate by means of
analytical isoelectrofocusing, in the presence or not of NP40
(globin had been purified by haptoglobin-Sepharose affinity chromatography). Preliminary results indicate that the IDA line shows
spontaneous and induced synthesis of embryonic ζ- and ε-chains,
but apparently not of fetal (α, γ) and adult (β) globin. Further
experiments are now in progress to confirm and extend these
observations.

In conclusion, the IDA line may provide a unique experimental
model to investigate erythropoietic differentiation, at both
cellular and molecular level, with particular focus on embryonic
globin production.

ACKNOWLEDGEMENTS

This work has been partially supported by CNR grants to C.
P., Progetti Finalizzati "Ingegneria Genetica" (Contract
No.83.001019.51) "Controllo Crescita Neoplastica" (No.
83.00908.96), and "Medicina Preventiva e Riabilitativa" (No.
83.02772.56).

REFERENCES

1) Ferrero, D. and Rovera, G. (1984) Clinics in Hematology,
    in press.
2) Lozzio, C.B. and Lozzio, B.B. (1975) Blood, 45, 321-330.
3) Martin, P. and Papayannopoulou, T. (1982) Science 216,
    1233-1235.
4) Lozzio, B.B., Lozzio, C.B., Bamberger, E.G. and Felin, A.S.
    (1981) Proc. Soc. Exp. Biol. Med. 166, 546-550.
5) Reuben, R.C., Rifkind, R.A., Marks, P.A. (1980) BBA Rev.
    Cancer 605, 325-331.
6) Anderson, I.C., Jokinen, M. and Gahmberg, C.G. (1979)
    Nature, 278, 364-366.
7) Rutherford, T.R., Clegg, J.B. and Weatherall D.J. (1979)
    Nature, 280, 164-165.
8) Cioè, L., McNab, A., Hubbell, H.R., Meo, P., Curtis, P. and
    Rovera, G. (1981) Cancer Res. 41, 237-247.
9) Rutherford, T., Clegg, J.B., Higgs, D.R., Jones, R.W.,

Thompson, J. and Weatherall, D.J. (1981) Proc. Natl. Acad. Sci. USA 78, 348-352.

10) Charnay, P., Maniatis, T. (1983) Science 220, 1281-1283.

11) Marie, J.P., Izaguirre, C.A., Civin, C.I., Mirro, J. and McCulloch, E.A. (1981) Blood 58, 708-711.

12) Gewirtz, A.M., Burger, D., Rado, T.A., Benz, E.J. and Hoffman,R. (1982) Blood 60, 785-789.

13) Sandoz, S.A., Bale, Atlas of Hematology, 1972.

14) Gianni, A.M., Presta, M., Polli, E., Saglio, G., Lettieri, F., Peschle, C., Comi, P., Giglioni, B. and Ottolenghi, S. (1982) In "Advances in Red Cell Biology" Weatherall, D.J. et al., eds., Raven Press, New York, pp.279-287.

PRESENCE OF ONCOGENES IN SPONTANEOUS RAT TUMORS

Oliviero E. Varnier[1], Giorgio Ivaldi[2], Proto Pippia[2], Olimpio Muratore[1], Stephen P. Raffanti[1] and Suraiya Rasheed[3]

1. Institute of Microbiology, School of Medicine, Genova, Italy; 2. Institute of General Physiology and Biological Chemistry, Sassari, Italy, 3. Department of Pathology, Cancer Research, Los Angeles, California

The origin of cancer seems to be the consequence of some variation that results in uncontrolled cellular proliferation. Exciting discoveries have led to the concept that a cellular genetic element, an oncogene, is responsible for initiation or maintenance (or both) of the transforming state. Cellular DNA contains a highly conserved battery of potential transforming genes, called c-onc, that could be activated in a variety of ways (Bishop, 1982). Genomic DNA-transfection studies have shown that 30% of the DNA from many human tumors possess transforming activity (Krontiris, 1983). Several of these oncogenes are homologous to the transforming genes of two acute transforming retroviruses, the Harvey and Kirsten strains of murine sarcoma viruses (HaMSV and KiMSV, respectively; Cooper, 1982). The oncogenes of HaMSV and KiMSV were derived from rat normal cellular sequences during in vivo passage of murine leukemia viruses.

This oncogene family, called ras, is a rather divergent group, which includes the oncogenes of HaMSV and KiMSV (Ha-v-ras and Ki-v-ras) and a third related rat oncogene (Ra-v-ras), isolated from the purely rat Rasheed strain of rat sarcoma viruses (RaSV; Rasheed et al., 1983). Four different human cellular homologues have been characterized (Chang et al., 1982); two (Ha-c-ras^1 and Ha-c-ras^2) are more closely related to the Ha-v-ras, while the others (Ki-v-ras^1 and Ki-c-ras^2) are similar to Ki-v-ras. A fifth possible member of this family was recently isolated from a human neuroblastoma. DNA sequence analysis of these rat and human oncogenes indicate that a single base change, corresponding to amino acid 12 of the encoded protein, confers transforming activity to the ras gene (Tabin et al., 1982; Reddy et al., 1982).

Spontaneous rat tumors are rare and oncogenes have not been identified from any of the naturally occuring malignancies of rats. Solimano (1924) observed a solid tumor in a Rattus norvegicus, var. albus, Galliera strain. The tumor, designated Sarcoma Galliera (SG), has been maintained for over 60 years as a transplanted tumor in the same rat strain (Pippia et al., 1978). The exceedingly long in vivo passage history makes the SG a unique candidate for the study of the rat cellular sequences involved in the development of spontaneous tumors.

Finely minced SG preparations induce non-invasive tumors in 25-30 days in 90% of the inoculated Galliera rats (Table 1) with a remarkable host specificity In fact other rat strains, mouse and guinea pigs were not susceptible (data not shown). No immunosoppression was required for tumor induction in Galliera rats and tumors grew rapidly even when tumor preparations were inoculated in over 4 month old rats. We have established and characterized a tumor cell line (SGS) from this spontaneous sarcoma (Pippia et al., 1978). The SGS cell line consists of mixed cell populations ranging from fusiform to somewhat rounded and epithelial type. Several cultures were derived from single cell clones of the parental SGS line. They differ in cell morphology, adhesion and growth rate. In contrast to the original SG tumor, they induce tumor formation in 100% of the inoculated rats with a very short latency period of only 3 to 6 days (Table 1).

The SGS culture fluids showed high levels of reverse transcriptase activity at a density of 1.14-1.15 g/ml in sucrose-density gradients and a protein cross-reactive with the rat leukemia virus core antigen of about 27.000 (data not shown). No transforming virus was recovered, even after chemical

Table 1.   In vivo and in vitro characteristics of Sarcoma Galliera

Cells	Growth rate	Tumorigenicity[a] positive rats/ inoculated rats	induction time (days)
SG tumor	–	90/100	25–30
SGS	moderate	50/50	4–6
SGS,C–10	high	20/20	3–5
SGS,C–4	moderate	20/20	3–5
FG	very low	0/20	–

a. 200 mg of finely minced tumor preparations or 2×10^5 cultured cells were inoculated subcutaneously in 2-4 month old male Galliera rats.

induction or cocultivation with chemically or DNA virus transformed rat cells (Rasheed et al., 1978). The virus was capable of rescuing defective sarcoma virus from both Ki-MSV and Ra-SV transformed non producer cells. These results indicate that SGS cells but not the normal Gallicra rat embryo fibroblasts (FG) spontaneously release an endogenous ecotropic rat retrovirus, designated SG-RaLV, which does not carry an oncogene in its genome.

Preliminary experiments indicate that transfection in mouse 3T3 cells of DNA from two SG tumors and not that from the spleen of a control animal results in transformation of the recipient cells with an average number of 3 foci per plate, corresponding to 0.15 foci per microgram of DNA (Table 2). This indicates that the oncogenic sequences from SG tumors have been transferred to

Table 2.   Transforming activity od Sarcoma Galliera DNA

Donor DNA	Average number of foci per plate	Foci per ug of DNA
SG-RaLV positive tumor 3	3	0.15
SG-RaLV positive tumor 11	3	0.15
SG-RaLV negative spleen	0	<0.005
RaSV-ras	1000	200

NIH 3T3 cells were exposed to 20 ug of donor DNA per recipient culture and foci of transformed cells were counted 12-15 days after transfection (Shih et al., 1979).

NIH 3T3 cells. Analysis of the transformed cellular DNA is now underway to further characterize the genes involved in the spontaneous development of Sarcoma Galliera.

Since normal embryo fibroblasts from Galliera rats do not express detectable endogenous rat retrovirus (Varnier et al., 1983), it is possible that the replicating SG-RaLV may have activated the expression of a rat cellular oncogene in this rat strain.

ACKNOWLEDGEMENTS

This work was partially supported by the grant CA 27246 of the National Cancer Institute and by CNR, Special Project "Control of Neoplastic Growth", grant n. 82.00221.96.

REFERENCES

Bishop, J.M., 1982, Oncogenes, Sci. Amer., March:81.
Chang, E.H., Gonda, M.E., Ellis, R.W., Scolnick, E.M., and Lowy,
    D.R., 1982, Human genome contains four genes homologous to
    transforming genes of Harvey and Kirsten murine sarcoma
    viruses, Proc. Natl. Acad. Sci. USA, 79:4848.
Cooper, G.M., 1982, Cellular transforming genes, Science,
    217:801.
Krontiris, T.C., The emerging genetics of human cancers,
    New Engl. J. Med., 309:404.
Pippia, P.,. Tilloca, G., Vargiu, F., Cherchi, G.M., Coinu, R.,
    and Ivaldi, G., 1978, Colture continue di cellule di Sarcoma
    Galliera, Pathologica, 70:19.
Rasheed, S., Gardner, M.B., and Huebner, R.J., 1978, In vitro
    isolation of stable rat sarcoma viruses, Proc. Natl. Acad.
    Sci. USA, 75:2972.
Rasheed, S., Norman, G.L., and Heidecker, G., 1983, Nucleotide
    sequence of the Rasheed rat sarcoma virus oncogene : new
    mutations, Science, 221:155.
Reddy, E.P., Reynolds, R.K., Santos, E., and Barbacid, M.,1982, A
    point mutation is responsible for the acquisition of
    transforming properties by the T24 human bladder carcinoma
    oncogene,Nature, 300:149.
Shih, C., Shilo, B.Z., Goldfarb, M.P., Danneberg, A., and
    Weinberg, R.A., 1979, Passage of phenotypes of chemically
    transformed cells via transfection of DNA and chromatin,
    Proc. Natl. Acad. Sci. USA, 76:5714.
Solimano, G., 1924, Studi di sistematica oncologica. Nota I[a]:
    caratteri discriminativi e trapiantabilità di un sarcoma
    spontaneo del "Mus norvegicus" (Sarcoma Galliera), Patholo-
    gica, 16:615.
Tabin, C.J., Bradley,S.M., Bargmann, Weinberg, R.A., Papageorge,
    A.G., Scolnick, E.M., Dhar, K., Lowy, D.R., and Chang, E.M.,
    1982, Mechanism of activation of a human oncogene, Nature,
    300:143.
Varnier, O.E., Raffanti, S.P., Muratore, O., Ivaldi, G., Pippia,
    P., Meloni, M.A., and Rasheed, S., 1983, Isolation of an
    endogenous rat retrovirus from an highly tumorigenic Sarcoma
    Galliera (SGS) cell line, in "Symposium on Oncovirology",
    Bratislava, 3:9.

MOLECULAR BIOLOGY OF HTLV

F. Wong-Staal, G. Franchini, B. Hahn, S. Arya,
E. P. Gelmann, V. Manzari* and R. C. Gallo

Laboratory of Tumor Cell Biology, National Cancer
Institute, National Institutes of Health, Bethesda
Maryland 20205

INTRODUCTION

HTLV is a family of related, human T-cell tropic retroviruses,
consisting of at least two distinct subgroups, HTLV-I and HTLV-II.
The biology, seroepidemiology and protein biochemistry of HTLV are
presented by R. C. Gallo et al. elsewhere in this symposium. This
paper will present only molecular biological studies on HTLV,
focusing on two aspects:

(1) A molecular epidemiological survey of human leukemias
using cloned HTLV probes. Seroepidemiological studies have already
defined geographical areas where HTLV is endemic or present spor-
adically, as well as shown an association of HTLV with a subtype
of mature T-cell malignancy now collectively called adult T-cell
leukemia-lymphoma (ATLL). When molecular clones of the two HTLV
subgroups became available, we conducted a survey of DNA from
different leukemic cells, both fresh and cultured, for the presence
of HTLV sequences. This analysis will allow detection of HTLV
infection even in the absence of viral antigens or antibodies. In
seropositive cases where the patient's diseases are not ATLL, this
analysis may indicate whether HTLV plays a direct role in these
diseases.

(2) The molecular mechanism of transformation by HTLV in vivo
and in vitro. We approach this by examining the state of the
provirus in fresh ATLL cells, primary T-cell lines established

---

*Present address: Istituto di Patologia Generale III Cattedra
Università degli Studi di Roma

from these, and normal cord blood T-cell lines transformed in vitro
with HTLV and the mode of expression of viral and some relevant
cellular genes in different HTLV-infected cells.

MATERIAL AND METHODS

   Fresh peripheral blood leukocytes and tissues of leukemic
patients were obtained from the clinicians. Tissue culture cells
were harvested by centrifugation. DNA was isolated by standard
phenol extraction, and RNA was isolated by the guanidine-
hydrochloride procedure (Westin et al., 1982). Derivation of
molecular clones (Manzari et al., 1983; Gelmann et al., in press)
and procedures for screening and Southern and Northern blot
hybridization have been described (Wong-Staal et al., 1983;
Westin et al., 1982).

RESULTS AND DISCUSSION

Molecular Epidemiology of HTLV and Human Leukemias

   We have used the cloned genomes of HTLV-I and HTLV-II (Manzari
et al., 1983a; Gelmann et al., in press) to survey fresh cells
and tissues of patients with various hematologic malignancies. A
summary of these results is presented in Table 1. All of the
typical ATLL samples as well as a few cases of more benign
cutaneous T-cell lymphoma were positive. All of these contain
closely related, if not identical, proviruses of the HTLV-I subgroup. All other malignancies including acute and chronic myel id
leukemias, acute lymphocytic leukemias and hairy cell leukemia
were negative. Thus, HTLV-I is tightly associated with mature
T-cell malignancies, and HTLV-II is an extremely rare variant of
HTLV, obviously not the agent associated with hairy cell leukemia
in general. With one exception, all fresh tumor cells appear to
be clonally infected. One patient (H T) with ATL who migrated
to London from the Caribbean was unique in that his cells were
polyclonally infected. More detailed analysis of this case is
underway. The other leukemic cells contained 1 to 3 copies of
proviruses that are either complete or defective. A patient
(JM) who was seronegative for HTLV antigens contained a single
defective provirus in their leukemic cells.

   Autopsy tissues from two patients showed that the level of
detectable HTLV sequences correlated with the degree of infiltration of the leukemic cells, while noninvolved tissues were negative.

Table 1. HTLV-I and HTLV-II Proviruses in Human Hematopoietic
          Neoplastic Fresh Cell DNAs

Disease	Number of Cases	HTLV Positive	Average Copy Number
ATLL[a],[b] (USA)	3	3	1.5
ATLL[b] (Japan)	8	8	1.5
ATLL[b] (Caribbean)	2	2	3 or more
ATLL[b] (Brazil)	1	1	3
AML	31	0	–
AMML	3	0	–
CML	9	1[c]	?
ALL	8	0	–
CTCL	8	0	–
Others	25	0	–
HCL	5	0	–

[a]ATLL, adult T-cell leukemia-lymphoma; AML, acute myeloid
leukemia; AMML, acute myelomonocytic leukemia; CML, chronic
myeloid leukemia; CTCL, cutaneous T-cell lymphoma; HCL, hairy
cell leukemia.

[b]Many more cases of ATLL have been found positive for the presence
of HTLV by various criteria: virus isolation, immunofluorescence,
etc., but the proviral DNA has not been studied in such cases,
usually for the lack of sufficient amount of fresh cells.

[c]This case contains sequences distantly related to HTLV-I.

     Leukemic cells of two patients who were seropositive for HTLV
but whose diseases were not ATLL were examined. Both samples, a
T ALL and a B-CLL, did not contain detectable HTLV sequences,
although cultured T-cells of the latter did contain HTLV. This
result indicates that HTLV does not have a direct role in these
patients' disease. However, since it has been observed that in
HTLV endemic regions, a higher percentage of HTLV positivity was
found in patients with lymphoid malignancies in general than
normal, it is possible that HTLV-infected T-cells in some patients
can secrete a protein, e.g., a growth factor that stimulates the
abnormal proliferation of B cells or immature T cells secondarily.
Alternatively, HTLV-infected individuals may be immune compromised
and more prone to develop other malignancies.

Clonal Selection of HTLV-Infected Cells In Vivo and In Vitro

All ATL leukemic cells as well as established T-cell lines
from HTLV-positive individuals are mono- or oligo-clonally derived
as analyzed by provirus integration (Wong-Staal et al., 1983;
Yoshida et al., 1982). While peripheral blood cells from healthy
seropositive individuals are polyclonally infected (Yoshida et al.,
personal communication), cell lines established from normal
people also appear to be clonally derived (Hahn et al.,
unpublished). These observations suggest that clonal selection
occurs in vivo in the leukemic patient and in vitro for cells
established from nonleukemic individuals.

To determine whether fresh and cultured cells represent
similar infected cell populations, we compared DNA from fresh
peripheral blood cells of a patient SK and his cultured T cells.
In this experiment, a probe containing the entire HTLV genome was
used. As shown in Fig. 1, fresh SK cells contained one predominant
cell clone as reflected by the 17 Kb EcoRI bands. The predominant
clone in the fresh cells was present at best as a rare clone in
the cultured SK cell line, which contained multiple copies of
HTLV provirus, some of which are defective. Comparison of several
other pairs of primary and cultured leukemic cells consistently
showed 1-2 copies of HTLV in the fresh cells and increased copies
in the cultured cells (Wong-Staal et al., 1983). Digestions with
PstI, BamHI and SstI revealed conserved internal bands between SK
fresh cells and cell lines but noncorresponding junction bands.
The most clear-cut result was with XbaI which cuts once in the
HTLV genome. The two junction bands in fresh SK cells do not
comigrate with any of the junction bands of the SK cell line.

These results suggest that the clonally expanded leukemic
cells lost their proliferative advantage so that the normal T
cells infected in vivo or during culture grow out and the cells
may initially go through a polyclonal phase. However, a specific
cell population eventually dominates in the culture. The apparent
clonality of the infected cell lines established from normal people
may have been a progression of this selection process in vitro.
Examination of primary infected cells or cultured cells at different
time intervals from these individuals is necessary to address this
possibility.

Normal T cells infected and immortalized by HTLV in vitro
are also clonal and we consider them to be equivalent to the
established cell lines from ATLL patients. These newly infected
cells resemble primary transformed cells in many respects (Popovic
et al., 1983) and provides a good model for studying the process
of initiation of transformation. The circulating leukemic cells,

on the other hand, provide a good system of studying maintenance
of the leukemic state. We shall examine the role of viral and
some cellular genes in these two separate cell systems.

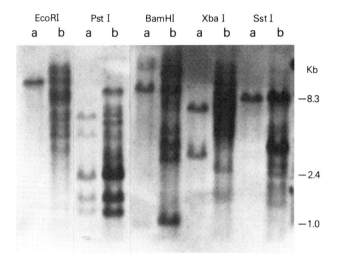

Fig. 1. Comparison of HTLV proviruses in primary leukemic cells
         and an established cell line of an ATLL patient.

         High molecular cellular DNA was digested with the enzymes
         as indicated, electrophoresed in 0.8% agarose gels,
         transferred to metrocellulose and hybridized with a
         complete HTLV-I genomes probe. The conditions for
         hybridization, washing and autoradiography were as
         described (Wong-Staal et al., 1983) (a) fresh leukemic
         cells of SK (b) the SK line.

Detection of Viral Transcripts in HTLV-Infected Cell Lines and Fresh Leukemic Cells of ATL Patients

RNA obtained from the fresh lymphocytes of five ATL patients
and five established cell lines were hybridized to specific probes
of HTLV including LTR, gag, pol, env and pX sequences. Several
species of viral mRNA were detected in all cell ines and one of
the five fresh cell samples, including a 9.0 Kb mRNA corresponding
to the HTLV genomic size which must encode for the gag and pol
proteins and a four Kb species which appears to be the mRNA for
the env protein. Furthermore, a smaller mRNA species (2.0-2.5
Kb) hybridized specifically to LTR and a pX probe, suggesting
that the pX region is transcribed separately from env sequences
as a subgenomic mRNA. Other mRNA species of variable size between
3.0 and 4.0 Kb have also been observed.

RNA from four fresh samples did not hybridize to any viral probes. Thus it appears that expression of viral proteins, including pX, may be necessary for the initiation but not for maintenance of transformation.

Mode of Expression of the T-Cell Growth Factor Gene and Some Cellular onc Gene Homologues

The clonality of the HTLV in vivo and in vitro transformed cells, the presence of defective virus genomes and the lack of necessity of viral gene expression are features that resemble the avian leukosis virus-bursal lymphoma system (Neel et al., 1981). In the latter, activation of a cellular proto-oncogene c-myc is known to be responsible for neoplastic transformation. We therefore examined the possibility of gene activation as a possible mechanism of leukemogenesis by HTLV. The most obvious candidates are growth factor genes and cellular homologues of retroviral onc genes. All HTLV-infected cells express a high density of T-cell growth factor (TCGF) receptors (Waldmann et al., 1983) and a gene HT-3 which may be the gene for the receptor is expressed at high levels in all HTLV-infected cells (Manzari et al., 1983b). Therefore, an attractive model would be expression of TCGF in these same cells resulting in autostimulation. Using a cloned TCGF gene (Clark et al., in press) as a probe, we detected only an extremely low level of transcripts in a few HTLV-positive cell lines and not in most. Neither is TCGF expressed in the fresh leukemic cells. Therefore, a simple autostimulation mechanism cannot be operative either in initiation or maintenance of the leukemic state. However, it is possible that the TCGF receptor expressed on these cells has been altered so that it now recognizes another growth factor or that in its altered state, it is activated without binding to any factor. There is some evidence that the TCGF receptor expressed in HTLV infected T cells may be qualitatively different from that of normal cells (W. Greene, personal communication). Therefore, the receptor for TCGF is a natural focus for future efforts to understand the mechanism of transformation by HTLV.

We have also examined the posibility of onc gene activation after HTLV infection. Using cloned probes of sis, myc, myb, fes, abl, src, H-ras, K-ras, we failed to find consistent activation of any onc gene in either the in vitro infected cells or fresh leukemic cells, thus negating a requisite role of the onc gene tested in either initiation or maintenance of transformation. However, it is of interest to note that a significant number of HTLV-infected cell lines express c-sis, (Westin et al., 1982; and our unpublished data) a gene not normally expressed in hematopoietic cells. Since c-sis is now known to code for a growth factor (PDGF), which normally acts on fibroblasts, smooth muscle cells and glial cells, it would be of interest to see if the sis product produced in these cells can aberrently stimulate their proliferation.

SUMMARY

The molecular biology of HTLV has progressed since the cloning of the viral genomes was accomplished. We now know that HTLV consists of two distinct subgroups. Members of subgroup I are highly conserved if not identical isolates obtained worldwide, while subgroup II consists of only two isolates so far. HTLV-I infection is tightly associated with adult T-cell leukemia-lymphoma, but the disease spectrum of HTLV-II has not been defined.

HTLV does not carry an onc gene and is associated with tumors that are clonally derived. Therefore, it falls into the class of chronic leukemia viruses. However, it is the only known chronic leukemia virus that can efficiently immortalize fresh human cells in vitro. We believe that in vitro immortalization represents a first stage (initiation) of neoplastic transformation while the circulating leukemic cells represent a later stage involving maintenance of the transformed state. We found that viral expression may be necessary for inititation, but not maintenance of transformation. A simple autostimulation mechanism involving TCGF production in the transformed cells has been ruled out at both early and late stages, and there is no evidence of consistent activation of a known onc gene. However, the TCGF receptor and c-sis are genes we want to further investigate. Whether HTLV activates these other cellular gene(s) by provirus insertion during the initiation phase and the kind of events that lead to establishment of leukemia are questions of great interest.

REFERENCES

Clark, S. C., Arya, S. K., Wong-Staal, M., Matsumoto-Kobayashi, R. M., Kay, R. J., Kaufman, E. L., Brown, C., Shoemaker, T., Copeland, T., Oroszlan, S., Smith, K., Sarngadharan, M. G., Linder, S. G., and Gallo, R. C., in press, Human T-cell growth factor: partial amino sequence of the proteins expressed by normal and leukemic cells, molecular cloning of the mRNA from normal cells, analysis of gene structure and expression in different human cell types, Proc. Natl. Acad. Sci., U.S.A.

Gelmann, E. P., Franchini, G., Manzari, V., Wong-Staal, and Gallo, R. C., in press, Molecular cloning of a new unique T-leukemia virus (HTLV-II$_{Mo}$), Proc. Natl. Acad. Sci. U.S.A.

Manzari, V., Wong-Staal, F., Franchini, G., Colombini, S., Gelmann, E. P., Oroszlan, S., Staal, S. P., and Gallo, R. C., 1983, Human T-cell leukemia-lymphoma virus, HTLV: Molecular cloning of an integrated defective provirus and flanking cellular sequences, Proc. Natl. Acad. Sci. U.S.A., 80:1574.

Manzari, V., Gallo, R. C., Franchini, G., Westin, E., Chccherini-Nelli, L., Popovic, M., and Wong-Staal, F., 1983, Abundant transcription of a cellular gene in T-cells infected with human T-cell leukemia-lymphoma virus (HTLV), Proc. Natl. Acad. Sci. U.S.A., 80:1574.

Neel, B. G., Hayward, W. S., Robinson, H. L., Fang, J., and Astrin, S. M., 1981, Avian leukosis virus induced tumors have common proviral integration sites and synthesize discrete new RNA's: oncogenes by promoter insertion, Cell 23:323.

Popovic, M., Lange-Wantzin, G., Sarin, P. S., Mann, P., and Gallo, R. C., 1983, Transformation of human umbilical cord blood T-cells by human T-cell leukemia/lymphoma virus, Proc. Natl. Acad. Sci., U.S.A. 80:5402.

Seiki, C., Hattori, S., Hirayama, Y., and Yoshida, M., 1983, Human adult T-cell leukemia virus: Complete nucleotide sequence of the provirus genome integrated in leukemia cell DNA. Proc. Natl. Acad. Sci. U.S.A., 88:3618.

Waldmann, T., Broder, S., Greene, W., Sarin, P. S., Goldman, C., Frost, K., Sharrow, S., Depper, J., Leonard, W., Uhiyama, T., and Gallo, R. C., 1983, A comparison of the function and phenotype Sezary T-cells with human T-cell leukemia/lymphoma virus (HTLV) associated with adult T-cell leukemia cells, Clin. Res., 31:547A.

Westin, E. H., Wong-Staal, F., Gelmann, E. P., Dalla=Favera, F., Papas, T. S., Lautenberger, J. A., Eva, A., Reddy, E. P., Tronick, S. R., Aaronson, S. A., and Gallo, R. C., 1982, Expression of cellular homologues of retroviral onc genes in human hematopoietic cells, Proc. Natl. Acad. Sci. U.S.A., 79:2490.

Wong-Staal, F., Hahn, B., Manzari, V., Colombini, S., Franchini, G., Gelmann, E. P., and Gallo, R. C., 1983, A survey of human leukemias for sequences of a human retrovirus, Nature, 302: 626.

Yoshida, M., Miyoshi, I., and Hinuma, Y., 1979, Isolation and characterization of retrovirus from cell lines of human adult T-cell leukemia and its implication in the disease. Proc. Natl. Acad. Sci. U.S.A., 79:2031.

HIGH LEVEL TRANSCRIPTION OF A HUMAN GENE IN HTLV POSITIVE

T-CELLS: cDNA CLONING AND CHARACTERIZATION

Vito M. Fazio, Vittorio Manzari, Luigi Frati,
Genoveffa Franchini, Flossie Wong-Staal and
Robert C. Gallo

Istituto di Patologia Generale, Policlinico Umberto I
Universita' degli Studi di Roma, Italy
Laboratory of Tumor Cell Biology, NCI, NIH
Bethesda Md, USA

Human T-cell Leukemia Lymphoma Virus is associated with ATL (Acute T-cell Leukemia) or related diseases (Sezary syndrome, mycosis fungoides) (1-4): in a very high percentage its provirus genome is integrated in human DNA in one or more copies, with complete or defective sequences (5). The genome of HTLV contains two LTR sequences at 3' and 5' ends with an unusually long R sequence, the regions that code for viral proteins "gag", "pol", "env", and a region called "pX" constituted of small reading frames with no homology with the normal human DNA. It doesn't seem to contain any typical "onc" gene (11,12) (fig.1).

To date, the site of provirus integration in human genome was found to be random in different patients but common in all the leukemic T-cells of the same patients (5). The HTLV can also be isolated from neoplastic T-cell lines grown in suspension culture by addition of TCGF (13,14). By cocultivation with a cell line producing HTLV (HUT 102), it is possible to immortalize normal cord blood T lymphocytes "in vitro" (15,16): the resulting cell cultures are completely or partially independent of TCGF.

345

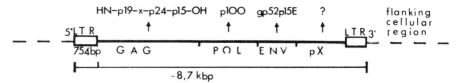

Fig. 1. HTLV viral genome and known products of viral genes.

These results seem to suggest a role of HTLV infection in modulation of specific steps in T-cell proliferation, especially if directly or indirectly related to TCGF. To investigate the influence of HTLV integration in neoplastic transformation and proliferation of T-cells, and to detect gene/s expressed at high levels in these cells, we analyzed the transcription of human T lymphocytes infected by HTLV. mRNA was extracted and selected from a T-cell line actively producing HTLV (HUT 102): using this mRNA as a template, we constructed a cDNA library, and a clone, hybridizing specifically with HUT 102 c-DNA and not to HUT 78 (18,19), which was isolated and characterized to analyze HUT 102 expression (17).

cDNA LIBRARY CONSTRUCTION

RNA from HUT 102 (1) was poly(A)selected by oligo(dT)cellulose column chromatography and transcribed by reverse transcriptase. The second strand was constructed by E. Coli DNA polymerase I (large fragment) and single stranded regions were eliminated by S1 nuclease. The double stranded cDNA obtained was fractionated and selected on a Bio-Gel A 150 m column and the excluded material was precipitated by ethanol and washed with 70% ethanol. The selected cDNA was tailed with poly(dC) by deoxynucleotidyltransferase, and the reaction was stopped after 8-12 nucleotides. This cDNA was annealed to plasmid pBR322, cleaved with Pst I, and tailed with poly(dG) in the same way, and then it was cloned in MC1061 as recipient cells.

ANALYSIS OF cDNA LIBRARY

The cDNA library was analyzed by differential screening with two different probes:
- homologous radiolabeled cDNA
- a labeled cDNA obtained from mRNA of HUT 78 (a cutaneous T-cell lymphoma line negative to HTLV).

Clones containing inserts hybridizing only to HUT 102 cDNA and not HUT 78 cDNA were selected. One of these clones, HT-3 clone, in particular hybridized strongly to HUT 102 cDNA, suggesting that this clone could be a very frequent mRNA in HUT 102. Further analysis and the restriction map of the clone showed the length of 1.37 kb of the insert. To verify the specificity of the clone HT-3 to HUT 102 mRNA, the insert was isolated, labeled by nick-translation, and used as a probe for a RNA gel blot containing mRNA from HUT 78 and from two cell lines producing HTLV (HUT 102, MO). HT-3 hybridizes specifically to a single species mRNA of 2.3 kb in HUT 102 and MO (20) but not in HUT 78 (fig. 2). The upper band corresponds to an aspecific interaction between ribosomal RNA (28S) and the labeled plasmid DNA, and it was eliminated after poly(A) selection of RNA. Other HTLV producing cell line RNAs (M.J., M.I., Sez. 2) (2, 16) were tested and hybridized to radiolabeled HT-3, confirming the specificity of the clone for HTLV infected and virus producing T-cells. Comparing with HTLV transformed cells containing a known number of viral transcripts, it was possible to estimate that HT-3 mRNA is contained in several hundred copies in HTLV infected T-cells.

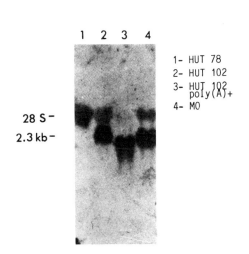

Fig. 2. Screening by HT-3 probe of mRNA
from two HTLV positive T-cell lines

ACTIVATION OF HT-3 GENE

   To analyze the correlation between HTLV infection and HT-3
activation we tested the amount of transcription of HT-3 gene in
normal cord blood T lymphocytes maintained in short-term culture
with TCGF and the same cells infected by HTLV. A whole cell
blotting assay was developed to analyze the transcription of HT-3
in the small number of cells obtainable from cord blood: this
technique allows us to study the T-lymphocytes expression by less
than 10 cells. The infected and non infected cells were collected
by low speed centrifugation, washed by phosphate buffered saline,
and diluted to 5 x10 cells per ml in PBS. From this concentration
a two-fold serial dilution was prepared and 200 1 of each cell
dilution were applied on a nitrocellulose sheet by using a 96-well
filtration manifold. Then, each well was washed, air dried, baked
for two hours in a vacuum oven, and prehybridized. The
hybridization was carried out with radiolabeled HT-3 probe and
labeled ribosomal cDNA as control. After hybridization, the
filters were washed with 2x NaCl/Cit/0.1 % NaDodSO two times for 5
minutes each with constant agitation, then with 0.1x NaCl/Cit/
0.1% NaDodSO two times at 42 C for 15' each. HTLV infected cells
are shown to hybridize strongly to HT-3 probe and to express high
levels of HT-3 transcripts (1, lanes A-B), while non-infected
cells do not express detectable levels (1, lane C) (fig. 3).

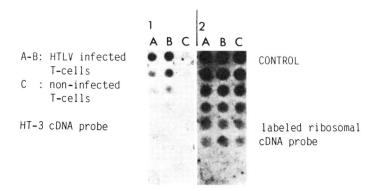

Fig. 3. HT-3 activation in cord blood T-lymphocytes
       infected with HTLV by cocultivation.

CELLULAR HT-3 GENE LOCUS ON HUMAN GENOME

     To better characterize the HT-3 gene, the DNAs extracted from
HUT 102 and from normal leukocytes of three patients were cleaved
by two restriction enzymes: EcoR I (lanes 1-4) and Pst I (lanes
5-8), and hybridized to p-labeled HT-3 probe. In all the DNAs
digested by EcoR I we found hybridization with only one band
corresponding to a length of 7.3 kb, and the signal intensity
seemed to be identical in HUT102 and in other normal T-cells,
showing that no amplification of HT-3 gene occurs in HUT102 cells
(fig. 4). Genomes digested by Pst I has two different kind of
hybridization and two allelic genotypes for HT-3 gene:

- HUT102 and other cell lines hybridize with a single band of 2.8
  Kb
- other cell lines show two bands of 2.8 and 3.4 Kb.

     These results suggest that HT-3 is a cellular gene, not
amplified in HTLV infected T-cells, with two allelic genotypes, as
Pst I cleavage indicates.

SCREENING OF HUMAN HEMATOPOIETIC CELLS FOR HT-3 GENE EXPRESSION

     The data obtained indicate a close correlation between HTLV
infection, T-cells activation and HT-3 expression, but they do not
explain the function of HT-3 RNA production in cell proliferation
and transformation. To investigate HT-3 function and expression,
we screened a survey of human hematopoietic cells of myeloid,
erythroid and lymphoid lineages. The results can be so summerized
according to the level of HT-3 transcription:

- in lymphoid precursor cells, REH (pre-T), KM 3 (pre-B), in EBV
  transformed B cell lines (IM-9, Raji, Daudi, and NC37) (22), in
  the myeloid cell line HL 60 (22), in the erythroid line K562,
  derived from chronic myelogenous leukemia (24), in immature
  t-cell lines (Jurkat, HSB-2, RPMI 8402, MOLT 4, CCRF-CEM)
  (21,22), and in mature T-lymphocytes, the expression is very low
  or undetectable.
- fresh lymphocytes and the cell lines Jurkat and HSV-2, if activated by lectins (PHA or PHA and TPA), become producers of high
  levels of transcription of HT-3 gene.

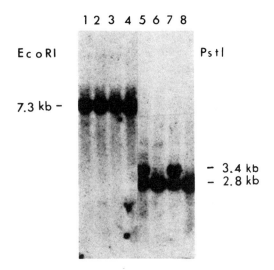

Fig. 4. Identification of the cellular HT-3 gene locus.

One gibbon T-cell line infected by GaLV and constitutively
producing TCGF, UCD144 (25,26), show also high levels of HT-3
transcription while 6G-1 cells, derived from the same origin
but not producing detectable levels of TCGF (27), have very
moderate levels of HT-3 transcription.
- in T-cells infected with HTLV by cocultivation, and in HTLV
  positive T cell lines (HUT102, Sez. 2, MO, MJ) the expression
  of HT-3 gene reaches the highest peak with several hundred
  copies of transcript.

Since HT-3 gene is not amplified in HTLV infected T
lymphocytes and it corresponds to a single species mRNA of about
2.3 Kb, we can suppose that the high levels of HT-3 mRNA depends
on transcriptional efficiency of the gene.

DISCUSSION

Seroepidemiological studies and molecular biological analysis (5,6) from all over the world are consistently confirming the association and correlation between a malignant lymphoma of T-lymphocytes with some particular features (28), and the human T-cell leukemia virus. The role of HTLV infection in cell transformation and in the genesis of the disease is still unknown, but many recent interesting data are available. Studying the expression of HTLV positive neoplastic T-cells, we identified a human gene with specific high levels of transcription in cells infected by HTLV.

A cDNA clone (HT-3), derived from mRNA of HTLV positive tumor cell line (HUT102), was obtained from a cDNA library by differential screening with homologous cDNA probe made from a cutaneous T-cell lymphoma line HTLV negative (HUT78).

This cDNA clone hybridizes to a cellular single copy gene present in all human genomes and identified a single species mRNA of about 2.3 Kb produced at detectable levels in lectin-activated T-cell and at very high levels only in HTLV infected T-cells.

Of interest is that the Jurkat T-cell line activated by lectins becomes a producer of a high level of TCGF and of TCGF receptors. Moreover, a gibbon T-cell line (UCD 144), infected by GaLV and producing constant high levels of TCGF, also transcribes actively the HT-3 gene while a homologous gibbon T-cell line not producing TCGF (6G-1) does not. According to these results we could suppose that HT-3 gene corresponds to TCGF gene, but recent data absolutely remove this hypothesis:

- HUT78, a HTLV negative lymphoma T-cell line that presents a
  stage of differentiation similar to the HTLV infected T-cell
  lines, produces low levels of TCGF but does not transcribe
  HT-3 gene at detectable levels (18,19).
- the production rate of TCGF is not always correlated to HT-3
  levels of transcription.
- the recent identification and cloning of TCGF gene which
  appears to be completely different from HT-3 gene (29).

A possible correlation between HT-3 product and TCGF receptors is today an appealing idea: in fact, the rate and the activation of TCGF production seems to be similar to HT-3 transcriptional activation (30).

HT-3 cDNA clone sequence will give us a better way to characterize HT-3 product and to construct an aminoacid sequence to analyze and to compare with.

In conclusion, although we cannot indicate any certain candidate to HT-3 gene product identification, we can say that HT-3 may be involved in at least one of the steps related to TCGF production. Another problem associated with HT-3 expression is: how can the high level of transcription of this gene be determined? As our data suggest, HT-3 gene is a cellular gene and not a proviral sequence, present in all human DNAs as a single copy per haploid genome with at least two allelic genotypes among individuals.
In the cells with high levels of HT-3 transcription it is not amplified compared with cells not detectably expressing HT-3: these results suggest that HT-3 high expression is related only to transcriptional efficiency of the gene.

At last, we must investigate the correlation between HTLV infection and HT-3 high levels of transcription: is the HT-3 increased expression related to infection and integration of HTLV directly or indirectly? As many reports suggest (5), the integration site of HTLV provirus in human genome is not constant in different patients, but the infected T-cells in the same patient are of clonal origin; moreover, the genome of HTLV provirus does not seem to contain any typical "onc" gene. A peculiar characteristic of the virus is the fact that the "R" sequence at both ends of viral RNA present an unusual length of 228+/-1bases (12), much longer than other retroviruses and similar only to BLV.

Furthermore in the HTLV genomic there is a region (pX) that contains small reading frames with no homology with normal human DNA: but the role of this viral gene is not yet known. We can only speculate that these unusually long R sequences could provide fuctions fundamental expression of some human genes (promotion, initiation, and polyadenylation of transcripts) (31) or that the pX products could interact with human genome, but until now we do not have any certain data. Since HTLV transforms human mature T-cells, the integration of its proviral sequence in human DNA induces transformation and T-cell proliferation, but we still do not know whether it is a direct or indirect mechanism, and if HTLV is involved in maintenance of neoplastic status. These differences between HTLV proviral genome and other retroviruses, although very interesting in investigating the implication in human T-cell transformation, do not allow us to compare the mechanism of other retroviruses with HTLV. We are going on studying HTLV genome and the cellular integration sites to obtain further data about HTLV provirus interaction with cellular human DNA and to explain the role of HT-3 and its activation in cells infected by HTLV.

REFERENCES

1. Poiesz, B.J., Ruscetti, F.W., Gazdar, A.F., Bunn, P.A., Minna, J.D. and Gallo, R.C. Proc. Natl. Acad. Sci. USA 77, 7415-7419 (1980)
2. Poiesz, B.J., Ruscetti, F.W., Reitz, M.S., Kalyanaraman, V.S. and Gallo, R.C. Nature (London) 294, 268-271 (1981)
3. Reitz, M.S., Poiesz, B.J., Ruscetti, F.W. and Gallo, R.C. Proc. Natl. Acad. Sci. USA 78, 1887-1891 (1981)
4. Kalyanaraman, V.S., Sarngadharan, M.G., Poiesz, B.J., Ruscetti, F.W. and Gallo, R.C. J. Virol. 38, 906-913 (1981)
5. Wong-Staal, F., Hahn, B., Manzari, V., Colombini, S., Franchini, G., Gelman, E.P. and Gallo, R.C. Nature 302, 626-628 (1983)
6. Posner, L.E., Robert-Guroff, M., Kalyanaraman, V.S., Poiesz, B.J., Ruscetti, F.W., Fossieck, B., Bunn, P.A., Minna, J.D. and Gallo, R.C. J. Exp. Med. 154, 333-346 (1981)
7. Kalyanaraman, V.S., Sarngadharan, M.G., Bunn, P.A., Minna, J.D. and Gallo, R.C. Nature (London), 294, 271-273, (1981)
8. Kalyanaraman, V.S., Sarngadharan, M.G., Nakao, Y., Ito, Y., Aoki, T. and Gallo, R.C. Proc. Natl. Acad. Sci. USA 79, 1653-1657 (1982)
9. Robert-Guroff, M., Nakao, Y., Notake, K., Ito, Y., Sliski, A. and Gallo, R.C. Science 215, 975-978 (1982)

10. Catovsky, D., Greaves, M.F., Rose, N., Galton, D.A.G., Golden, A.W.G., McCluskey, D.R., White, J.M., Lampert, I., Bourikas, G, Ireland, R., Brownell, A.I., Bridges, J.M., Blattner, W.A. and Gallo, R.C. Lancet i, 639-643 (1982)

11. Manzari, V., Wong-Staal, F., Franchini, G., Colombini, S., Gelman, E.P., Oroszlan, S., Staal, S. and Gallo, R.C. Proc. Natl. Acad. Sci. USA 80, 1574-1578 (1983)

12. Seiki, M., Hattori, S. and Yoshida, M. Proc. Natl. Acad. Sci. USA 79, 6899-6902 (1982)

13. Morgan, D.A., Ruscetti, F.W. and Gallo, R.C. Science 193, 1007-1008, (1976)

14. Gootemberg, J.E., Ruscetti, F.W., Mier, J.W., Gazdar, A. and Gallo, R.C. J. Exp. Med 154, 1403-1418 (1981)

15. Miyoshi, I., Kubonishi, I, Yoshimoto, S., Akagi, T., Ohtsuki, Y., Shiraiski, Y., Nagota, K. and Hinuma, Y. Nature (London), 294, 770-771 (1981)

16. Gallo, R,C., Popovic, M., Wantzin, G.L., Wong-Staal, F. and Sarin, P.S., in "Hematopoietic Stem Cells", eds. Kilman, S.A., cronkite, E.P. and Muller-Beratt, C.N. (Munksgaard, Copenhaghen) (1983)

17. Manzari, V., Gallo., R.C., Franchini., G., Westin, E., Ceccherini-Nelli, L., Popovic, M. and Wong-Staal, F., Proc. Natl. Acad. Sci. USA 80, 11-15, (1983)

18. Gazdar, A.F., Carney, D.N., Bunn., P.A., Russel., E.K., Jaffe, E.S., Schecter, G.P. and Guccion, J.G. Blood 55, 409-417, (1980)

19. Poiesz, B.J., Ruscetti, F.W., Mier, J.W., Woods, A.M. and Gallo, R.C. Proc. Natl. Acad. Sci. USA 77, 6815-6819, (1980)

20. Saxon, A., Stevens, R.H. and Golde, D.W. Ann. Int. Med. 88, 323-326, (1978)

21. Kaplan, J., Tilton, J. and Peterson, W.D., Jr. Am. J. Hemat. 1, 219-225 (1976)

22. Minowada, J., Sagawa, K., Lok, M.S., Kubonishi, I., Nakazawa, S., Tatsumi, E., Ohnuma, T. and Goldblum N. in "International Symposium on new Trands in Human Immunology and Cancer Immunotherapy", eds., Serrou, B. and Rosenfield, C., (Doin, Paris) pp 189-199, (1980)

23. Collins, S.J., Gallo, R.C. and Gallagher, R.E. Nature (London) 270, 347-349 (1977)

24. Lozzio, C.B. and Lozzio, B.B. Blood 45, 321-334 (1975)

25. Kawakami, T.G., Huff, S.D., Bukley, B.M., Dungworth, D.L., Snyder, S.P. and Gilden, R.W. Nature (London) New Biol. 235,

170-171 (1972)
26.Rabin, H., Hopkins, R.F., Ruscetti, F.W., Neubauer, R.H.,
   Brown, R.L. and Kawakami, T.G. J. Immunol. 127, 1852-1856
   (1981)
27.Gallo, R.C., Gallagher, R.E., Wong-Staal, F., Aoki, T.,
   Markham, P.D., Schetters, H., Ruscetti., F.W., Valerio, M.,
   Walling, M., O'Keefe, R.T., Saxinger, W.C., Smith, R.G.,
   Gillespie, D.H. and Reitz, M.S. Virology 84, 359-373 (1978)
28.Bunn, P.A. Jr., Schecter, G.P., Jaffe, E., Blayney, D., Young,
   R. C., Matthews, M.G., Blattner, W., Broder, S., Robert-Guroff,
   M. and Gallo, R.C. N. Engl. J. Med. 309, 257-264 (1983)
29.Clark, S.C., Arya, S.K., Wong-Staal, F., Matsumato-Kobayashi,
   M., Kay, R.B., Kaufman, R.J., Brown, E.L., Shoemaker, C.,
   Copeland, and Gallo, R.C. "Human T-cell Growth Factor: cloning
   and expression of the gene and characterization and sequencing
   of the purified protein from normal and leukemic cells",
   in preparation
30.Lando, Z., Sarin, P., Megson, M., Greene, W.C., Waldman, T.A.
   Gallo, R.C. and Broder, S. Science 216, 812-820 (1983)

CLINICAL FEATURES OF HUMAN T-CELL LEUKEMIA/LYMPHOMA VIRUS

(HTLV) ASSOCIATED T-CELL NEOPLASMS

Hiroaki Mitsuya and Samuel Broder

Clinical Oncology Program
Mational Cancer Institute
Bethesda, MD 20205

Approximately seven years ago clinical investigators in Kyoto reported a rapidly fatal T-cell lymphoproliferative syndrome, which seemed to affect adult populations born in the Southwestern part of the Japanese archipelago, even though the population may have migrated to another area of Japan. They referred to this disease as adult T-cell leukemia, and to date over 300 patients have been described by several groups in Japan. The syndrome is characterized by the presence of pleomorphic neoplastic cells with the membrane markers of mature T-lymphocytes. Several other findings are common at presentation including lymphadenopathy, hepatomegaly, splenomegaly, cutaneous infiltration with neoplastic T cells, hypercalcemia (with or without lytic bone lesions), and interstitial pulmonary infiltrates. Characteristically, there was an absence of mediastinal tumor involvement.

The striking geographic distribution of these patients induced these Japanese clinical investigators to conclude that adult T-cell leukemia represented a new category of T-cell malignancy. However, it was not possible to ascribe an etiology for this newly recognized, endemic form of cancer.

At approximately the same time, clinical investigators within the intramural National Cancer Institute began studying American patients who carried the diagnosis of cutaneous T-cell lymphoma (mycosis fungoides/Sezary syndrome) but who had the clinical and laboratory features of adult T-cell leukemia in Japan. In 1978, Gallo and his co-workers were able to identify a human type-C-RNA tumor virus in these patients. This retrovirus was referred to as

HTLV (human T-cell leukemia-lymphoma virus). HTLV was shown to be a
unique, exogenously acquired retrovirus that is not closely related
to any of the known animal retroviruses in terms of antigenicity,
amino-acid sequence, and nucleic-acid sequence homology.

The identification of HTLV in patients seen at the National
Cancer Institute lead to the discovery of HTLV-infection in patients
from Japan and subsequently from other countries where adult T-cell
leukemia was being recognized as a new entity. The recognition
that HTLV-infection is closely correlated with an independently
defined clinical syndrome represents a dramatic advance in cancer
research.

The purpose of this chapter is to summarize certain clinical
and laboratory features of the adult T-cell leukemia/lymphoma
syndrome and HTLV.

At the outset, we would like to present a case history of a
patient with this syndrome recently admitted to the Clinical Oncology
Program of the National Cancer Institute.

The patient was a 23-year-old Black mother of one from Florida
when she developed a cough productive of a small amount of white
sputum late in January 1983. A week later the cough had worsened,
and over the next 3 weeks she developed nausea and vomiting, head-
ache, dizziness, lower abdominal pain, fever, and cervical
adenopathy. She sought medical attention from her personal
physician at the beginning of March. At that time it was found
that her last menstrual period had been in December 1982. Physical
examination revealed bilateral 2x1 cm cervical adenopathy, an
inflamed oropharynx with enlarged tonsils, slightly enlarged liver
and spleen, and a small midline lower abdominal mass. Laboratory
examination showed a hematocrit of 36% with an MCV of 71, 6500
WBC/mm^3 with 20% neutrophils, 76% lymphocytes, 1% metamyelocytes,
and 3% eosinophils. Liver function tests were abnormal: LDH 485,
alkaline phosphatase 1594, and SGOT 440. On 3/9/83, her WBC count
had risen to 60,000/mm^3 with numerous abnormal lymphocytes, and she
was referred to another Florida hospital. On 3/17/83, she developed
shortness of breath with patchy infiltrates in both lung fields
and hypoxemia. She underwent bronchoscopic lung biopsy which
revealed interstitial pneumonitis with no organisms identified.
She was placed on trimethoprim/sulfamethoxazole empirically and her
condition improved over the next week. She was found to have a
positive pregnancy test on 3/23, underwent a therapeutic abortion
and an abdominal hysterectomy. Her adenopathy progressed, fevers
persisted, and her peripheral WBC count continued to rise. On the
evening of 4/5/83, she was referred to the National Institutes of
Health.

At that time she had lost 10 kg of body weight (to 44 kg) and
complained of weakness, somnolence, shortness of breath, and had
noticed a skin rash on her face, upper extremities and trunk that
had progressed over the previous three weeks. On physical examination, she had a diffuse papular rash over her face, back, chest,
and upper extremities. She had enlarged tonsils and bilateral
cervical, axillary, inguinal, and femoral adenopathy. She had
decreased breath sounds at both lung bases, a 2/6 systolic ejection
murmur at the base of the heart without radiation, total liver span
of 16 cm and a 3 cm spleen tip palpable. Radiographic exam showed
abruptly worsening bilateral interstitial pulmonary infiltrates
despite the use of prophylactic trimethoprim/sulfamethaxazole.
Laboratory examination upon admission revealed 145,000 WBC/mm^3
with 71% lymphoblasts with bizarre cloven multilobed nuclei, 5%
neutrophils, 23% lymphocytes, and 1% monocytes, hematocrit 27%,
and platelet count of 613,000/mm^3. Serum chemistry profile showed
alkaline phosphatase 835, SGOT 101, LDH 1485, calcium 7.6 mEq/L,
and albumin 3.4 gms%. Urinalysis was benign, cerebrospinal fluid
showed 28 WBC/mm^3, 57% malignant lymphocytes, 18 RBC/mm^3, glucose
74 mg%, and protein 22 mg%. Bilateral bone marrow aspirates and
biopsies showed hypercellular marrow consisting of nearly 80%
malignant lymphocytes. Iron was present. Open biopsy of the lingula
revealed that the abnormal radiographic findings were leukemic cell
infiltrates. No microorganisms were seen.

Analysis of surface markers on the malignant lymphocytes
revealed them to be OKT 3$^+$, 4$^+$, 8$^-$ T lymphocytes. They also
expressed the T-cell growth factor (interleukin 2) receptor as
measured by their staining with anti-Tac antibody. The patient had
high titers of serum antibody directed against proteins of the
human T cell leukemia/lymphoma virus (HTLV), a unique human RNA-tumor
virus with tropism for cells of T-cell origin, which we will take
up in detail later.

In summary, this 23-year-old Black woman had a 2 month history
of weight loss, fatigue, and lymphadenopathy. She developed hypercalcemia, interstitial pulmonary infiltrates responding initially
to antibiotic therapy suggesting opportunistic infection, and a
clonal T cell malignancy eventually involving bone marrow, peripheral
blood, lymph nodes, tonsils, liver and spleen, central nervous
system, lung and skin and associated with high titers of antibody
to the human retrovirus HTLV.

Her hypercalcemia was initially managed with natriuresis and
after plasmapheresis, which reduced her peripheral WBC count from
210,000/mm^3 to 98,000/mm^3, she was begun on combination chemotherapy
for her malignancy and cranial irradiation with intrathecal methotrexate for her malignant leptomenigitis on 4/8/83. The response

of the malignancy to cyclophosphamide, 650 mg/M^2 IV, doxorubicin
25 mg/M^2 IV, and VP-16 120 mg/M^2 IV was prompt and gratifying
with virtual complete disappearance of palpable lymph nodes, the
skin rash and all malignant cells from the peripheral blood and
normalization of serum calcium levels by 4/15; however, malignant
cells were again noted in the peripheral blood on 4/20. She was
then given vincristine, daunorubicin, prednisone and L-asparaginase
as an antileukemic regimen without discernible response. There was
no demonstrable anti-tumor effect. She died of progressive leukemia
and pneumonia on 5/17.

Post mortem examination revealed extensive pneumonia in the
right lung and HTLV-associated adult T cell leukemia involving the
bone marrow, peripheral blood, lymph nodes, liver, spleen, kidneys,
and lungs.

With this case in the background, we would now turn to a general
discussion of T-cell lymphoproliferative disorders. T cell
malignancies are heterogeneous in their cell of origin, their
histologic pattern, and their clinical spectrums of disease. In
order to understand the diversity of T cell malignancies, some
discussion of the normal T cell differentiation pathway might be
useful.

Normal T cell precursors in the bone marrow (termed prothymocytes) bear the T9 and T10 differentiation antigens which are also
present on marrow cells of other lineages.[1] The prothymocytes
migrate to the thymus where they account for about 10% of all
cells in the thymus. Over time, these prothymocytes lose T9,
retain T10 and acquire T6 (an antigen present only on thymocytes),
T4, and T8. These T4, T6, T8, T10 positive thymocytes account for
about 70% of the cells in the thymus. With further maturation, T6
is lost, T1 and T3 are strongly expressed, and individual cells
retain either T4 or T8 but normally not both.[2] These cells egress
from the thymic medulla to the periphery as functional T lymphocytes
and tend to lose T10. About 2/3 of peripheral T cells are T1, T3,
and T4 positive and 1/3 are T1, T3, and T8 positive. The T4 positive
population often recognizes antigens in association with class II
histocompatibility antigens (HLA-DR) also called Ia antigens, and
function predominately as helper cells in B cell responses and as
inducer cells that aid the maturation of suppressor and cytotoxic T
cells. The T8 positive population often recognizes antigens in
association with class I histocompatibility antigens (HLA-A, B, C)
and functions predominately as cytotoxic effector cells and
suppressor cells.[3]

Other cell surface structures are also useful in distinguishing
T cells from other lymphoid and nonlymphoid cells. T lymphocytes
generally appear to have a receptor capable of binding to sheep

erythrocytes and form so-called E rosettes in which several red
cells surround a central lymphocyte. This T cell receptor reacts
with OKT 11 monoclonal antibody.[4] Two other markers are found on
activated proliferating T lymphocytes, Ia antigen and the receptor
for T cell growth factor (TCGF). There are a variety of monoclonal
antibodies specific for nonpolymorphic Ia determinates which can
be used to identify Ia antigens as a general class. Anti-Tac is a
monoclonal antibody specific for the TCGF receptor.[5] Resting T
cells fail to express either Ia or Tac antigen; however, normal T
cells activated by any of several processes express both.

The T cell malignancies generally conform to the notion that
lymphocyte malignancies represent arrest of development at a
particular stage of the normal differentiation pathway. Furthermore,
it has been taught that the more mature the stage of development
at which the predominate malignant cell is arrested, the more
indolent the course of the disease. For example, the malignant
cell of the ordinary cutaneous T cell lymphomas (Sezary syndrome
and mycosis fungoides) is a T1, T3, T4 positive T lymphocyte and
many patients have malignant cells that retain helper T cell function in assays of T dependent immunoglobulin synthesis.[6] The
clinical course of the average patient with cutaneous T cell lymphoma
is indolent with median survival being about 10 years.[7]. The
malignant cells of T cell chronic lymphocytic leukemia, hairy cell
leukemia of T cell type, and other neoplasms in a family called
peripheral T cell lymphoma are similarly more mature in phenotype
(usually being either T1, T3, T4, T11 positive or T1, T3, T8, T11
positive), and the natural history of patients with these diseases
is often moderately long. On the other hand, although there is
some marker heterogeneity, T cell acute lymphoblastic leukemia
cells are usually T4, T6, T8, T10, T11 positive cells characteristic
of cortical (immature) thymocytes. The natural history of T cell
ALL is aggressive and it is rapidly fatal unless multi-drug chemotherapy is successful at inducing complete remission. Similarly,.
T cell lymphoblastic lymphoma cells are usually T6 negative, T1
and T3 positive and express either T4 or T8, placing the malignant
cell slightly more mature among thymocytes than the T cell ALL
cell.[8]. T cell lymphoblastic lymphoma is also a rapidly fatal
disease without the use of effective combination chemotherapy
regimens. Both the malignant cell phenotypes and the clinical
syndromes of T cell ALL and lymphoblastic lymphoma may overlap
considerably, however, they clearly arise from cells of thymocyte
origin and behave aggressively.

An exception to this schema relating maturity of cell phenotype
to clinical pace of disease is the HTLV-associated adult T cell
leukemia (ATL). (We will discuss HTLV itself further below.) As
was demonstrated by the clinical course of the patient under
discussion, the malignancy associated with HTLV can be exceedingly

aggressive, yet the cell of origin appears to be a peripheral T lymphocyte characterized by T1, T3, T4 and T11 positivity. An important distinction between HTLV-associated ATL and other peripheral T cell malignancies is that the majority of ATL cells readily express the T cell growth factor (TCGF) receptor as revealed by reactivity with anti-Tac antibody.[9]. Some cell lines derived from HTLV associated ATL produce and respond to TCGF.[10] Thus, the autocrine effects of a tumor-produced growth-promoting factor or perhaps heightened sensitivity to exogenous TCGF might be related to the accelerated rate of growth of some ATL cells in vivo. (However, autocrine TCGF production per se is not felt to be essential to the neoplastic process.) Certainly among the peripheral T cell lymphomas there is a spectrum of growth rates of the malignant cells, but the HTLV-associated ATL can be among the most aggressive cancers clinicians may face.

As we have already touched upon, the evolution of our current understanding of HTLV-associated ATL was accelerated by an international collaboration between researchers in Japan and at the National Cancer Institute. To re-capitulate, in 1977, Uchiyama et al[11] reported on a syndrome they observed in southern Japan which they called adult T cell leukemia/lymphoma. The syndrome was characterized by leukemia of T lymphocytes, adenopathy, liver and spleen enlargement, and skin involvement. Hypercalcemia and opportunistic infections were also commonly seen. The median survival of the disease was about 8 months. Poiesz et al. in Robert Gallo's laboratory isolated a retrovirus termed human T cell leukemia/lymphoma virus or HTLV[12] from a cell line derived from a Black patient with what was thought to be an atypical form of mycosis fungoides. The patient had lymphomatous meningitis, hypercalcemia, and lytic bone lesions[13] and, in retrospect, his clinical course resembled the ATL described in Japan. The virus HTLV was unique in its nucleic acid sequences,[14] its major core proteins p24[15] and p19[16], and its reverse transcriptase.[17] Subsequent clinical study of Japanese ATL revealed a clustering of cases in the Kyushu and Shikoku provinces suggesting the possibility of a transmissable agent playing an etiologic role.[18] Using reagents developed in Gallo's laboratory, it was found in 1981 that HTLV was associated with the endemic ATL of Japan[19] and more recently, a virus closely related or identical to HTLV has been isolated from Japanese patients.[20] Last year a group of patients with a syndrome similar to ATL was reported in Black Caribbean patients who had migrated to England[21] and they, too, showed evidence of HTLV association.[22] In the United States, a group of cases has been identified in the southeastern region,[23,24] and one must include this region in the list of endemic areas. A disproportionate number of HTLV-associated neoplasms occur in Blacks. Sporadic cases of HTLV-associated neoplasms can occur outside known endemic areas, and sometimes HTLV-associated tumors have clinical and histologic features consistent with a range of non-Hodgkin's

lymphomas other than ATL. It is worth stressing this point since a
pre-occupation with certain histopathologic features can theoretically
obscure the recognition of HTLV as a cause of several kinds of
lymphoma.

The study of cells from patients with HTLV-associated ATL
reveals that the virus genome is acquired by the malignant cells
and is not incorporated into the germ line DNA.[25] Finally,
coculture experiments of HTLV-associated malignant cells clearly
indicate that the virus can transform suitable normal target cells
into permanent exogenous T-cell growth factor-independent cell
lines.[26] While HTLV acts as a T-cell tropic virus, non-T cells
can bear HTLV in some settings.

In summary, HTLV is a unique human retrovirus that is endemic
in several parts of the world and may be significantly linked to
non-Hodgkin's lymphomas in certain regions. Actually, the term
HTLV denotes a family of closely related viruses. For the most
part, we are discussing viruses belonging to the HTLV-I strain.

The full spectrum of diseases associated with HTLV is not known.
There are data supporting the hypotheses that certain patients with
the recently defined acquired immunodeficiency disease syndrome
(AIDS)[27,28] either have an increased risk of infection with viruses
in the HTLV-family or become infected with a strain of HTLV as the
precipitating event of their disease.[29-32] There are clear
precedents in animal systems in which a retrovirus can have both
leukemogenic and immunosuppressive capacities. The possibility
that HTLV or some variant of this virus can cause acquired immunodeficiency disease is one of the most important areas of clinical
investigation, and we will return to this concept later.

Histopathological features of HTLV-associated lymphomas are
somewhat variable when classified by the Rappaport or other conventional lymphoma schemas. Lymph nodes are generally classified
as being diffuse aggressive lymphomas but the histologic subtype
may be immunoblastic, large cell, or mixed. Pautrier's microabcesses
and many other features suggesting mycosis fungoides to the patholo-
gist are not rare (vide infra). The malignant cells may be pleomorphic in size and shape and may have bizarre cloven nuclei.
There are no morphologic features that are pathognomonic for HTLV-
associated ATL, although experienced pathologists can make this
diagnosis rather reliably in the relevant clinical setting. As
new molecular techniques are adopted by clinical laboratories,
in situ hybridization and other recombinant DNA technologies may
add reliability and precision to the histopathologic diagnosis.

Clinical features of ATL can also be somewhat variable,[24] but
cases seen in the United States have uniformly had circulating
malignant cells. Ninety-three percent have had hypercalcemia of

unknown etiology that responds well to anti-tumor treatment but responds rather variably to conventional treatments like natriuresis and corticosteroids. Life threatening hypercalcemia can dominate the clinical picture. At some medical centers patients have been mistakenly diagnosed as having hyperparathyroidism and have been referred for parathyroidectomies. Lytic bone lesions may be seen in 50% of patients but biopsies of such lesions usually show no evidence of malignancy. The lesions often contain activated osteo-clasts, but further efforts to clarify the etiology are necessary. Adenopathy is seen in over 90% of patients and about 50% have hepatosplenomegaly. There is no obvious pattern of lymph node involvement. Half of the patients have skin lesions characterized as a papular rash usually on the face, chest, and back. In 2/3 of patients with skin involvement, epidermal infiltration was observed which resembled the Pautrier's micro-abscesses usually associated with cutaneous T cell lymphomas (mycosis fungoides). Thus, distinguishing these two entities on morphologic grounds alone is sometimes difficult. About 30% of patients developed malignant leptomeningitis and over half developed interstitial pneumonitis during the course of their illness either from opportunistic infection (e.g., with Pneumocystis carinii), lymphoma cell infil-tration, or both. Clinicians frequently face serious diagnostic dilemmas regarding a patient's pulmonary status.

It is of interest that ATL patients seem to be at increased risk of developing opportunistic infection, particularly Pneumocystis carinii, even before chemotherapy. This is somewhat similar to the clinical situation seen in the acquired immunodeficiency syndrome (AIDS) seen in the United States.[27,28] We have already touched on this point. It is possible that ATL and AIDS represent two ends of a spectrum of HTLV-related disease: the former resulting when cells are transformed by HTLV and the latter when cells are somehow lytically infected by HTLV. (Indeed both processes could conceivably occur together in some settings.) Such events could be mediated by immune response gene phenomena or additional environ-mental factors.

The management of patients with ATL has not been as successful as the management of other aggressive forms of malignant lymphoma.[33] The Japanese have extensive experience, but consistent long-term disease-free survival has not been attained with any known treatment. Matsumoto et al[34] treated 28 patients with various anti-leukemia regimens made up of 2 to 5 drugs. No complete responses were seen and the median survival was 2 months. Fouteen patients died of interstitial pneumonitis, 9 from sepsis, and 4 from progressive malignancy. The Lymphoma Study Group of Japan[35] treated 12 patients with a four-drug regimen consisting of vincristine 1 mg IV weekly x 6 weeks, cyclophosphamide 300 mg IV days 1, 8, 22, and 29, prednisolone 40 to 60 mg daily by mouth for the first 3 days of each week, and adriamycin 40 to 60 mg IV days 1 and 22. The

regimen was called VEPA and was given in a 6 week cycle. Six of
the 12 patients with ATL achieved a complete response but the
median duration of remission was 2 months. In England, Catovsky
et al[21] treated 6 Caribbean ATL patients with CVP (cyclophosphamide
200 mg/M^2 orally qd x 5, vincristine 1.4 mg/M^2 IV day 1, prednisone
100 mg/M^2 orally qd x 5, cycle repeated every 21 days), or CHOP
(cyclophosphamide 750 mg/M^2 IV day 1, adriamycin 50 mg/M^2 IV day 1,
vinristine 1.4 mg/M^2 IV day 1, and prednisone 100 mg orally qd x 5,
cycle repeated every 21 to 28 days) or both. Of the three patients
treated initially with CVP, two achieved partial responses. Both
of the CVP-induced partial responders and two other previously
untreated patients were given CHOP and all 4 patients had partial
responses. The median response duration was 4 months. There have
been no long-term remissions off therapy.

At the NCI Clinical Oncology Program, we have had the oppor-
tunity to treat 11 patients with typical features of ATL. Our
approach has been somewhat more intensive than that employed by
investigators in Japan and England largely because of the striking
successes we have had in inducing long-term disease-free survival
in patients with another aggressive lymphoma, the once uniformly
fatal diffuse histiocytic lymphoma.[36] Six of 11 patients were
given ProMACE-MOPP combination chemotherapy (Prednisone 100 mg/M^2
orally days 1-14, cyclophosphamide 650 mg/M^2 IV days 1 and 8,
doxorubicin 25 mg/M^2 IV days 1 and 8, VP-16 120 mg/M^2 IV days 1 and
8, methotrexate 1500 mg/M^2 IV day 15 with leucovorin rescue given
in 3 monthly cycles followed by 3 cycles of MOPP chemotherapy and
3 maintenance cycles of ProMACE), and three of the six achieved
complete remissions lasting 2, 3, and 26 months. All patients for
whom we have adequate followup have relapsed. Three other patients
had dramatic but exceedingly short-lived responses. Three patients
were given CHOP as their primary therapy and two others received
CHOP at their first relapse. Two complete and two partial responses
were seen, the longest of which was 12 months. Several other
regimens have been tried in relapsed patients without success. The
major problems facing the clinician managing HTLV-associated ATL
patients at this time are (1) we have not found an anti-tumor
regimen routinely capable of achieving durable complete remissions
(of course since HTLV infection can be a persistent process, it is
theoretically possible that some relapses following chemotherapy
represent a different oncogenic event associated with the retrovirus); (2) there is a high incidence of interstitial pneumonitis
which may be due to lymphoma, Pneumocystis carinii, both or some
other opportunistic pathogens (3) there is a high incidence of
sepsis; (4) malignant leptomeningitis is common and may be
complicated by CNS infection; and (5) a variety of metabolic
complications, chiefly hypercalcemia, may require aggressive
intervention. We believe that the treatment of ATL should be
undertaken in referral centers equipped to provide experimental
therapies and laboratory support. New therapies are needed.

Attempts to improve the treatment of HTLV-associated lymphomas of leukemias are underway at the National Cancer Institute taking advantage of some new information on synergy between certain anti-tumor agents and employing drugs known to be more toxic to T cells than B cells (e.g. asparaginase, 2 deoxycoformycin). We are also exploring biologic response modifiers such as interferon. In addition, we are testing a new concept in monoclonal antibody immuno-therapy of ATL in collaboration with Dr. Thomas Waldmann. In the several clinical trials of monoclonal antibodies that have been reported,[37-40] antibodies directed at differentiation antigens on normal and/or malignant cells have been administered and have resulted in variable antitumor responses. One of the mechanisms by which tumors have escaped antibody-mediated cytotoxicity is by shedding the target antigen from cell surfaces, an event sometimes referred to as antigenic modulation. We are using anti-Tac to treat selected patients with HTLV-associated ATL. It will be recalled that anti-Tac binds the TCGF receptor, a target which is readily expressed on malignant T cells infected with HTLV. In vitro tests have shown that anti-Tac can prevent the growth of certain cell lines even in the absence of complement by blocking the TCGF from gaining access to the TCGF receptor. Furthermore, should antigenic modulation of the TCGF receptor occur in vivo, it would be expected that tumor cell growth would be affected in some cases by the absence of a target through which TCGF might induce proliferation. Thus, anti-Tac might exert antitumor activity through at least three mechanisms: (1) antibody-mediated lysis of cells to which the antibody binds, (2) blocking access of TCGF to the TCGF receptor, and (3) antigenic modulation of the TCGF receptor resulting in refractoriness to TCGF. Eventually, it might be possible to con-struct regimens combining chemotherapy with monoclonal antibodies.

As important as clinical research in the management of HTLV-associated ATL patients is, an equally important area for research is the potential for developing a vaccine that might prevent the disease if administered to selected people in endemic areas. Precedent exists for preventing retrovirus induced malignancy by vaccination.[41] However, three immunologic properties of HTLV could add an unforeseen layer of complexity in this area of research, and should be borne in mind in discussing new immunologic strategies: First, the p19 gag protein of HTLV appears to cross-react with a determinant expressed in normal human thymic epithelium.[42] Secondly, it has recently been learned that there is nucleic acid homology between the HTLV envelope gene region (env) and class I histo-compatibility genes.[43] Also, HTLV-infected cells appear to express alien histocompatibility antigens.[44] Finally, there is a preferen-tial association of purified (extra-cellular) HTLV virions with the receptor for human T-cell growth factor (TCGF).[45] The role of cell mediated immunity in the control of HTLV-associated neoplasia has been suggested by a recent study in which we were able to establish a long-term HTLV-specific cytotoxic T cell line in vitro.[46] We were also able to develop various T-cell clones with defined functional and phenotypic properties.

Our efforts to establish comparable T cell lines in HTLV+ patients with residual or relapsed malignancy or short remissions were unsuccessful. The only cytotoxic line successfully established to date was from a patient with an unusually durable remission. It is tempting to suggest that our success in establishing a cyto- toxic T cell line and T-cell clones from the patient that could kill his own tumor in vitro is related to the high frequency of such T cells in the patient and that, in turn, they are playing an important role in the maintenance of his disease-free status. Yet this hypothesis is offered with certain reservations: The patient's malignancy was atypical for HTLV-associated lymphomas and more strongly resembled ordinary cutaneous T cell lymphoma in the pace of disease and the absence of the usual findings of hypercalcemia, interstitial pneumonitis, or malignant leptomeningitis. Further studies are underway to correlate host immune factors with clinical disease status. Nevertheless, we feel that adoptive cellular therapy using cytotoxic HTLV-specific T cells is a realistic possibility in the near future.

The reader can expect new applications of monoclonal antibody technologies in diagnosis (and perhaps assisting in the therapy) of HTLV-associated lymphoproliferative diseases. For example, activated adult T-cell leukemia cells have recently been shown to express the marker OKT 17 suggesting an origin from a particular subset of activated OKT 4+ T-cells.[47]

Finally, in HTLV research we feel it is important to re- emphasize that the current state of knowledge has come about because of a close collaboration between clinician and basic scientist, each of whom has illuminated the path taken by the other. Continued progress will require the same collaboration.

REFERENCES

1. E. L. Reinherz, P. C. Kung, G. Goldstein, R. H. Levey, and S. F. Schlossman, Discrete stages of human intrathymic differentiation: Analysis of normal thymocytes and leukemic lymphoblasts of T cell lineage, PNAS 77:1588 (1980).
2. E. L. Reinherz, P. C. Kung, G. Goldstein, and S. F. Schlossman, A monoclonal antibody with selective reactivity with functionally mature human thymocytes and all peripheral human T cells, J. Immunol. 123: 1312 (1979).
3. E. L. Reinherz and S. F. Schlossman, The characterization and function of human immunoregulatory T lymphocyte subsets, Immunology Today 2: 69 (1981).

4. W. Verbi, M. F. Greaves, C. Schneider, K. Koubeck, G. Janossy,
    H. Stein, P. Kung, and G. Goldstein, Monoclonal antibodies
    OKT11 and OKT11A have pan-t reactivity and block sheep
    erythrocyte "receptors." Eur. J. Immunol 12:81 (1982).

5. T. Uchiyama, S. Broder, and T. A. Waldmann, A monoclonal
    antibody (anti-Tac) reactive with activated and functionally
    mature T cells. I. Production of anti-Tac monoclonal anti-
    body and distribution of Tac T cells, J. Immunol. 126:
    1393 (1981).

6. S. Broder, R. L. Edelson, M. A. Lutzner, D. L. Nelson, R. P.
    MacDermott, R.P., M. E. Dunn, C. K. Goldman, D. B. Meade,
    and T. A. Waldmann, Sezary syndrome: A malignant prolifera-
    tion of helper T cells, J. Clin. Invest. 58:1297 (1976).

7. P. A. Bunn and S. I. Lamberg, Report of the committee on staging
    and classification of cutaneous T-cell lymphomas, Cancer
    Treat. Rep. 63:725 (1979).

8. J. Cossman, T. M. Chused, R. I. Fisher, I. Magrath, F. Bollum, and
    E. S. Jaffe, Diversity of immunologic phenotypes of lympho-
    blastic lymphoma, Cancer Res. 43:4486 (1983).

9. T. A. Waldmann, S. Broder, W. C. Greene, P. S. Sarin, D. Blayney,
    C. K. Goldman, K. Frost, S. Sharrow, J. Depper, W. Leonard,
    T. Uchiyama, and R. Gallo, A comparison of the function and
    phenotype of Sezary T cells with human T cell leukemia/
    lymphoma virus (HTLV)-associated adult T cell leukemia,
    (submitted) (1983).

10. J. F. Gootenberg, F. W. Ruscetti, J. W. Mier, A. Gazdar, and
    R. C. Gallo, Human cutaneous T-cell lymphoma and leukemia
    cell lines produce and respond to T cell growth factor,
    J. Exp. Med. 154:1403 (1981).

11. T. Uchiyama, J. Yodoi, K. Sakawa, K. Takatsuki, and H. Uchino,
    Adult T cell leukemia: Clinical and hematologic features of
    16 cases, Blood 50:481 (1977).

12. B. J. Poiesz, F. W. Ruscetti, A. F. Gazdar, P. A. Bunn, J. D.
    Minna, and R. C. Gallo, Detection and isolation of type C
    retrovirus particles from fresh and cultured lymphocytes
    of a patient with cutaneous T cell lymphoma, Proc. Natl.
    Acad. Sci. USA 77:7415 (1980).

13. B. A. Brigham, P. A. Bunn, J. E. Horton, G. P. Schechter, L. M.
    Wahl, E. C. Bradley, N. R. Dunnick, and M. J. Matthews,
    Skeletal manifestations in cutaneous T cell lymphomas,
    Arch. Dermatol. 118:461 (1982).

14. M. S. Reitz, B. J. Poiesz, F. W. Ruscetti, and R. C. Gallo,
    Characterization and distribution of nucleic acid sequences
    of a novel type C retrovirus isolated from neoplastic
    human T lymphocytes, Proc. Natl. Acad. Sci. USA 78:1187
    (1981).

15. V. S. Kalyanaraman, M. G. Sarngadharan, B. J. Poiesz, F. W. Ruscetti, and R. C. Gallo, Immunologic properties of a type C retrovirus isolated from a cultured human T-lymphoma cells and comparison to other mammalian retroviruses, J. Virol. 38:906 (1981).

16. M. Robert-Guroff, F. W. Ruscetti, L. E. Posner, B. J. Poiesz, and R. C. Gallo, Detection of the human T-cell lymphoma virus p19 in cells of some patients with cutaneous T cell lymphoma and leukemia using a monoclonal antibody, J. Exp. Med. 154:1957 (1981).

17. H. M. Rho, B. J. Poiesz, F. W. Ruscetti, and R. C. Gallo, Characterization of the reverse transcriptase from a new retrovirus (HTLV) produced by a human cutaneous T cell lymphoma cell line, Virology 112:355 (1981).

18. K. Tajima, S. Tominaga, T. Kuroishi, H. Shimizu, and T. Suchi, Geographical features and epidemiological approach to endemic T cell leukemia/lymphoma in Japan, Jpn. J. Clin. Oncol. 9(suppl):495 (1979).

19. R. C. Gallo, G. B. deThe, and Y. Ito, Kyoto Workshop on some specific recent advances in human tumor virology. (Meeting report), Cancer Res. 41:4738 (1981).

20. M. Popovic, M. S. Reitz, M. G. Sarngadharan, M. Robert-Guroff, V. S. Kalyanaraman, Y. Nakao, I. Miyoshi, J. Minowada, M. Yoshida, Y. Ito, and R. C. Gallo, The virus of Japanese adult T cell leukaemia is a member of the human T cell leukaemia virus group, Nature 300:63 (1982).

21. D. Catovsky, M. F. Greaves, M. Rose, D. A. G. Galton, A. W. G. Goolden, D. R. McCluskey, J. M. White, I. Lampert, G. Bourikas, R. Ireland, J. M. Bridges, W. A. Blattner, and R. C. Gallo, Adult T cell lymphoma-leukemia in Blacks the West Indies, Lancet i:639 (1982).

22. W. A. Blattner, V. S. Kalyanaraman, M. Robert-Guroff, T. A. Lister, D. A. G. Galton, P. Sarin, M. H. Crawford, D. Catovsky, M. F. Greaves, and R. C. Gallo, The human type C retrovirus, HTLV, in Blacks from the Caribbean region and relationship to adult T-cell leukemia/lymphoma, Int. J. Cancer 30:257 (1982).

23. W. A. Blattner, D. W. Blayney, M. Robert-Guroff, M. G. Sarngadharan, V. S. Kalyanaraman, P. S. Sarin, E. S. Jaffe, and R. C. Gallo, Epidemiology of the human T cell leukemia/ lymphoma virus (HTLV), J. Infect. Dis. 147:406 (1983).

24. D. W. Blayney, E. S. Jaffe, W. A. Blattner, J. Cossman, M. Robert-Guroff, D. L. Longo, P. A. Bunn, and R. C. Gallo, The human T-cell leukemia/lymphoma virus) HTLV defines a distinct clinical entity, Blood 62:401 (1983).

25. R. C. Gallo, D. Mann, S. Broder, F. W. Ruscetti, M. Maeda, V. S. Kalyanaraman, M. Robert-Guroff, and M. S. Reitz, Human T-cell leukemia-lymphoma virus (HTLV) is in T- but not B-lymphocytes from a patient with cutaneous T-cell lymphoma, Proc. Natl. Acad. Sci. USA 79:5680 (1982).

26. R. C. Gallo and F. Wong-Staal, Retroviruses as etiologic agents of some animal and human leukemias and lymphomas and as tools for elucidating the molecular mechanism of leukemogenesis, Blood 60:545 (1982).
27. J. Vieira, E. Frank, T. J. Spira, and S. H. Landesman, Acquired immunodeficiency in Haitians: Opportunistic infections in previously healthy Haitian immigrants, N. Engl. J. Med. 308:125 (1983).
28. D. Mildvan, V. Mathur, R. W. Enlow, P. L. Romain, R. J. Winchest C. Colp, H. Singman, B. R. Adelsberg, and I. Spigland, Opportunistic infections and immune deficiency in homosexual men, Ann. Int. Med. 96:700 (1982).
29. M. Essex, M. F. McLane, T. H. Lee, L. Falk, C. W. S. Howe, J. I. Mullins, C. Cabradilla, and P. P. Francis, Antibodies to cell membrane antigens associated with human T-cell leukemia virus in patients with AIDS, Science 220:859 (1983).
30. E. P. Gelmann, M. Popovic, D. Blayney, H. Masur, G. Sidhu, R. H. Stahl, and R. C. Gallo, Proviral DNA of a retrovirus, human T-cell leukemia virus, in two patients with AIDS, Science 220:862 (1983).
31. R. C. Gallo, P. S. Sarin, E. P. Gelmann, M. Robert-Guroff, E. Richardson, V. S. Kalyanaraman, D. Mann, G. D. Sidhu, R. E. Stahl, S. Zolla-Pazner, J. Leibowitch, and M. Popovic, Isolation of a human T-cell leukemia virus in acquired immune deficiency syndrome (AIDS), Science 220:865 (1983).
32. M. Essex, M. F. McLane, T. H. Lee, T. Jachibana, J. I. Mullins, J. Kreiss, C. K. Kasper, M. C. Poon, S. Landay, S. F. Stein, D. P. Francis, C. Cabradilla, D. N. Lawrence, and B. L. Evatt, Antibodies to human T-cell leukemia virus membrane antigens (HTLV-MA) in hemophiliacs, Science 221:1061 (1983).
33. P. A. Bunn, G. P. Schechter, E. Jaffe, D. Blayney, R. C. Young, M. J. Matthews, W. Blattner, S. Broder, M. Robert-Guroff, and R. C. Gallo, Clinical course of retrovirus-associated adult T cell lymphoma in the United States, N. Engl. J. Med 309:257 (1983).
34. M. Matsumoto, K. Nomuia, T. Matsumoto, K. Nishioka, S. Hanada, H. Furusho, H. Kikuchi, Y. Kato, A. Utsunomiya, T. Uematsu, M. Iwahashi, S. Hashimoto, and K. Ydenoki, K., Adult T-cell leukemia-lymphoma in Kagoshima District, Southwestern Japan: Clinical and hematological characteristics, Jpn. J. Clin. Oncol. 9(suppl):325 (1979).
35. Lymphoma Study Group, Combination chemotherapy with vincristine, cyclophosphamide (Endoxan), prednisolone, and adriamycin (VEPA) in advanced adult non-Hodgkin's lymphoid malignancies: Relation between T-cell and non-T-cell phenotype and response Jpn. J. Clin. Oncol. 9(suppl):397 (1979).

36. R. I. Fisher, V. T. DeVita, Jr., S. M., Hubbard, D. L., Longo,
    R. L. Wesley, B. A. Chabner, and R. C. Young, Diffuse
    aggressive lymphomas: Increased survival after alternating
    flexible sequences of ProMACE and MOPP chemotherapy, Ann.
    Int. Med 98:304 (1983).
37. L. M. Nadler, M. Stashenko, R. Hardy, W. D. Kaplan, L. N. Button,
    D. W. Kufe, K. H. Antman, and S. F. Schlossman, Serotherapy
    of a patient with a monoclonal antibody directed against a
    human lympohoma-associated antigen, Cancer Res. 40:3147
    (1980).
38. R. A. Miller, D. G. Maloney, J. McKillop, and R. Levy, In vivo
    effects of murine hybridoma monoclonal antibody in a patient
    with T cell leukemia, Blood 58:78 (1981).
39. J. Ritz, J. M. Pesando, S. E. Sallan, L. A. Clavell, J.
    Notis-McConarty, R. Rosenthal, and S. F. Schlossman, Sero-
    therapy of acute lymphoblastic leukemia with monoclonal
    antibody, Blood 58:141 (1981).
40. R. A. Miller and R. Levy, Response of cutaneous T cell lymphoma
    to therapy with hybridoma monoclonal antibody, Lancet
    ii:226 (1981).
41. C. K. Grant, F. de Noronha, C. Tusch, M. T. Michalek, and M. F.
    McLane, Protection of cats against progressive fibrosarcomas
    and persistent leukemia virus infection by vaccination with
    feline leukemia cells, J. Natl. Cancer Inst. 65:1285 (1980).
42. B. F. Haynes, M. Robert-Guroff, R. S. Metygar, G. Franchini,
    V. S. Kalyanaraman, T. J. Palker, and R. C. Gallo, Monoclonal
    antibody against human T cell leukemia virus p19 defines a
    human thymic epithelial antigen acquired during ontogeny,
    J. Exp. Med. 157:907 (1983).
43. M. F. Clarke, E. P. Gelmann, and M. S. Reitz, Jr., Homology of
    human T-cell leukemia virus envelope gene with class I HLA
    gene, Nature 305:60 (1983).
44. D. L. Mann, M. Popovic, P. Sarin, C. Murray, M. S. Reitz, D. M.
    Strong, B. F. Haynes, R. C. Gallo, and W. A. Blattner, Cell
    lines producing human T-cell lymphoma virus show altered
    HLA expression, Nature 305:58 (1983).
45. Z. Lando, P. Sarin, M. Megson, W. L. Greene, T. A. Waldmann,
    R. C. Gallo, and S. Broder, Association of human T-cell
    leukemia/lymphoma virus (HTLV) with the Tac antigen-marker
    for the receptor T-cell growth factor, Nature, in press
    (1983).
46. H. Mitsuya, L. A. Matis, M. Megson, P. A. Bunn, C. Murray,
    D. L. Mann, R. C. Gallo, and S. Broder, Generation of an
    HLA-restricted cytotoxic T-cell line reactive against
    cultured tumor cells from a patient infected with human
    T-cell leukemia/lymphoma virus (HTLV), J. Exp. Med. 158:994
    (1983).

47. H. Tsuda and K. Takatsuki, Adult T-cell leukemia cells
     expressing OKT 17 antigen in the activated state,
     Hematological Oncology 1:263 (1983).

PARTICIPANTS

AARONSON S.A.
Laboratory of Cellular
and Molecular Biology, NIH
Bethesda Md. - USA

ARYA S.
Lab. of Tumor Cell Biology NCI
NIH - Bethesda Md. - USA

AUSIELLO C.
Ist. Tipizzazione Tissutale
L'Aquila - Italy

BARNABEI O.
Ist. Fisiologia Generale
Univ. di Bologna - Italy

BIANCO A.R.
Dip. di Oncologia
II Univ. di Napoli - Italy

BISTONI F.
Ist. di Microbiologia
Univ. di Perugia - Italy

BONMASSAR E.
Ist. di Farmacologia
II Univ. di Roma - Italy

BRODER S.
Clinical Oncology Program
NCI Bethesda Md. - USA

CAPOBIANCHI M.R.
Ist. di Virologia
Univ. di Roma - Italy

CAPUZZO A.
Ist. di Fisiologia Generale
Univ. di Ferrara - Italy

CASSONE A.
Lab. di Microbiologia e Micologia
Ist. Sup. di Sanita' Roma - Italy

CECCHERINI-NELLI L.
Cattedra di Patologia Medica
Univ. di Milano - Italy

CHIARUGI V.
Ist. di Patologia Generale
Univ. di Firenze - Italy

CHIRIGOS M.A.
Lab. of Immunopharmacology
NCI - FCRF
Frederick Md. - USA

CIMINO F.
Ist. di Scienze Biochimiche
II Univ. Napoli - Italy

COLCHER D.
Lab. of tumor Immunology
NCI NIH Bethesda Md.- USA

373

COLNAGHI M.I.
Ist. Naz. Tumori
Milano - Italy

COMOGLIO P.M.
Ist. Istologia
Univ. Torino - Italy

CONFORTI A.
Ist. Patologia Generale
Univ. Roma - Italy

DI FIORE P.P.
Centro Endocrinologia e
Oncologia Sper. CNR
II Univ. di Napoli - Italy

DOLEI A.
Ist. Virologia
Univ. Roma - Italy

EVA A.
Lab. of Cellular and Molecular
Biology NCI - NIH
Bethesda Md. - USA

FAGGIONI A.
Ist. di Patologia Generale
Univ. Roma - Italy

FAZIO V.M.
Ist. Patologia Generale
Univ. Roma - Italy

FIBBI G.
Ist. Patologia Generale
Univ. Firenze - Italy

FISHER P.
Lab. of Tumor immunology
NCI - NIH
Bethesda Md. - USA

FORNI G.
Dip. Microbiologia
Univ. Torino - Italy

FRANCHINI G.
Lab. of Tumor Cell Biology
NCI - NIH
Bethesda Md. - USA

FRATI L.
Ist. Patologia Generale
Univ. Roma - Italy

FUSCO A.
Centro Endocrinologia ed Oncologia
Sper. CNR
II Univ. di Napoli - Italy

GALLO R.C.
Lab.of Tumor Cell Biology
NCI - Bethesda Md. - USA

GAZZANIGA P.P.
Ist. di Patologia Generale
Univ. Roma - Italy

GELMAN E.P.
Lab. of Tumor Cell Biology
NIH - Bethesda Md. - USA

GIANCOTTI F.G.
Ist. Istologia
Univ. Torino - Italy

GOL R.
Lab. of Cellular and Molecular
Biology
NCI - Bethesda Md. - USA

GRAZIANI G.
Dip. Medicina Sperimentale
II Univ. Roma - Italy

GREINER J.
Lab. of Tumor Immunology
N.C.I Bethesda Md. - USA

GULINO A.
Ist. di Patologia Generale
Univ. Roma - Italy

HAHN B.
Lab. of Tumor Cell Biology
NCI Bethesda Md. - USA

HAND P.
Lab. of Tumor Immunology
NCI Bethesda Md. - USA

HERBERMAN R.B.
Frederick Cancer Center
NCI - Frederick - USA

KATOPODIS N.
Sloan-Kettering Inst. for
Cancer Research N.Y. - USA

MANDELLI F.
Dip Ematologia
Univ. Roma - Italy

MANZARI V.
Ist. Patologia Generale
Univ. Roma - Italy

MARCHETTI P.
Ist. Patologia Generale
Univ. Roma - Italy

MARCONI P.
Ist. Microbiologia
Univ. Perugia - Italy

MIGLIACCIO G.
Dip. Ematologia
Univ. Roma - Italy

MITSUYA H
Clinical Oncology Program
NCI Bethesda Md. - USA

MURARO R.
Lab. Of Tumor Immunology
NCI - Bethesda Md.- USA

NOGUCHI P.
Lab. of Tumor Immunology
NCI - Bethesda Md.- USA

PASQUALINI J.R.
CNRS Steroid Hormone
Research Unit
Paris - France

PESCHLE C.
Dip Ematologia
Univ. Roma - Italy

PESTKA S.
Lab. of Tumor Immunology
NCI - Bethesda Md.- USA

PICCOLI M.
Ist. Patologia Generale
Univ. Roma - Italy

PONTIERI G.M.
Ist. Patologia Generale
Univ. Roma - Italy

RASHEED S.
Dept. of Pathology
Cancer Research
Los Angeles Ca.- USA

RICCARDI C.
Ist. Farmacologia
Univ. Perugia - Italy

RICCIARDI I.
Dip. Oncologia
Univ. Napoli - Italy

ROBBINS K.C.
Lab. of Cellular and Molecular
Biology
NCI - Bethesda - USA

RUGGIERO M.
Ist. Patologia Generale
Univ. Firenze - Italy

SALVATORE F.
Ist. Chimica Biologica II
II Univ. Napoli - Italy

SANTAMARIA L.
Ist. Patologia Generale
Univ. Pavia - Italy

SANTONI A.
Ist. Patologia Generale
Univ. Roma - Italy

SCHLOM J.
Lab. of Tumor Immunology
NCI - Bethesda Md. - USA

STOCK C.C.
Sloan-Kettering Inst. for
Cancer Research, N.Y. - USA

TOMASI V.
Ist. Fisiologia Generale
Univ. Bologna - Italy

TREVISANI A.
Ist. Fisiologia Generale
Univ. Ferrara - Italy
(Deceased June 1983)

TRONIK S.R.
Lab. of Cellular and Molecular
Biology
NCI Bethesda Md. - USA

VARNIER O.E.
Ist. Microbiologia
Univ. Genova - Italy

VECCHIO G.
Ist. Patologia Generale
II Univ. Napoli - Italy

VERNA R.
Ist. Patologia Generale
Univ. Roma - Italy

WONG-STAAL F.
Lab. of Tumor Cell Biology
NCI - Bethesda Md.- USA

WUNDERLICH D.
Lab of Tmor Immunology
NCI - Bethesda Md.- USA

YUASA Y.
Lab. of Cellular and Molecular
Biology NCI
Bethesda Md.- USA

INDEX